EMOTION, MISSION, ARCHITECTURE

To my mum

And, for a friend

EMOTION, MISSION, ARCHITECTURE

Building Hospitals in Persia and British India, 1865–1914

Sara Honarmand Ebrahimi

EDINBURGH
University Press

Edinburgh University Press is one of the leading university presses in the UK. We publish academic books and journals in our selected subject areas across the humanities and social sciences, combining cutting-edge scholarship with high editorial and production values to produce academic works of lasting importance. For more information visit our website: edinburghuniversitypress.com

© Sara Honarmand Ebrahimi, 2023, 2024

Edinburgh University Press Ltd
13 Infirmary Street
Edinburgh EH1 1LT

First published in hardback by Edinburgh University Press 2023

Typeset in 11/15 Adobe Garamond by
IDSUK (DataConnection) Ltd

A CIP record for this book is available from the British Library

ISBN 978 1 4744 8657 6 (hardback)
ISBN 978 1 4744 8658 3 (paperback)
ISBN 978 1 4744 8659 0 (webready PDF)
ISBN 978 1 4744 8660 6 (epub)

The right of Sara Honarmand Ebrahimi to be identified as author of this work has been asserted in accordance with the Copyright, Designs and Patents Act 1988 and the Copyright and Related Rights Regulations 2003 (SI No. 2498).

Supported by the Paul Mellon Centre for Studies in British Art

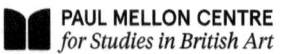

CONTENTS

List of Figures vi
Acknowledgements ix
Note on Abbreviations and Transliteration xii

Introduction: Medical Mission Work and Building Trust 1

1 Life Before and Outside the Mission Hospitals 34

2 Missionaries and the Development of Novel Hospital Designs 67

3 Hospital Visitors and a Hospital for a Whole Family 114

4 Female Missionaries and the Architecture of Women's Hospitals 148

5 Medical Missions and the Anglo-Russian Rivalry 182

Conclusion: Affecting Bodies, Saving Souls 216

Bibliography 224

Index 246

FIGURES

I.1	The entrance to the CMS hospital in Kerman	2
I.2	The Mohammedan Lands of the East, 1896	8
I.3	The entrance to Nūrīe hospital in Kerman	20
I.4	The narrow blind alley leading to the entrance of the CMS hospital in Kerman	21
1.1	Map of Baluchistan showing the places where missionaries visited while itinerating	43
1.2	Itinerating Medical Work	47
1.3	The caravanserai that was converted to the hospital in Yazd	53
1.4	The house that was converted to the hospital in Kerman	53
1.5	The caravanserais that were converted to the hospital in Peshawar	54
1.6	Patients gathered around the fountain in front of the doctor's private room and veranda, Peshawar hospital	56
2.1	Isfahan's new women's hospital	68
2.2	The first purpose-built structures in Kashmir	71
2.3	A ward in Kashmir hospital	72
2.4	Ground plan of Dera Ismail Khan hospital	75

2.5	Dera Ismail Khan medical mission	76
2.6	Plan of the eye ward at Bannu hospital	77
2.7	The eye ward at Bannu hospital	79
2.8	Abulcasis (936–1013), Islamic Spanish physician in the hospital at Cordoba, Spain	80
2.9	Peshawar hospital, view from the main entrance	81
2.10	Inside of one of the large wards at Peshawar	82
2.11	The outpatient block, Peshawar hospital	83
2.12	Plan of the new men's hospital in Isfahan	86
2.13	Old villager and his daughter, Isfahan hospital	88
2.14	A ward in rented buildings, Isfahan women's hospital	89
2.15	A ward in Isfahan new hospital	90
2.16	The new outpatient department with workmen at Yazd	91
2.17	Plan of the new hospital at Yazd	92
2.18	Men's hospital in Yazd	94
2.19	Section and elevation of the proposed hospital in Mosul	94
2.20	The narrow blind alley run between men's and women's hospitals at Kerman	95
2.21	Sketch plan of the men's hospital in Kerman	97
2.22	Floor plan of one of the wards in Kerman hospital	98
2.23	The men's hospital in Kerman	99
2.24	Kerman hospital game	101
2.25	Kerman hospital site	102
3.1	Realistic hospital sense	122
3.2	A Shahzada with his children, friends and servants in Yazd hospital	127
3.3	Plan of the new hospital at Peshawar	132
3.4	The James Serai	134
3.5	A caravanserai in Peshawar	135
3.6	The inpatient building in the adapted caravanserais	136

3.7	The veranda of the inpatient serai, Peshawar hospital	136
3.8	Plan of the Bannu hospital	138
3.9	Rough plan of the Seth Hiranand hospital's inpatient serais	139
3.10	Two cubicles in the inpatient department in the Seth Hiranand hospital	139
4.1	The Islamabad hospital	160
4.2	The medical mission at Multan	162
4.3	Rough plan of the Multan hospital	162
4.4	Part of inner section of the Multan hospital	163
4.5	Serai outside the Multan hospital which accommodated patients' families	164
4.6	Inside of a ward in Multan hospital	165
4.7	Friends of Hindu patients cooking in the hospital	167
4.8	New block of ward at Peshawar	169
4.9	Plan of the entrance to the Isfahan's women's hospital	170
5.1	Dr Pennell siting on the right	189
5.2	Dr Pennell in a ward in the Bannu hospital	192
5.3	Reading the Quran to the sick	193
5.4	The Punjab, Western Himalaya, &c., distinguishing the routes of the Rev. Clark and Lieut Colonel Martin and of the Rev. Dr Prochnow	198
5.5	Pennell of the Indian Frontier	203

ACKNOWLEDGEMENTS

I want to thank several colleagues, mentors and friends whose support and encouragement were influential in the development and completion of this book.

First, I owe a special debt to Samantha Martin, who supervised my PhD dissertation and has supported me ever since. I am also grateful to Leslie Topp and Kathleen James-Chakraborty for their enduring belief in me; they have kept me going. I am thankful to Catherine Cox for welcoming me to the UCD Centre for the History of Medicine in Ireland (CHOMI). This book reminds me how good an idea it was to take the module Gender and Medicine in the first year of my PhD. I also learned a lot from the CHOMI seminars. I am very grateful to my colleagues at the School of Architecture, Planning and Environmental Policy and the Humanities Institute, University College Dublin. The interdisciplinary research environment of the UCD Humanities Institute left its mark on this project. I am also indebted in various ways to Jennifer Bond, Josh Doble, Maja Hultman, Lily Rice, Katherine Vyhmeister and especially James Grannell and Ismay Milford, who have been my rock.

I wrote parts of this book while being a visiting postdoctoral researcher at the School of Architecture and Landscape Architecture, University of Edinburgh. I am very grateful to Alex Bremner for supporting me during my tenure and having been an inspirational mentor and friend ever since. Alex has completed friendship for me, as we say in Farsi.

I would also like to thank the speakers of the 'Worrying about the Field of the History of Emotions in Ireland' event series, held in 2019–20 at UCD, especially Monique Scheer and Rob Boddice. Writing this book became possible due to their influential works (and many others) under the umbrella term the history of emotions. I also thank Rob for reading parts of this book, answering my many questions over email and being so incredibly generous with his knowledge. My special thanks also go to Katherine Fama for supporting me in the organisation of this event series. Our conversations about the history of the relationship between architecture and emotions have been most stimulating.

For their financial support, I would like to thank the Irish Research Council, Osler Library of the History of Medicine, McGill University and especially the Paul Mellon Centre for Studies in British Art, which supported this book initially through a research support grant and subsequently through a postdoctoral fellowship and a publication grant. I would not have been able to complete this book without their support.

I am grateful to the staff in the Cadbury Research Library at the University of Birmingham, who helped me to track down materials regarding the architecture of the CMS medical missions. In particular, Ivana Frlan was as enthusiastic as me about the architecture of mission hospitals. Her knowledge of the materials helped me find certain details that I would not have been able to otherwise. In addition, staff at the National Library and Archive of Iran and the Osler Library of the History of Medicine, McGill University, were extremely helpful. Unfortunately, I had to cancel my visit to the Osler Library of the History of Medicine due to the Covid pandemic. However, Mary K. K. Hague-Yearl kindly provided me with digital copies of the materials.

Some parts of this book have previously been published as journal articles. Sections from Chapters One and Two were published as '"Ploughing before Sowing": Trust and the Architecture of the Church Missionary Society (CMS) Medical Missions', in *Architecture and Culture* 7, no. 2 (2019): 197–217. Parts of Chapter Five appeared as 'The Church Missionary Society (CMS) and Anglo-Russian Rivalry, 1865–1914' in *Interventions: International Journal of Postcolonial Studies* 24, no. 1 (2022): 12–30. And, sections of Introduction and Chapter Three were published as 'Medical Missionaries and the Invention of the "Serai Hospital" in North-western British India'. *European*

Journal for the History of Medicine and Health 79, no. 1 (2022): 67–93 (Open Access). They are produced here with Taylor & Francis's permission. I would like to thank the journal editors and anonymous reviewers for their helpful comments, suggestions and criticism on these articles.

To editorial team at Edinburgh University Press, I offer my gratitude for their editorial expertise. I am most grateful to my parents, Shahin and Mehdi, and my sister and brothers. Thanks to dad who made me study architecture. Sadly, he did not live to see the culmination of those years of study. My mum has always been an example to me; I could not have written this book without her strength. While I have rarely seen my family over the last nine years, I have started every day with their texts. My sister, and most recently her son, have given me lots of energy. And I should thank Amber, Gary and Hazel who made me so welcome in their house while I was finishing this book. In many ways, they became a second family to me. This book is dedicated to my mum; it is also for a friend.

NOTE ON ABBREVIATIONS AND TRANLITERATION

ABCFM American Board of Commission for Foreign Mission
BMS Baptist Missionary Society
CEZMS Church of England Zenana Missionary Society
CIM China Island Mission
CMMA China Medical Missionary Association
CMS Church Missionary Society
CS Church of Scotland
EIC East India Company
FES Society for Promoting Female Education in China, India and the East
LMS London Missionary Society
MMA Medical Mission Auxiliary
PWD Public Work Department of the Government of India
RGS Royal Geographical Society
SPCK Society for Promoting Christian Knowledge
SPG Society for the Propagation of the Gospel

* * *

I have used IJMES transliteration conventions with some modifications. I have chosen to write names of certain places and people as they appear in archival sources without diacritic marks to facilitate research.

INTRODUCTION
MEDICAL MISSION WORK
AND BUILDING TRUST

In 2011, I visited the Morsalīn hospital in Kerman (southern Persia) for the first time. I intended to work on the revitalisation plan of a historic hospital, and I was advised to focus on this particular hospital – I was told that the Morsalīn hospital was the first contemporary hospital of Kerman. I was born, grew up, and studied architecture in Kerman, yet I was not aware of this hospital, and my advisor had failed to mention that it was established and built by British missionaries. On my first visit, the hospital did not appear to me to be British at all, or foreign for that matter I felt that I was in a familiar place. I only learned that the hospital was built by British missionaries after my third visit; approaching the main entrance of the hospital (which is now closed) I noticed the sign at the top of the entrance, which reads 'CMS Hospitals' (Figure I.1). Upon further reading, I realised that the CMS stands for the Church Missionary Society (CMS), which built more than seventy hospitals in Asia and Africa between 1865 and 1939. The first impression that the buildings of the Kerman hospital left with me did not diminish in time, and ultimately it informed the direction of my project – I constantly asked myself how patients felt when visiting the hospitals or, to use Sara Ahmed's words, how the hospital impressed patients and impressed upon patients.[1]

In 1864 Reverend Robert Clark, a CMS missionary in Punjab, and his wife, Elizabeth Mary Browne, visited Kashmir to find an 'opening' for evangelistic

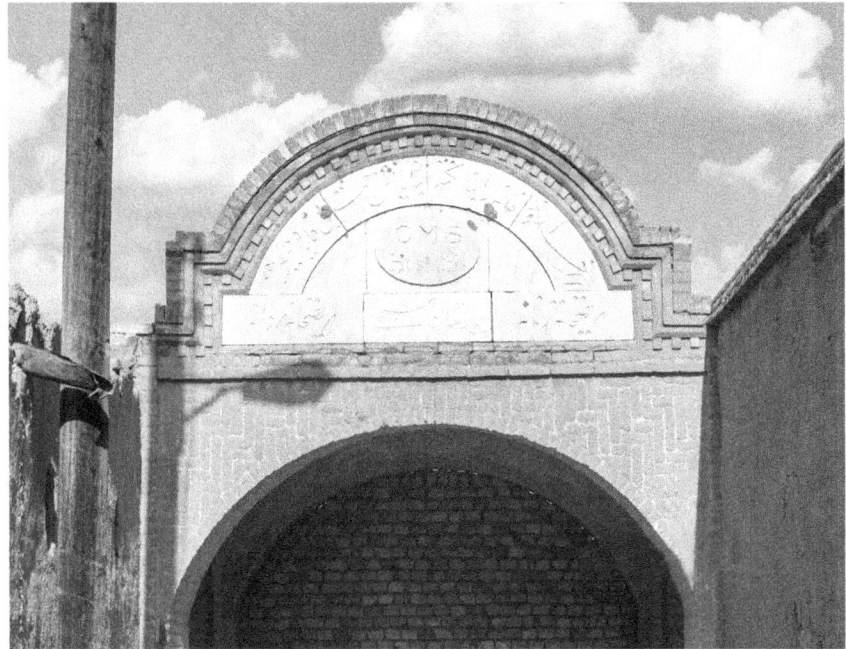

Figure I.1 The entrance to the CMS hospital in Kerman.
Photo by author.

work. They were greeted with 'opposition' by the officials of the Maharajah and by 'the masses' who showed 'Mr. and Mrs. Clark that neither they nor their religion was welcome in Kashmir'. Despite these obstacles, Mrs Clark opened a dispensary that 'was largely attended', and this signified the need for a medical mission. Subsequently, the CMS Committee passed a resolution, and Dr William Jackson Elmslie, a medical graduate of the University of Edinburgh, was appointed to Kashmir to start a medical mission.[2] On 9 May 1865, Elmslie wrote, 'to-day is memorable in the history of the Kashmir Medical Mission from the fact that I opened my dispensary this morning.' The dispensary was in a small veranda in Elmslie's bungalow, which had been 'rudely fitted up'. He then altered another veranda for inpatients and wrote that he had opened his 'small hospital'.[3]

Obliged to leave Kashmir for the winter upon the order of the Maharajah, Elmslie returned the following spring to find that the landlord of his old quarters 'had been forbidden to let the house to the Padre Doctor Sahib, on the excuse that it was too near the city'. After some negotiations, a dispensary was built for him near the city. Again 'in spite of sepoys placed at the different avenues leading to his house to prevent people coming to him', Elmslie wrote a 'few days ago I had as many as a hundred and eighty patients in a morning, and at this moment a fine-looking elderly Mussulman of rank, from the east end of the valley, has called to ask my advice'. Then came an outbreak of cholera, which 'opened many doors to his western skills and his message of Christianity, which otherwise might have remained closed from fear of persecution'. While the opposition of authorities persisted, Elmslie not only reported an increase in the number of patients but also stated that 'the people are much less bigoted than formerly . . . and a very large number of the inhabitants of the valley now look upon us as their friends, and in their difficulties and sorrows come to us for advice and sympathy'.[4]

Upon his return to Kashmir in 1871, after two years on leave, Elmslie reported:

> I am thankful to say that the native authorities seem less hostile than formerly. Not that they are friendly and smile upon our work – that we do not expect from heathen – but so far as I have been able to ascertain, they do not throw obstacles in the way of the sick coming to us.

Elmslie died in 1872 and was succeeded by Dr Theodore Maxwell and his wife, Elizabeth Eyre, who arrived in Kashmir in autumn 1873. They managed to gain permission from the Wazir (Governor) to build a hospital. The number of patients grew in subsequent years, and the hospital was enlarged by Maxwell's successors, Dr Arthur Neve and Dr Ernest Neve, and became one of the biggest medical missions of the CMS.[5]

This narrative summary, extracted from a series of articles published in the first volume of *Mercy and Truth*, a CMS medical magazine, is a testimony to how the publications of different Protestant missionary organisations represented medical missions as instrumental in opening the door to evangelistic work. With few exceptions, published letters and reports uniformly discuss how, after experiencing a series of ups and downs, medical missionaries overcame the distrust of the local people, who would otherwise be unreceptive of the missionaries, and gained access to their homes.

To be sure, views of this nature had been expressed since at least the early nineteenth century. For example, Abdul Masih (Abdool Messeh), a catechist of the CMS, administrated medicine in the Agra mission station in 1816–17. His letters were subsequently published declaring that 'daily, many poor, destitute, sick people attend'.[6] In 1834, the American Board of Commission for Foreign Mission (ABCFM) sent Dr Peter Parker to China to establish a hospital as the only feasible avenue of access to the Chinese. This initiative eventually led to the establishment of the Medical Missionary Society.[7] Nevertheless, these and similar efforts were short-lived; Protestant missionary organisations seldom sought the talents of medical doctors until the 1870s.[8] Mission historians have identified two main reasons for this: one was the 'primitive', 'unregulated' and 'community-based' state of medicine in Europe and North America in the late eighteenth and the start of the nineteenth centuries, and thus its inefficiency in colonies. As David Hardiman puts it, 'the treatment resorted to by [physicians, surgeons and apothecaries] was frequently more iatrogenic than curative'.[9] Moreover, depicting 'paganism' as a sickness of both mind and body, late eighteenth- and early nineteenth-century Evangelical missionaries' conceptualisations of illness had little room for medical doctors.[10] In Britain, even after the Medical Act of 1858, which regulated the qualifications of practitioners in medicine, actions to recognise medical mission work were still slow to emerge.[11] Missionaries had doubts about the advantage of medical mission work and thus demonstrated a lack of commitment to invest in establishing medical missions. Between 1851 and 1870 the CMS recruited seven doctors out of a total of 107 new missionaries and founded only two medical missions.[12]

The 1870s brought new promises, however. The conviction, raised by some missionaries, that medical work could purchase 'friendship' from people who would otherwise be 'hostile', and the heightening of philanthropic concerns in the late nineteenth century, brought medical work increasingly to the fore as a 'benevolent' and 'sentimental' practice with persuasive power.[13] The North American missionaries of a variety of denominations, along with Scottish doctors, were particularly driven by these concerns and took the lead in adopting medical work.[14] Elmslie was of the Free Church of Scotland. Although opposition among Anglican missionaries, such as the Universities'

Mission to Central Africa, persisted, the CMS had grown enthusiastic about medical work by the 1890s. Speaking at the CMS Medical Mission Auxiliary (MMA) annual meeting in 1898, Dr Arthur Neve of the Kashmir medical mission argued for 'practical Christianity', encouraging churches and hospitals to be built side by side.[15] Protestant missionary organisations (in particular, British and North American) founded and built many hospitals in colonial territories in the late nineteenth and early twentieth centuries and became one of the primary providers of the so-called western biomedical services if not the only one in some regions.[16]

While the medical missionaries were supposed to succeed through serving others, as historians such as Emrah Şahin and Terence O. Ranger highlight, they would struggle in maintaining their fragile relationship with the local population, which could be endangered by a failure in treatment.[17] To this must be added that while the missionaries' deployment of 'love' could result, from their point of view, in 'emotional ties' and a high rate of conversion,[18] local populations could perceive the relationship differently, and the outcomes were diverse. Indigenous people might well have attended the medical missions or were receptive to the missionaries for their own various personal reasons.[19] Therefore, mission hospitals inspired and were sites for the practice of mixed feelings.

In certain regions such as the Belgian Congo, the medical missionaries used coercive techniques.[20] In other words, violence and cruelty became constitutive aspects of missionary medicine's benevolent sensibility.[21] Although, as Hardiman notes, '[t]o what extent this harsh side of medical mission was a product of the particular colonial history of the Congo' remains to be determined.[22] In many places, however, obtaining trust gained an importance of its own apart from mission medicine's sensibility as the fundamental act of missionary business – an essential first step for a given mission. As noted in 1905 by Dr F. O. Lasbery, a medical missionary in Egypt, gaining trust was 'the ploughing time before the sowing'.[23]

It is essential not to make a false equivalence between present configurations of trust and friendship and the stated feelings of historical missionaries situated in different places. It is equally important not to readily translate these terms to 'pacifying' or 'solidifying' and assume that the missionaries understood them in a way similar to other colonial actors across time and space.[24]

As Rob Boddice states, there is nothing 'intrinsic, objective or timeless' about emotion words.[25] To understand the meaning of these terms in the context of medical mission work, we should return to the establishment story of the Kashmir medical mission and consider what changed with the introduction of medical work. Missionaries, who were not allowed to preach (and were greeted with stoning according to some accounts[26]) or failed to reach diverse people through Bible sales and distributions and schools,[27] could, through medicine, get closer to a larger and more varied group of local people and visit them at their homes. In other words, these terms imply a change in the sensory relationship between missionaries and local people. They emerged out of a century of mission work marked by frustration and failure to reach a large audience. There were differences in how building trust was understood and practised based on the medical missionaries' gender, national affiliation and the country they worked in. For example, building trust did not carry the same colonial weight for North American missionaries as for British missionaries. Moreover, it was seen as particularly important in the Muslim World. Despite these differences, coming into close contact with indigenous people was embedded in medical work of many Protestant missionary organisations.

The Focus of this Book

The motto 'healing bodies, saving souls' might be rendered 'affecting bodies, saving souls'. This book contemplates the missionary side of this motto through the locus of the CMS medical mission work in Persia and north-western British India, building upon existing scholarship on Protestant mission work in the Middle East and British India. This change is interpretive and captures my argument; that is, medical missions should be viewed as 'emotional set-ups' that served to change the sensory relationship between missionaries and local people. Missionaries spent a great deal of time contemplating their own and prospective converts' emotions. The medical missionaries' practice of obtaining people's trust is an integral part of this history, which has recently gained a new impetus due to the growing attention to the role of emotions in the making of history. Studies have gone beyond seeing emotions as limited to the private sphere of missionary family interactions and intimacy,[28] and have shown that we need to investigate emotions if we are to understand colonial missions and colonialism fully.[29]

This book offers additional answers to questions of why medical missions developed in a specific way, why the missionaries opted for one region, and city or town over another, why certain architectural forms were privileged over others. While the focus of the book is on missionaries' side of the story, it also discusses, to some extent, how it felt to stay in a mission hospital, showing we can speculate about indigenous perspectives by focusing on emotions.

The study covers a span of nearly fifty years, from the foundation of the Kashmir medical mission in 1865 to the start of the First World War. Medical mission work was at its peak during this period. It focuses primarily on Persia and north-western British India because they are part of a block of territory defined by missionaries as the 'Moslem Lands' (Figure I.2).[30] They felt the need to establish medical missions in the Muslim lands the most keenly. In other words, medical work was considered as the most potent instrument for attracting people in 'Mohammedan cities'.[31] Moreover, British medical missionaries predominantly worked among Muslims in these two regions, with the CMS being the most active society.

The story of Protestant mission work among Muslims began with Henry Martin. An East Indian Company (EIC) chaplain and a member of the CMS, Martin translated the New Testament into Urdu and revised the Persian and Arabic translations of the same work after travelling to British India in 1806 and spending almost a year in Shiraz (Persia) before his eventual death of disease in Ottoman East.[32] The next step was taken when the CMS established a mission in Malta, then a British possession, in 1815, and from there started working in Syra (Syros) (1828), Egypt (1825) and Smyrna (Izmir) (1830),[33] followed by the ABCFM in Palestine 1819 and the Basil Mission in the Caucasus in 1821.[34] It was not the CMS but rather the ABCFM that commenced the first mission in Persia, in Orūmīyeh in 1834, where they directed their activities mainly to the members of the Church of the East. Nor was the CMS the first British missionary society that showed interest in mission work in Persia. Several missionaries of the Society for Promoting Christian Knowledge (SPCK) and the Society for the Propagation of the Gospel (SPG) undertook expeditions in Orūmīyeh and the surrounding regions in the first half of the nineteenth century.[35] The CMS was the first to commence work among Muslims in Persia by opening the Isfahan (Julfā) mission in 1869. The ABCFM followed suit and opened

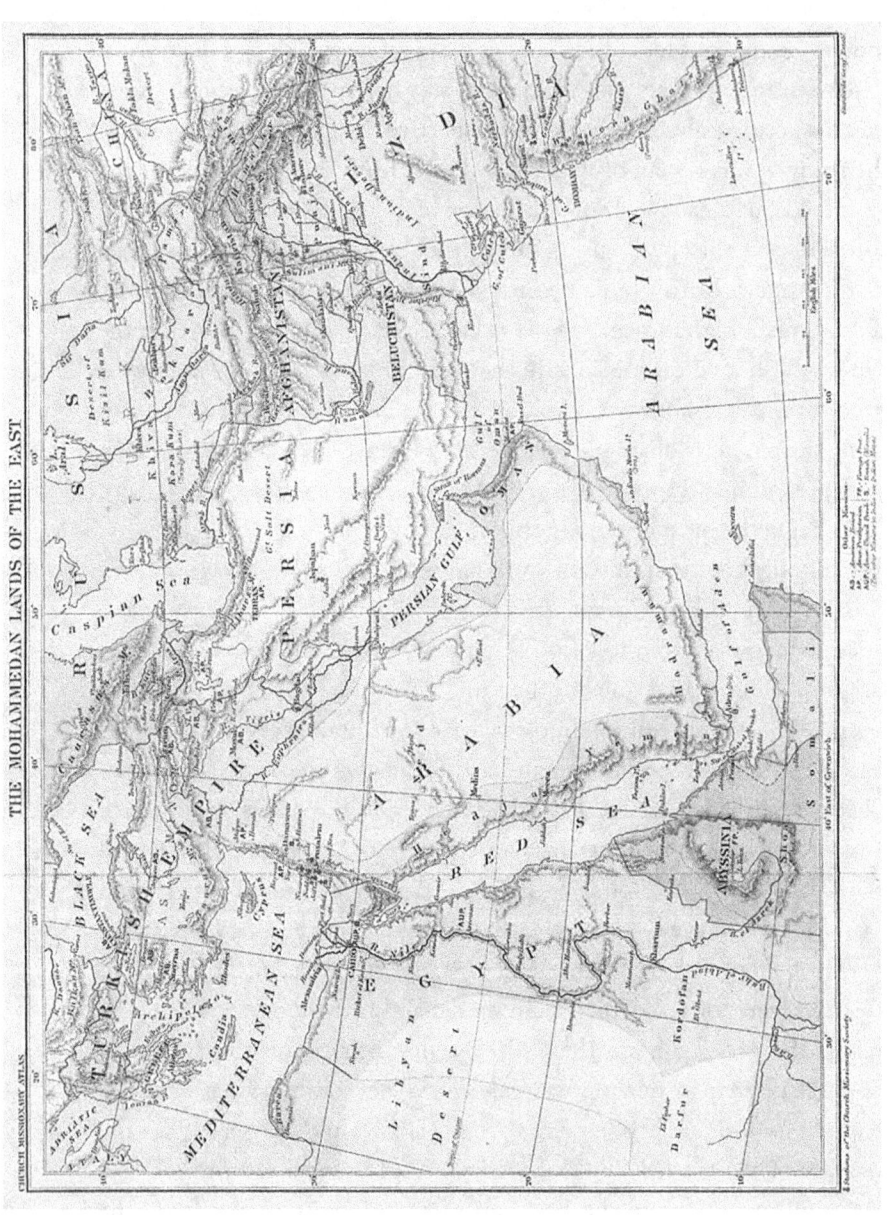

Figure I.2 The Mohammedan Lands of the East, 1896. Note the CMS stations in north-western British India. *CMS Atlas*, Church Missionary Society Archive, Cadbury Research Library, Special Collections, University of Birmingham.

missions in Tehran (1872), Tabriz (1873), Hamadan (1881), Kermanshah (1894), Rasht (1902) and Mashhad (1911).[36]

The ABCFM also preceded the CMS in starting mission work in Punjab and north-western British India by opening the Ludhiana mission in 1833.[37] It would be almost twenty years before the CMS would start a regular mission in Punjab. Reverend Robert Clark opened this mission in Amritsar in 1852. Apart from the ABCFM and the CMS, representatives of the Baptist Missionary Society (BMS), the Church of Scotland (CS), the Church of England Zenana Missionary Society (CEZMS) and the Salvation Army, to name but a few, were active in Punjab and its Himalayan hinterlands.[38]

Among the first group of missionaries that the ABCFM sent to Persia was a doctor, Asahel Grant, who arrived in the country with his wife, Judith Campbell, in 1835.[39] We can also find a few references to medical work in the letters that Reverend William Krusé, a Lutheran clergyman, sent from Jaffa in the 1860s.[40] Nonetheless, no permanent medical mission work was started, especially among Muslims, until the CMS commenced the Kashmir medical mission in 1865 and the Isfahan medical mission in 1869.[41] Over the next fifty years the CMS expanded its medical work in north-western British India and Persia, eventually establishing the following ten medical missions: Dear Ghazi Khan (1879), Amritsar (1882), Quetta (1885), Bannu (1894), Peshawar (1898), Dera Ismail Khan (1899), Multan (1899), Yazd (1899), Islamabad (1901) and Kerman (1901), each with several branch dispensaries. While the CMS took the claim of medical mission work later than certain British missionary societies,[42] it was the first to open medical missions among Muslims in Persia and north-western British India. In time, it became the largest and most important British mission in both regions. By 1900, missionaries had identified Egypt as a 'strategic centre' for Muslim evangelisation worldwide,[43] yet the CMS only opened two hospitals in Egypt.[44] It was in southern Persia and north-western British India that British medical missionaries worked primarily among Muslims. The ABCFM founded more medical missions than the CMS in the Muslim world. For example, they had twenty hospitals in the Ottoman Empire by 1909[45] and were the most prominent Protestant mission in Egypt.[46] Medical missions that were founded in the late Ottoman Empire, Egypt, Palestine and north-west Persia were partly missions to Muslims as a focus on members of the Eastern church persisted in these regions. The ABCFM worked among Muslims in Tehran, Rasht and Mashhad in the north and north-east Persia and Basra (1891), and Bahrain (1900).[47] I will refer to some of these medical missions throughout this book, but my focus will remain on the CMS medical missions in Persia and north-western British India.

From the 1910s onwards missionaries increasingly faced new challenges relating to emerging nationalistic consciousness, the First World War and the collapse of the Ottoman Empire. These changes, along with concerns regarding the low conversion rate, caused missionaries to propose new approaches to missionary work, including missionary work among Muslims.[48] According to Catriona Laing, one such approach identified a 'kinship' between Islam and Christianity and called for 'prayer, print and presence among Muslims'.[49] Although new hospitals were founded after the war, including the CMS hospital in Shiraz (1923) and the hospital of the United Presbyterian Church in the USA (PCUSA) in Mashhad, ongoing mission work in many cases became difficult, and many hospitals were closed down as a result. The nature of mission work also changed due to the increasing involvement of indigenous churchmen and women in the leadership of the churches.

Focusing on the CMS medical missions in Persia and north-western British India is crucial. Additionally, it is essential to consider these hospitals jointly because they were supposed to form a chain for political and practical reasons. Nevertheless, the book does not aim at examining the histories of these medical missions in all their nuances. Although histories of missionaries and their medicine and architecture in the British Empire have both splintered into a variety of approaches, they have not been combined. This book brings these histories together and engages with the field of the history of emotions to contribute a new (architectural) history of Christian mission and imperialism.[50]

Researching the History of Emotions and Christian Missions

Throughout this book, I engage with methodological approaches offered by the field of the history of emotions. There are two central claims upon which emotion history has been grounded. The first one warns against the temptation to translate historical emotion terms, arguing that emotions are not universal, but rather are intertwined in the dynamics of the cultural presence.⁵¹ Some historians, such as Ute Frevert, have gone so far as to illustrate that some emotions have even been 'lost'.⁵² Scholars of Christian mission have responded to this call by analysing feelings, such as Christian love, fear, pity, hatred or happiness, in their specific and changing cultural contexts.⁵³ For example, Claire McLisky demonstrates that 'Evangelical Love' took on many forms: 'constraining, compassionate, controlling, unreciprocated, and even on occasions, violent'.⁵⁴ As stated above, this book takes care not to make a false equivalence between present configurations of trust, friendship and affection and the stated feelings of historical missionaries. Of foremost importance is how the introduction of medical mission work influenced missionaries' sensory experience of the local people and vice versa.*

The second convention of emotion history rejects the restrictive dichotomy between reason/emotion, head/heart and public/private, seeing them instead bundled together to define, (re)produce and refine social, political and scientific histories. As Boddice puts it, emotions are far from 'mere fleeting passages of irrational behaviour'; they 'are at once the effect of historical circumstances and a cause of their changes'.⁵⁵ A variety of methodological approaches has been developed to address the historical role of emotions, among which concepts of 'emotional practices' and 'emotional communities' have shown to be particularly useful for studying emotions in the Christian mission contexts.⁵⁶ A clarification about the adjective 'emotional' and the word 'emotion' is in order before discussing these concepts. 'Emotional' and 'emotion' are not always representative of historical usage, which is crucial to bear in mind. Moreover, they have been keywords 'in crises' since their adaptation as fully-fledged theoretical terms since the nineteenth century. There is little agreement among emotion scientists on what they mean. Historians of emotions have often used them for the sake of convenience and sometimes interchangeably with other terms, including feeling, passion, sentiment and affect⁵⁷ while showing how they are not merely mental states with an outward bodily expression.⁵⁸

At its core, this book draws on the concept of emotional practices, which Monique Scheer has developed in detail. It emphasises that emotions are

---

* Missionaries used these terms interchangeably. I will use them interchangeably throughout this book too.

connected closely to bodily practices.[59] In other words, far from being prior to, they are produced through practices or performances. Thus, to study emotions, one also must examine the practices in which they were experienced. The practice theory deconstructs the binaries between mind and body, expression and experience and subject and object by emphasising their interrelations.

Bettina Hitzer, Scheer, Rebecca Swartz and Jacqueline van Gent, among others, have highlighted how songs, hymns, prayers, rhetorical style of preachers and so on were negotiated as emotional practices in missionaries' endeavours.[60] These emotional practices are mobilising practices that evoke and change emotions. Indeed, Scheer recognises four types of emotional practices: mobilising, naming, communicating and regulating.[61] Mobilising emotions, with which I am concerned in this book, include media, habits, rituals and everyday pastimes. They involve the self (as both body and mind) as well as others, language, material artefacts and the environment. According to Scheer, we can bring about an emotional state in ourselves by seeking certain spaces, sounds, companions and so on, or we can simply be confronted with an 'emotional set-up' (involving self, others, objects, sounds, smells, the environment).[62] Building on Scheer's approach, I speculate about the medical activities and infrastructures of the missionaries as emotional set-ups that served to change the sensory relationship between the missionaries and the local people. Thinking about medical missions in this way requires considering the missionaries, local people, objects, sounds, smells and the (built) environment side by side. This consideration, in turn, necessitates examining not only the making and remaking of metropolitan forms[63] but also the exploration of modes of occupation. Indigenous people did not passively feel certain emotions. Rather, the material arrangements facilitated certain habits and routines – such as observing a surgery, cooking in the hospital, drinking tea, interacting with family and friends – and thus 'doing emotions'. Although it is important to note that emotional practices could fail, leading to a form of 'feeling differently' or 'failing to feel correctly'.[64]

Moreover, the book's overall argument expands upon the concept of emotional communities. Barbara Rosenwein introduced this concept in her 2002 article and subsequent writings about medieval Early Middle Ages Europe.[65] Rosenwein compares emotional communities to social communities such as 'families, neighbourhoods, parliaments, guilds, monasteries, and parish church membership', encouraging researchers to uncover these communities' systems of feeling:

> what these communities (and the individuals within them) define and assess as valuable or harmful to them; the evaluations that they make about others' emotions; the nature of the affective bonds between people that they recognize; and the modes of emotional expression that they expect, encourage, tolerate and deplore.[66]

In other words, Rosenwein is concerned with how 'emotional standards' were formed at various social levels. In addition, she recognises that individuals can move between and live in different, yet relatively similar, communities, adjusting their emotional displays and judgements.

Rosenwein's formulation has been adopted widely. However, her argument that navigation among emotional communities is only possible if they are not radically different has been questioned. Mark Seymour has shown that, depending on circumstances, radically different emotional communities can overlap.[67] But, does sharing an emotional community mean integration? This question has particular implications concerning cross-cultural encounters. Historians of emotions and Christian mission have shown how missionaries, through re-working emotional behaviours and generating a 'fellow feeling', sought to integrate the (potential) converts into a diverse, sometimes imagined, emotional community with specific emotional styles. But the missionaries' efforts to transform and Christianise the 'other' involved maintenance of distance, resulting in complications and uncertainties for the converts as well as the missionaries themselves.[68] Many converts could also develop new emotional styles of their own. Karen Vallgårda, Kristine Alexander and Stephanie Olsen have defined these boundaries between different communities as 'emotional frontiers'.[69] They have devised 'emotional formations' instead of emotional communities to incorporate these boundaries. This concept accounts for a certain level of coherence in people's conception of appropriate emotional comportment in different situations as well as 'internal variations' within the same emotional formation based on ethnic, class, age and gender differences. It also signals a process where individuals not only adjust their emotion structures but also continually consolidate or alter them to align themselves with given hierarchies of emotion.[70]

The concept of emotional communities also does not elaborate enough on how power implements specific emotional styles. We may turn to William Reddy's 'emotional regimes' to consider how power works.[71] It discusses how 'any stable political regime' inculcates 'normative emotions'. Rosenwein introduced emotional communities partly in criticism of William Reddy's emotional regimes. She views Reddy's concept as a 'roadblock', arguing that it links regimes only to elites and political power.[72] Instead, emotional communities refer to the existence of multiple power structures within 'a seemingly hegemonic system'. However, as Boddice states, she understands regimes 'narrowly' and 'literally'; Reddy does not employ this term to refer only to the nation state.[73] These two concepts are more or less the same but, according to Boddice, emotional regimes offer greater scope for understanding how power influences how emotions work. Reddy talks about regimes that work through strict enforcement as well as 'loose regimes',[74] but he does not consider how a loose regime might contribute to the operation of a restrict regime.

Examining politics of emotions, conversion and childhood in the Danish Protestant Christian mission in twentieth-century colonial South India, Vallgårda has shown how missionaries treated children 'gently' to win their hearts for Christ. This strategy was as much a religious as a political vision because they sought to change emotional norms while reconfiguring the social landscape at large. Vallgårda rethinks the idea of emotional communities to 'capture the dynamic force of emotions not only in mobilising or regulating individual emotional comportment within a community but also in forging the very community'.[75] She also gives some thought to mobilising emotions through gentleness. This is where we need to expand upon emotional communities – and regimes – further. The medical missionaries did not always expect local people to develop new emotional structures.[76] This point is nowhere more noticeable than in 'family wards' (which I will examine in Chapter Three). The missionaries often interfered in indigenous family structures. Children, who attended missionary schools, were sometimes separated from their family members. Conversely, patients, including children, could stay with their family and friends in a family ward. They could also bring their belongings, including cooking utensils and beddings, and thus live in the hospital as they would in their homes. The missionaries hoped to gain local people's trust and affection in this way. Their reluctance to interfere in local people's emotional formations was also a means to 'sustain relations of power'.[77] As will be discussed in Chapter Five, British medical missionaries in north-western British India viewed gaining trust, friendship or affection as a way of altering the feeling of the very community in favour of the colonial establishment.

Architecture and the History of Emotions

This book also engages with arguments regarding the history of the relationship between space, objects and emotions. Examining emotions as culturally and temporally specific has also provided an impetus to consider the history of the relationship between architecture and emotions afresh. Studies have questioned the premises of neuroarchitecture and affect theory. The former assumes an ahistorical relationship between body, mind and the built environment.[78] And the latter, even when attending to temporal and cultural varieties, considers space and its objects as mere producers of affect.[79] Margrit Pernau, among others, argues for 'temporalization' as the 'central category to link materiality with knowledge and practice'.[80] Building on Andreas Reckwitz's work regarding a 'praxeological' understanding of emotions, Pernau asserts that insofar as bodies are culturally and socially constructed, they cannot be affected by a space in any unequivocal or straightforward way.[81] Boddice further argues for a body, mind and world model, emphasising that the connection between a space and emotions does not take place against 'stable backgrounds' of experiential feelings that existed 'out there'; this connection can change over time, and the same space can trigger different emotions in various people.[82] The emotional appeal of architecture should be examined through careful consideration of the ongoing changes in norms, rules and regulations.[83]

Architectural historians of British imperialism have been slow to respond to emotions history promises. They have acknowledged emotions; for example, they have seen adaptation to local contexts as a sign of 'respect' for indigenous traditions, discussed how buildings were designed to inculcate 'adoration' and interpreted 'awe' as a local reception. But they have not paid attention to emotions' temporal and cultural variety.[84] Moreover, they have perceived the relationship between emotions and architecture as a 'static' rather than a 'dynamic' process.[85] As Razak Khan states in the context of South Asia, 'emotional and spatial categories are not only deeply entangled with, but constitutive of, imperial, colonial, postcolonial, and contemporary local and global spatial imagination'.[86] However, the interconnection between architecture, emotions and British imperialism is yet to be examined. A few studies have highlighted the importance of emotions to the British empire building,[87] but, as Khan's statement suggests, it is imperative to talk about the intersection between emotional and architectural histories of British imperialism.

Examining emotions as culturally and temporally situated could unbalance previously established views. Medical missions as emotional set-ups questions the extent to which they impressed upon local people Western medical ideas, institutions and practices.[88] Emotional set-ups in this respect might resemble Mary Louise Pratt's 'contact zones', Anthony King's 'third culture' or, as regards mission hospitals more specifically, Samir Boulos's 'culturally entangled space'.[89] These concepts highlight the zones where 'the cultures came into collision' and show that the imposition of colonial order and control occurred primarily at an ideological level. Yet, examining medical missions as emotional set-ups demands understanding the cultural histories and memories of objects (and spaces) to uncover their emotional charges. In this regard, it is essential to examine how patients encountered and evaluated spaces[90] because the potential of a space to evoke emotions largely depends on the 'specific cultural sensitivity and attentiveness' of the users. Affects only form when the users can practically appropriate the space. Pernau discusses the role of memory in this regard that 'spaces can be endowed with an emotional valence through practices and experiences repeated over a long time'.[91] For example, in arguing that surveillance by mapping in the early nineteenth-century Delhi 'might have been more of a colonial desire than a reality', Pernau draws on Mughal miniatures and demonstrates that the 'disciplining gaze might not have been as new as it seems at first sight'.[92] In a similar vein, I challenge the assumption that medical missions universally had a distinct 'disciplining' emotional affect. Even if missionaries hoped to teach patients to be punctual and self-disciplined through the spatial set-up of wards – beds in neat rows and with clean white sheets – their intention could have been sometimes misplaced.

Patients could re-appropriate the wards. But the argument here is different: the spatial arrangement may have appeared familiar to them.

As already emphasised, regarding medical missions as emotional set-ups also demands examining not only the buildings – their appearance and layout – but also the modes of occupation they engendered: how they were supposed to smell, how the beds were meant to feel and so on. There is a specific urgency to go beyond appearance and layout because histories of hospitals and colonial/imperial architecture have been extremely centred on visual perception and spatial experience. Michel Foucault's studies of prison, specifically the panopticon, and the rise of clinical medicine, placed visibility and control at the heart of scholarship. Although scholars have criticised Foucault's concentration on the technologies of visibility for failing to account for such concepts as class or actions as resistance, little attempt has been made to discuss the idea that people's (patients' as well as visitors' in the case of this study) senses and feelings were overtaken by conditions other than sight before and after they entered the buildings.[93] The missionaries permitted the patients to drink tea, cook food, bring certain utensils, smoke water pipes and so on in the hospitals. These conditions were influential in defining patients' experiences, conditioning emotive success – that is, feeling in accord with expectations and prescriptions.[94] Although there could have been various smells, tastes or noises in the hospitals, such as the smell of specific diseases or illnesses,[95] I am concerned with how patients were permitted to create certain smells and tastes while in the hospitals. I should emphasise that some patients might have found the buildings welcoming or have felt at home in the hospitals, but the extent to which they would have the same feelings towards missionaries is debatable.

Deploying Emotional Mode in Reading Historical Texts

I started the introduction by referring to my first visit to the CMS hospital in Kerman and how the buildings impressed me. I stated that this experience shaped the process of my research, which leads to the question of the place of emotions in the process of historical research and whether historians should pay attention to the emotional components of their work.

If the field of the history of emotions has unbalanced the strict dichotomy between emotion and reason, then viewing affective and unemotional ways of assessing the past as radically opposite is a pitfall.[96] Nevertheless, as Benno Gammerl states, the problem arises when a specific emotional style is celebrated in favour of others in historical writing.[97] For example, take Renée M. Sentilles' discussion about how experiencing a place where something happened can provide intellectual insight into an historical actor's life. While researching the American actress Adah Isaacs Menken's (1835–86) early life in East Texas, Sentilles drove to Livingston to check a few regional archives, a trip which helped her 'to understand her [Menken's] ongoing relationship with this part of the country'. Sentilles writes, 'driving through the lush but sparsely populated region, I realized that she was part of a glorious, mythological past.'[98] She does not elaborate on how such a realisation influenced her narrative, however, and, as a consequence, one may argue against her approach as being 'narcissistic' rather than based on 'a more communal sense'.[99] Moreover, it seems that she views Menken's experience as accessible insofar as it can be re-experienced, and this is the chief criticism that could be levelled at her approach. If, as Boddice and Mark Smith state, 'things like disgust, anger, fear, sympathy, empathy, and so on, are historically specific and contingent, then our own sensory and emotional reaction to the historical material we encounter cannot be permitted to be formative of historical analysis'.[100] The same criticism applies to Rachel Lee's account of her 'engagement' with the archive of the German architect, Otto Koenigsberger (1908–99), at the Swiss Institute for the Study of Egyptian Architecture in Cairo. Lee writes that she was able to 'share the physical experience of that private space [the Swiss Institute] of exposure with him [Koenigsberger] – albeit eighty years later'. But she could not have possibly 'stepped into a time machine', as she claims. Moreover, had the researcher been from Egypt, of different age, gender or background, they would have felt the 'cold', 'the flush mechanism' and 'the small sink' differently.[101]

The matter is not about being subjective or objective, but, as Sarah Tarlow discusses, is about making a clear distinction between 'past emotion as a subject of study and examination of subjectivity' of scholars as a 'method'. While our emotions can provide insight into feelings that motivated past actions, they should not be used to understand emotional experiences across time or space.[102] Boddice and Smith suggest that historians must consciously consider 'their own apparently automatic reactions to their sources' and 'cast them aside from their historical analysis'.[103] I suggest that historians should cast them aside, insofar as they should not draw a parallel between their impression of visiting a building and what historical actors experienced. I am not rejecting Jane Rendell's work on 'site-writing' or the author's position to the site of writing (on which Lee draws), but instead, I hope to see it from the vantage point of the history of emotions. Indeed, the history of emotions is an 'other' place from which it is possible to explore our position and the difference it makes to what we can know.[104]

The feelings implied in my encounter with buildings generated valuable insights[105] and thus, in a sense, remained inside the work. However, I do not draw a parallel between my first impression of visiting the buildings and what the patients experienced in the early twentieth century. The impression that the buildings left on me was an awakening call, which, to use Jane Hattrick's term, 'seduced' me.[106] 'Time and familiarity' might have woven specific colonial structures 'into the local fabric as if they had emerged from vernacular building traditions' as Peter Scriver and Vikramaditya Prakash state regarding the bungalows, barracks, institutional and technical infrastructures built in British India and Ceylon.[107] But my personal experience studying architecture in Kerman was crucial as I found a profound contrast between what I knew about the so-called Western architecture in early twentieth-century Persia and the buildings of the Kerman hospital. The entrance of the Nūrīe hospital, built by a local philanthropist a few years after the Morsalīn hospital, appeared more 'foreign' to me as it shows the same concern with external appearance as buildings constructed during the late Qajar dynasty under the influence of European architecture (Figure I.3).[108] By contrast, the entrance of the Kerman hospital is considerably smaller and might even be considered insignificant. Moreover, as I will discuss in Chapter Two, it is located at the end of a straight narrow blind alley, which resembles the blind alleys leading to houses in traditional cities in Persia, including Kerman (Figure I.4). This reaction made me pick up on the words trust, friendship and affection when reading the CMS materials and engage with the field of the history of emotions. Thus, to assert once more, these are not terms I am imposing here; they were regularly employed by the missionaries when reporting their activities or describing the buildings.

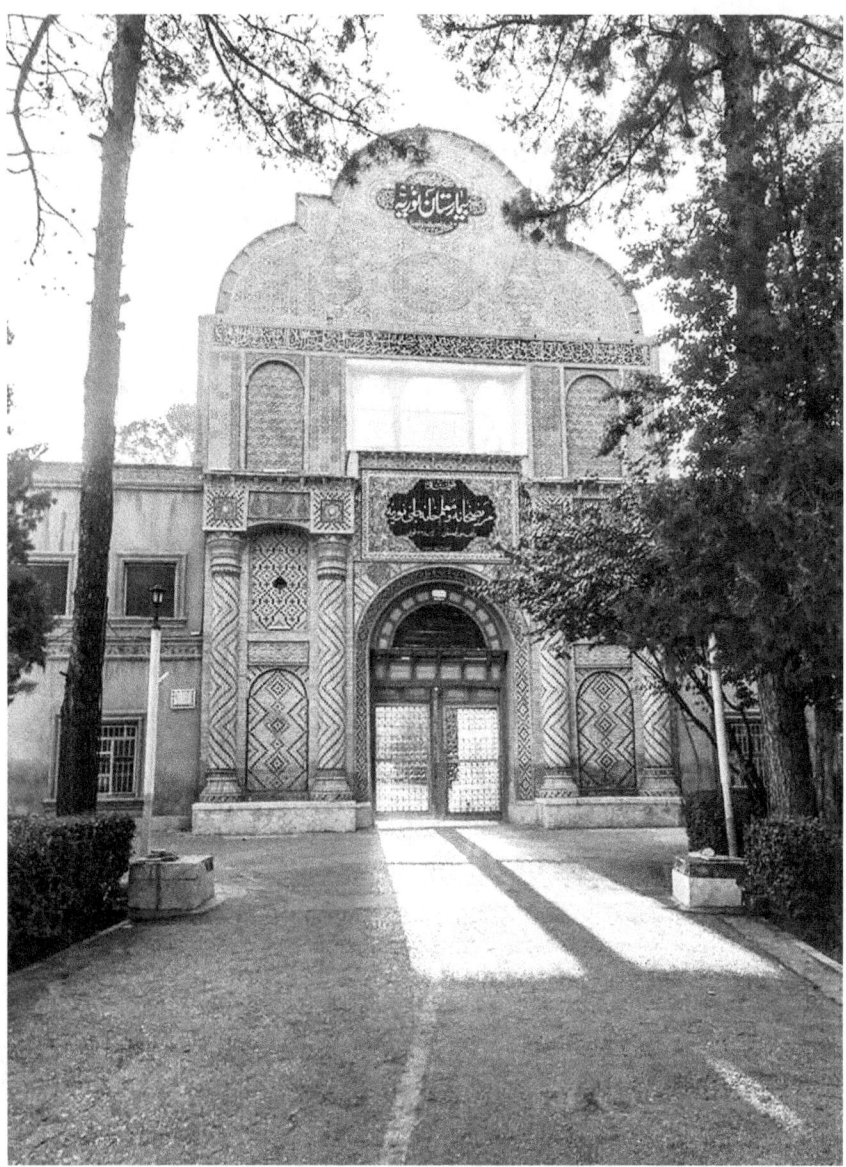

Figure I.3 The entrance to Nūrīe hospital in Kerman. Photo by author.

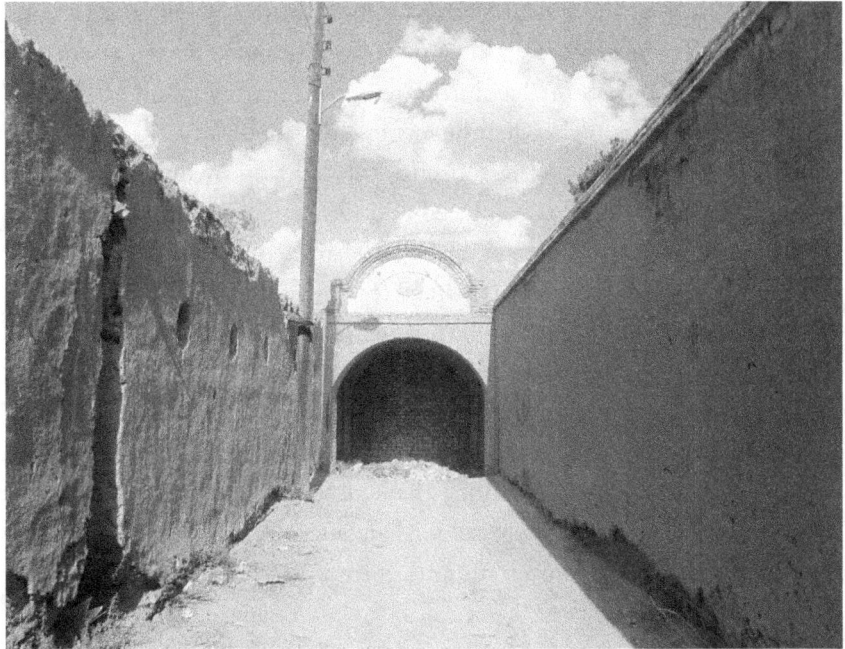

Figure I.4 The narrow blind alley leading to the entrance of the CMS hospital in Kerman.
Photo by author.

Outline

As mentioned above, this book aims at offering a new (architectural) history of Christian mission and imperialism. Thus, it is organised in such a way as to (re)examine some key (neglected) themes in the history of medical mission work and architecture through the issue of gaining trust. Chapter One examines missionaries' activities before the construction of and outside the mission hospitals. It shows that dispensaries, itineration tours and adapted existing buildings were viewed as instrumental in establishing contacts with larger numbers of people and thus in preparing the ground for hospital work. It expands existing studies that consider these activities at best ancillary to the development of medical missions and integrates them more fully into the story of the establishment of medical missions.

Chapter Two questions the assumption that mission hospitals universally demonstrated Christian order and cleanliness. It does so by examining the architecture of the medical missions and practices facilitated through architecture. It situates the architecture of the hospitals in the context of British imperial and hospital architecture in the nineteenth and early twentieth centuries. It highlights that the missionaries adopted local architectural forms and elements that were thoroughly caught up in the daily lives of the local people. They also employed and developed a wide range of construction methods and different types of hospital plans and ward designs, in contrast to the tendency in Britain to aim for standardisation among all wards and between hospitals. Missionaries drew on the architecture of Islamic four-part gardens or Persian courtyard houses and incorporated details and ornamentations associated with the Mughal era or used construction methods local to the respective regions and found in domestic spaces, such as the Kermanī arch. Adopting these local architectural forms and elements was neither a response to colonial anxieties around climate nor was it out of respect for indigenous traditions. Instead, it was a strategy to increase the number of patients.

The focus of Chapter Three is on hospital visiting, which is a largely neglected theme in the history of medicine, including imperial and missionary medicine. Various groups visited mission hospitals. This chapter identifies these groups, focusing on patients' visitors, namely family and friends. It presents hospitals as locations where boundaries between European and indigenous families were intentionally breached. From the 1880s onwards, visits from family and friends were increasingly policed in British hospitals due to fears that guests might introduce dirt and infection. By contrast, missionaries commonly allowed family and friends to visit the patients and even stay in the hospitals in the contexts described here. They developed a novel hospital design to host family and friends known as the 'serai-system', which was designed like a caravanserai, an inn for travellers built along the caravan routes in Central Asia. While missionaries observed that the presence of close associates was irksome, they allowed them to accompany the patients because this could bring the mission in contact with a larger number of people.

Chapter Four turns to female medical missionaries and builds upon scholarship concerning missionary women and women and architecture. The issue of gaining trust was relevant to activities of both male and female missionaries, but its manifestations differed according to gender. Female missionaries were seen as better suited for this task. Thus, a focus on female missionaries and hospitals for women is essential. This chapter provides a background of female (medical) missionary work and discusses how (medical) missions formed and were formed by diverse gender roles and expectations. It argues for another way in which female missionaries were active agents in the mission field by highlighting their involvement in the design process of the hospitals. A particular concern of the chapter is Dr Minnie Gomery, who was responsible for designing the Islamabad (Anantnag) hospital. Furthermore, the chapter shows that female medical missionaries did not universally and uniformly seek to modernise and enlighten women. This point is nowhere more evident than in the architecture of the medical missions. A specific type of hospital architecture, known as the 'Purdah hospital', was developed specifically for women according to Muslim and Hindu rules.

The focus of Chapter Five is on mission, emotions and imperialism. It examines the public views of the CMS missionaries in north-western British India concerning Anglo-Russian rivalry. In their reports, the missionaries recognised the value of their work as worth a 'regiment' to the British government. The chapter shows that this claim is comparable to the views of some of the early nineteenth-century missionaries, who talked about the providential purpose of the empire, arguing that the extension of the national church was beneficial culturally, religiously and politically. However, the CMS missionaries did not talk about the spread of Christianity per se, nor the dissemination of the English race or ethical values. Instead, they claimed their work was politically significant because it had been instrumental in obtaining people's trust or friendship. They justified this view on at least two grounds: firstly, they highlighted their ability to generate a new archive of knowledge about the region; secondly, they declared they were winning local people for the colonial establishment by changing their feelings.

These chapters illuminate the pivotal role of emotions in Christian medical mission endeavour. Moreover, they highlight how emotional prescriptions and set-ups are one thing, and emotional responses are another.[109] Delving on these points adds to our understanding of Christian missions, medicine, architecture and British imperialism. We still have a long way to go until the history of emotions becomes a way of writing histories of

Christian mission and architectural histories of British imperialism. I hope *Emotion, Mission, Architecture* inspires future enquiries into the relationship between architecture, emotions and British imperialism.

Notes

1. Sarah Ahmed, *The Cultural Politics of Emotion* (Edinburgh: Edinburgh University Press, 2004), 5–8.
2. A. W. F. H., 'The Opening of the Door in Kashmir, Part I', *Mercy and Truth* 1, no. 8 (1897): 174.
3. Ibid., 175.
4. Ibid., 176–7.
5. T. Maxwell, 'The Opening of the Door in Kashmir, 1873–1876', *Mercy and Truth* 1, no. 9 (1897): 199–203.
6. 'Church Missionary Society', *The Missionary Register* 4 (1816): 375; 'Reports of Societies', *The Missionary Register* 5 (1817): 425.
7. Michael C. Lazich, 'Seeking Souls through the Eyes of the Blind: The Birth of the Medical Missionary Society in Nineteenth-Century China', in David Hardiman (ed.), *Healing Bodies, Saving Souls: Medical Missions in Asia and Africa* (Amsterdam: Rodopi, 2006), 59–86; see also Theron Kue-Hing Young, 'A Conflict of Professions: The Medical Missionary in China, 1835–1890', *Bulletin of the History of Medicine* 47, no. 3 (1973): 250–72.
8. The Catholic Church did not become involved in medical mission work until the 1920s.
9. David Hardiman, 'Introduction', in *Healing Bodies* (see note 7), 11.
10. Ibid., 10–11; Peter Williams, 'Healing and Evangelism: The Place of Medicine in later Victorian Protestant Missionary Thinking', *Studies in Church History* 19 (1982): 272. doi:10.1017/S0424208400009414.
11. Although the Medical Act formally unified the medical profession in Britain, there were few immediate signs of uniformity up until 1886. See Michael Worboys, *Spreading Germs: Disease Theories and Medical Practice in Britain, 1865–1900* (Cambridge: Cambridge University Press, 2000), 20–8.
12. Williams, 'Healing and Evangelism', 271.
13. For example, the Members of the Lahore Missionary Conference of 1862 discussed that medical missionaries 'would prove very valuable auxiliaries to the direct work of propagating the Gospel, more especially in large cities, among the hill tribes, and in all places, as Cashmere [Kashmir], where medical aid is not available, and where deep prejudice may be removed by their means.' *Report of*

the Punjab Missionary Conference held at Lahore in December and January, 1862–63 (Lodiana: American Presbyterian Mission Press, 1863), 109; see also Rosemary Fitzgerald, '"Clinical Christianity": The Emergence of Medical Mission Work as a Missionary Strategy in Colonial India, 1800–1914', in Biswamoy Pati and Mark Harrison (eds), *Health, Medicine, and Empire: Perspectives on Colonial India* (New Delhi: Orient Longman, 2001), 101–2; Philippe Bourmaud, 'Public Space and Private Spheres: The Foundation of St Luke's Hospital of Nablus by the CMS (1891–1901)', in Heleen Murre-van den Berg (ed.), *New Faith in Ancient Lands: Western Missions in the Middle East in the Nineteenth and Twentieth Centuries* (Leiden and Boston: Brill: 2006), 133.
14. Hardiman, 'Introduction', 22–3.
15. A. Neve, 'Medical Mission Auxiliary Annual Meeting, May 5, 1898', *Mercy and Truth* 2, no. 10 (1898): 134.
16. Michael Jennings, '"Healing of Bodies, Salvation of Souls": Missionary Medicine in Colonial Tanganyika, 1870s–1939', *Journal of Religion in Africa* 38 (2008): 28. It was estimated in 1947 that there were 300 mission hospitals in China and 256 hospitals and 250 branch dispensaries in India: David Hardiman, 'The Mission Hospital, 1880–1960', in Mark Harrison, Margaret Jones and Helen Sweet (eds), *From Western Medicine to Global Medicine: the Hospital beyond the West* (Hyderabad: Orient BlackSwan, 2009), 198; see also Megan Vaughan, *Curing their Ills: Colonial Power and African Illness* (Cambridge: Polity Press, 1991), 56.
17. Emrah Şahin, *Faithful Encounters: Authorities and American Missionaries in the Ottoman Empire* (Montreal, Kingston, London and Chicago: McGill-Queen's University Press, 2018), 94–5; Terence O. Ranger, 'Godly Medicine: The Ambiguities of Medical Mission in Southeast Tanzania, 1900–1945', *Social Science and Medicine, Part B: Medical Anthropology* 15, no. 3 (1981): 261–77; see also Elizabeth Elbourne, 'Mother's Milk: Gender, Power, and Anxiety on a South African Mission Station, 1839–1940', in Patricia Grimshaw and Andrew May (eds), *Missionaries, Indigenous Peoples and Cultural Exchange* (Brighton, Portland and Toronto: Sussex Academic Press, 2010): 19–20; Michael Jennings, 'A Matter of Vital Importance: The Place of the Medical Mission in Maternal and Child Healthcare in Tanganyika, 1919–39', in *Healing Bodies* (see note 7), 245; David Hardiman, 'Christian Therapy: Medical Missionaries and the Adivasis of Western India, 1880–1930', in *Healing Bodies* (see note 7), 154.
18. Heleen Murre-van den Berg, '"Dear Mother of my Soul": Fidelia Fiske and the Role of Women Missionaries in Mid-nineteenth Century Iran', *Exchange* 30, no. 1 (2001): 33–48.

19. David Hardiman, *Missionaries and their Medicine: A Christian modernity for tribal India* (Manchester: Manchester University Press, 2017); Adam H. Becker, *Revival and Awakening: American Evangelical Missionaries in Iran and the Origin of Assyrian Nationalism* (Chicago and London: The University of Chicago Press, 2015), 90–1; Heather J. Sharkey, *American Evangelicals: Missionary Encounters in an Age of Empire* (Princeton and Oxford: Princeton University Press, 2008), 76–7.
20. Nancy Rose Hunt, *A Colonial Lexicon of Birth Ritual and Mobility in the Congo* (Durham and London: Duke University Press, 1999), 161.
21. Ildiko Csengei, *Sympathy, Sensibility and the Literature of Feeling in the Eighteenth Century* (Basingstoke: Palgrave Macmillan, 2012); Kathleen Wilson, 'Empire, Gender, and Modernity in the Eighteenth Century', in Philippa Levine (ed.), *Gender and Empire* (Oxford: Oxford University Press, 2004), 20; Rob Boddice, *The Science of Sympathy: Morality, Evolution, and Victorian Civilization* (Urbana and Chicago: University of Illinois Press, 2016), 9–10.
22. Hardiman, 'Introduction', 8.
23. 'A Visit to the Old Cairo Hospital', *Mercy and Truth* 9, no. 104 (1905): 249.
24. Yasmina El Chami, 'An American "Garden" in an Oriental "Desert": The Modernity of Timber at the Syrian Protestant College of Beirut', *Architectural Theory Review* 25, no. 1–2 (2021): 199–215, 10.1080/13264826.2021.1958354; Fassil Demissie, 'Colonial Architecture and Urbanism in Africa: And Introduction', in Fassil Demissie (ed.), *Colonial Architecture and Urbanism in Africa: Intertwined and Contested Histories* (Oxford and New York: Routledge, 2012), 1.
25. Rob Boddice emphasises this by referring to 'happy', 'compassionate' and 'pain'. Rob Boddice, *A History of Feelings* (London: Reaktion Books, 2019), 19.
26. For example, see D. W. Carr, 'Progress in Persia', *Mercy and Truth* 11, no. 128 (1907): 238.
27. Missionaries were not successful in establishing educational institutions in the Arabian Gulf; Eleanor Abdella Doumato, 'An "Extra Legible Illustration" of the Christian Faith: medicine, medical ethics and missionaries in the Arabian Gulf', *Islam and Christian-Muslim Relations* 13, no. 4 (2002): 377. I should state that I disagree with Doumato's overall analysis, which presents the Gulf as a disease-driven region and missionaries as providers of health.
28. Emily J. Manktelow, *Missionary families: Race, gender and generation on the spiritual frontier* (Manchester: Manchester University Press, 2013), 6.
29. Claire McLisky, Daniel Midena and Karen Vallgårda (eds), *Emotions and Christian Missions: Historical Perspectives* (Basingstoke: Palgrave Macmillan, 2015); Rebecca

Swartz, 'Educating Emotions in Natal and Western Australia, 1854–65', *Journal of Colonialism and Colonial History* 18, no. 2 (2017) doi: 10.1353/cch.2017.0022; Tony Ballantyne, 'Moving Texts and "Humane Sentiment": Materiality, mobility and the emotions of imperial humanitarianism', *Journal of Colonialism and Colonial History* 17, no. 1 (2016) doi: 10.1353/cch.2016.0000; Karen Vallgårda, 'Tying Children to God with Love: Danish Mission, Childhood, and Emotions in Colonial South India', *Journal of Religious History* 39, no. 4 (2015): 595–613; see also chapters five and six of Jane Lydon, *Imperial Emotions: The Politics of Empathy across the British Empire* (Cambridge: Cambridge University Press, 2020); 123–63; Jacqueline Can Gent, 'Global Protestant Missions and the Role of Emotions', in Ulinka Rublack (ed.), *Protestant Empires: Globalizing the Reformations* (Cambridge: Cambridge University Press, 2020), 275–95; Stephen Cummins and Joel Lee, 'Missionaries: False Reverence, Irreverence and the Rethinking of Christian Mission in China and India', in Benno Gammerl, Philipp Nielsen and Margrit Pernau (eds), *Encounters with Emotions: Negotiating Cultural Differences since Early Modernity* (New York and Oxford: Berghahn, 2019), 37–60.
30. *The World Call to the Church: The Call from the Moslem World* (London: The Press and Publication Board of the Church Assembly, 1926).
31. Henry White, 'Medical Missions to Moslems', *Mercy and Truth* 18, no. 213 (2014): 310.
32. Hugh Goddard, *A History of Christian–Muslim Relations* (Edinburgh: Edinburgh University Press, 2000), 123.
33. Heleen Murre-van den Berg, 'The Middle East: Western missions and the Eastern churches, Islam and Judaism', in Sheridan Gilley and Brian Stanley (eds), *The Cambridge History of Christianity*, vol 8, World Christianities c. 1815–1914 (Cambridge: Cambridge University Press, 2005), 460.
34. Heleen Murre-van den Berg, 'Introduction', *New Faith in Ancient Lands* (see note 13), 3.
35. Becker, *Revival and Awakening*, 276.
36. Heleen Murre-van den Berg, *From a Spoken to a Written Language: The Introduction and Development of Literary Urmia Aramaic in the Nineteenth Century* (Leiden: Nederlands Instituut Voor Het Nabije Ossten, 1999), 69.
37. Lyle. L. Vander Werff, *Christian Mission to Muslims: The record: Anglican and Reformed Approaches in India and the Near East, 1800–1938* (Pasadena: William Carey Library, 1977), 82.
38. Jeffrey Cox, *Imperial Fault Lines: Christianity and Colonial Power in India, 1818–1940* (Stanford: Stanford University Press, 2002), 2.

39. H. L. Murre-van den Berg, 'Asahel Grant's The Nestorians or the Lost Tribes (1841)', in *The Nestorians or The Lost Tribe*, Piscataway (Piscataway: Gorgias Press, 2004), iv–vi, https://doi.org/10.31826/9781463209582-001
40. 'Mediterranean Mission', *Church Missionary Record* 5, no. 7 (July 1860): 218; 'Annual Letters of the Bishop of Jerusalem', *The Church of England Magazine* 50 (February 1861): 111.
41. The ABCFM was only 'anxious to associate a physician with the mission so that there would be someone to look after the health and medical needs of missionaries.' See Lydia Wytenbroek 'Generational Difference: American Medical Missionaries in Iran, 1834–1940', in David Bagot and Margaux Whiskin (eds), *Iran and the West: Cultural Perceptions from the Sasanian Empire to the Islamic Republic* (London: Bloomsbury, 2020): 180.
42. In 1838, the LMS recruited William Lockhart as a medical missionary to China. A. Wylie, *Memorials of Protestant Missionaries to the Chinese: Giving a List of their publications and obituary notice of the deceased* (Shanghai: American Presbyterian Mission Press, 1867), 112.
43. Sharkey, *American Evangelicals*, 49.
44. The Old Cairo and the Menouf medical missions.
45. Şahin, *Faithful Encounters*, xi.
46. Sharkey, *American Evangelicals*, 1.
47. Catherine Woodward, 'The Discourse and Experience of the Arabian Mission's Medical Missionaries: Part I 1920–39', *Middle Eastern Studies* 47, no. 5 (2011): 779–805.
48. Sharkey, *American Evangelicals*, 96–148.
49. Catriona Laing, 'Anglican Mission amongst Muslims, 1900–1940', in William L. Sachs (ed.), *The Oxford History of Anglicanism*, vol. V, Global Anglicanism, c. 1910–200 (Oxford: Oxford University Press, 2017), 367–91.
50. As G. A. Bremner states, 'We do not want *a* new history of British imperial architecture but many new architectural histories of empire'. See, G. A. Bremner, 'Architecture, Urbanism, and British Imperial Studies', in G. A. Bremner (ed.), *Architecture and Urbanism in the British Empire* (Oxford: Oxford University Press, 2020), 15.
51. While there is a broad literature to cite, the following are some of the most influential works: Barbara H Rosenwein, 'Worrying about Emotions in History', *The American Historical Review* 107, no. 3 (June 2002): 821–45; William M. Reddy, *The Navigation of Feeling: A Framework for the History of Emotions* (Cambridge: Cambridge University Press, 2001); Rob Boddice, *The History of*

Emotions (Manchester: Manchester University Press, 2018); Ute Frevert, *Emotions in History – Lost and Found* (Budapest: Central European University Press, 2011); Monique Scheer, 'Are Emotions a Kind of Practice (and is that what makes them have a history)? A Bourdieuian Approach to Understanding Emotion', *History and Theory* 51, no. 2 (2012): 193–220; Boddice, *A History of Feelings*.

52. Frevert, *Emotions in History*, 19–85.
53. For 'happiness' see Kathleen Vongsathorn, 'Teaching, Learning and Adapting Emotions in Uganda's Child Leprosy Settlement, c. 1930–1962', in Stephanie Olsen (ed.), *Childhood, Youth and Emotions in Modern History: National, Colonial and Global Perspectives* (Basingstoke: Palgrave Macmillan, 2015), 56–75.
54. C. McLisky, 'Professions of Christian Love: Letters of Courtship between Missionaries-to-be Daniel Matthews and Janet Johnston', in Amanda Barry, Joanna Cruickshank, Andrew Brown-May and Patricia Grimshaw (eds), *Evangelists of Empire? Missionaries in Colonial History* (Melbourne: University of Melbourne eScholarship Research Centre, 2008), 173–86.
55. Boddice, *The History of Emotions*, 18.
56. Bettina Hitzer and Monique Scheer, 'Unholy Feelings: Questioning Evangelical Emotions in Wilhelmine Germany', *German History* 32, no. 3 (2014): 371–92.
57. Stephanie Trigg, 'Introduction: Emotional Histories – Beyond the Personalization of the Past and the Abstraction of Affect Theory', *Examplaria* 26, no. 1 (2014), 3–15.
58. Thomas Dixon, *From Passions to Emotions: the Creation of a Secular Psychological Category* (Cambridge: Cambridge University Press, 2003); Thomas Dixon, '"Emotion": The History of a Keyword in Crisis', *Emotion Review* 4, no. 4 (2012), 338–44.
59. Scheer, 'Are Emotions a Kind of Practice', 193–220.
60. See note 27; see also Hitzer and Scheer, 'Unholy Feelings,' 371–92; Monique Scheer, 'Feeling Faith: The Cultural Practice of Religious Emotions in Nineteenth Century German Methodism', in Monique Scheer, et al. (eds), *Out of the Tower: Essays on Culture and Everyday Life* (Tubingen: Tubinger Vereinigung fur Volkskunde, 2013), 217–47.
61. Kate Davison, et al., 'Emotions as a Kind of Practice: Six Case Studies Utilizing Monique Scheer's Practice-Based Approach to Emotions in History', *Cultural History* 7, no. 2 (2018): 227.
62. Scheer, 'Are Emotions a Kind of Practice', 209.
63. Metropolis is taken to mean British nation state. See G. A. Bremner, 'The Metropolis: Imperial Buildings and Landscapes in Britain,' in *Architecture and*

Urbanism (see note 50), 125. For the making, remaking and unmaking of metropolitan forms, see the following studies: Elizabeth E. Prevost, *The Communion of Women: Missions and Gender in Colonial Africa and the British Metropole* (Oxford: Oxford University Press, 2010), 7–8; Narthex, a special device used in ancient Christian architecture, reinvented by High Church missionaries as an 'ecclesiologically correct method' to provide a space for non-Christians. G. A. Bremner, 'Narthex reclaimed: Reinventing disciplinary space in the Anglican mission field, 1847–1903', *Journal of Historical Geography* 51 (2016): 1–17; Walima T. Kalusa, 'Missionaries, African Patients, and Negotiating Missionary Medicine at Kalene Hospital, Zambia, 1906–1935', *Journal of Southern African Studies* 40, no. 2 (2014): 283–94; Habib Badr, 'American Protestant Missionary Beginnings in Beirut and Istanbul: Policy, Politics, Practices and Response', in *New Faith in Ancient Lands* (see note 14), 211–19; American missionaries adapted the Kuwaiti custom of care for a post-partum woman, Doumato, 'An "Extra Legible Illustration" of the Christian Faith', 384–5.
64. Benno Gammerl, Jan Simon Hutta and Monique Scheer, 'Feeling differently: Approaches and their politics', *Emotion, Space and Society* 25 (2017), 89.
65. Rosenwein, 'Worrying about Emotions in History'; Barbara H. Rosenwein, *Emotional Communities in the Early Middle Ages* (Ithaca and London: Cornell University Press, 2006).
66. Rosenwein, 'Worrying about Emotions in History,' 842.
67. Mark Seymour, 'Emotional Arenas: From Provincial Circus to National Courtroom in Late Nineteenth-century Italy', *Rethinking History: The Journal of Theory and Practice* 16, no. 2 (2012): 177–97.
68. Eliza F. Kent, *Converting Women: Gender and Protestant Christianity in Colonial South India* (Oxford: Oxford University Press, 2004), 113; Jacqueline Van Gent suggests that the concept of 'imagined community' is 'an excellent analytical tool with which to understand the nature of the global Moravian Church'. Van Gent, 'Global Protestant Missions and role of emotions', 276; Jacqueline Van Gent, 'Protestant Global Missions', in Susan Broomhall (ed.), *Early Modern Emotions: An Introduction* (Oxford and New York: Routledge, 2017), 313–16; Van Gent borrows this concept from Benedict Anderson: Benedict Anderson, *Imagined Communities: Reflections on the Origin and Spread of Nationalism* (London and New York: Verso, 2006).
69. Karen Vallgårda, Kristine Alexander and Stephanie Olsen, 'Emotions and the Global Politics of Childhood', in *Childhood, Youth* (see note 53), 20–1.
70. Ibid., 20.
71. Reddy, *The Navigation of Feeling*.

72. Barbara H. Rosenwein and Riccardo Cristani, *What is the History of Emotions* (Cambridge: Policy Press, 2019), 39–41.
73. Boddice, *The Science of Sympathy*, 13–15.
74. Reddy, *The Navigation of Feeling*, 124–6.
75. Vallgårda, 'Tying Children to God with Love', 601.
76. Ibid.
77. Ibid., 20.
78. Till Großmann and Phillip Nielsen, 'Introduction: Architectural History of Emotions – emotional history of democracy', in Till Großmann and Phillip Nielsen (eds), *Architecture, Democracy, and Emotions: The Politics of Feeling since 1945* (New York and London: Routledge, 2019), 5. It should be noted that the field of neuroarchitecture continues to assume an historical relationship between space and emotions.
79. Reckwitz, 'Affective Spaces: A Praxeological Outlook', 255.
80. Margrit Pernau, 'Space and Emotion: Building to Feel', *History Compass* 12, no. 7 (2014): 541.
81. Reckwitz, 'Affective Spaces'; Andrew Reckwitz, 'Towards a Theory of Social Practices: A Development in Culturalist Theorizing', *European Journal of Social Theory* 5, no. 2 (2002): 257–8.
82. As Boddice states, 'There is no experimental feeling inherent in events, in objects, in relations. They all have to be made.' Boddice, *The History of Emotions*, 162.
83. Gammerl, Hutta and Scheer, 'Feeling differently: Approaches and their politics', 90.
84. G. A. Bremner, 'The Architecture of the Universities' Mission to Central Africa: Developing a Vernacular Tradition in the Anglican Mission Field, 1861–1909', *Journal of the Society of Architectural Historians* 68, no. 4 (2009): 514–39; Maurice Amutabi, 'Buildings as Symbols and Metaphors of Colonial Hegemony: Interrogating Colonial Buildings and Architecture in Kenta's Urban Spaces', in *Colonial Architecture and Urbanism* (see note 21), 330; Preeti Chopra, *A Joint Enterprise: Indian Elites and the Making of British Bombay* (Minneapolis and London: University of Minnesota Press, 2011), 58–70.
85. Nida Kirmani, 'Fear and the City: Negotiating Everyday Life as a Young Baloch Man in Karachi', *Journal of the Economic and Social History* 58, no. 5 (2015): 735.
86. Razek Khan, 'The Social Production of Space and Emotions in South Asia', *Journal of the Economic and Social History* 58, no. 5 (2015): 614.
87. Margrit Pernau, *Emotions and Modernity in Colonial India: From Balance to Fervor* (Oxford: Oxford University Press, 2019); Margrit Pernau, 'Great Britain:

The Creation of and Imperial Global Order', in Margrit Pernau, et al. (eds), *Civilising Emotions: Concepts in Nineteenth-century Asia and Europe* (Oxford: Oxford University Press, 2015), 45–62; Lydon, *Imperial Emotions*.
88. Hardiman, 'Introduction', 18.
89. Mary Louise Pratt, *Imperial Eyes: Travel Writing and Transculturation* (London and New York: 1992); Sara Mills, *Gender and Colonial Space* (Manchester: Manchester University Press, 2013); Anthony D. King, *Colonial Urban Development: Culture, Social Power and Environment* (London, Hanley and Boston: Routledge & Kegan Paul, 2007); Samir Boulos, *European Evangelicals in Egypt (1900–1956): Cultural Entanglements and Missionary Spaces* (Leiden and Boston: Brill, 2016), 181.
90. Ahmed, *The Cultural Politics of Emotion*, 5–8.
91. Pernau, 'Space and Emotions', 542.
92. Margrit Pernau, 'Mapping Emotions, Constructing Feelings: Delhi in the 1840s', *Journal of the Economic and Social History of the Orient* 58, no. 5 (2015): 646.
93. Mark Crinson, 'The Powers that be: Architectural potency and spatialized power', *ABE Journal* [online] 4 (2013). DOI: https://doi.org/10.4000/abe.3389
94. For 'emotive', see Reddy, *The Navigation of Feeling*. Before recent turns to emotion and sensory history, Guenter B. Risse stated in the introduction of his important book that '. . . the crackling sounds emanating from the public paging system, and even the smells wafting from wards and kitchen combine to shape a hospital's distinctive ambiance and character, which have a powerful impact on newcomers and visitors alike.' Guenter B. Risse, *Mending Bodies, Saving Souls: A History of Hospital* (New York and Oxford: Oxford University Press, 1999), 4.
95. Johnathan Reinarz, 'Learning to Use Their Senses: Visitors to Voluntary Hospitals in Eighteenth-Century England', *Journal of Eighteenth-Century Studies* 35, no. 4 (2012): 505–20.
96. Benno Gammerl, 'Emotional Style – concepts and challenges', *Rethinking History* 16, no. 2 (2012): 169–70.
97. Ibid., 170.
98. Renée M. Sentilles, 'Toiling in the Archives of Cyberspace', in Antoinette Burton (ed.), *Archive Stories: Facts, Fictions, and the Writing of History* (Durham, NC and London: Duke University Press, 2005): 145.
99. Trigg, 'Introduction: Emotional Histories', 10. Trigg refers to D. Vance Smith's criticism of a number of medieval scholars who have deployed a personal or affective mode in their reading of medieval texts. D. Vance Smith, 'The Application of Thought to Medieval Studies: The Twenty-First Century', *Examplaria* 22, no. 1 (2010), 85–94.

100. Rob Boddice and Mark Smith, *Emotion, Sense, Experience* (Cambridge: Cambridge University Press, 2020), 28.
101. Rachel Lee, 'Engaging the Archival Habitant: Architectural Knowledge and Otto Koenigsberger's Effect', *Comparative Studies of South Asia, Africa and Middle East* 40, no. 3 (2020): 530.
102. Sarah Tarlow, 'The Archaeology of Emotion and Affect', *The Annual Review of Anthropology* 41, no. 1 (2012): 169–85.
103. Boddice and Smith, *Emotion, Sense, Experience*, 27.
104. Jane Rendell, 'Site-Writing: She is Walking about in a Town Which She does not Know', *Home Culture* 4, no. 2 (2007): 178.
105. Gammerl, 'Emotional style', 169–70.
106. Jane Hattrick, 'Seduced by the Archive: A Personal and Working Relationship with the Archive and Collection of the London Couturier, Norman Hartnell', in Anna Moran and Sorcha O'Brien (eds), *Love Objects: Emotion, Design and Material Culture* (London: Bloomsbury Academic, 2014), 75–86.
107. Peter Scriver and Vikramaditya Prakash, 'Between Materiality and Representation: Framing an Architectural Critique of Colonial South Asia', in Peter Scriver and Vikramaditya Prakash (eds), *Colonial Modernities: Building, dwelling and architecture in British India and Ceylon* (London and New York: Routledge, 2007), 3.
108. Talinn Grigor, *The Persian Revival: The Imperial of the Copy in Iranian and Parsi Architecture* (Pennsylvania: Pennsylvania State University Press, 2021).
109. Benno Gammerl, Philipp Nielsen and Margrit Pernau, 'Encountering Feelings – Feeling Encounters', in *Encounters with Emotions* (see note 27), 1 and 4.

1

LIFE BEFORE AND OUTSIDE THE MISSION HOSPITALS

> I need hardly to say that the details of the work vary in different countries, but as a rule, the Mission is commenced by the opening of an out-patient dispensary, the Gospel being preached to the patients who come together; then, sooner or later, an in-patient department is added.[1]

This statement, made by Dr Arthur Lankester of the Peshawar medical mission in 1900, suggests that medical missions were established in a step-by-step manner. First, the missionaries opened outpatient dispensaries, after which they started inpatient departments. Dr Urania Latham (Mrs Napier Malcolm) of the Yazd medical mission echoed this statement in her book, *Children of Persia*, in 1911; she asserted, '[a]s a rule a dispensary is started first, to which out-patients can come to get medicine and have their hurts attended to. Later a hospital is opened.'[2] Lankester and Latham's statements are comparable to John Barton's, the CMS's secretary in British India, in 1874:

> We do not care in India to have the material fabric until we first obtain the spiritual fabric, consisting of living stones. This has always been the principle of the Church Missionary Society, and I hope always will be. It is very easy to pull down a mud chapel and build a stone building in its place when your congregation has increased from 50 to 500, or from 500 to 1000.[3]

The CMS advocated modesty in architecture throughout the nineteenth century.[4] But Lankester and Latham's use of the term 'as a rule' was more complex than it might seem at first sight. They did not necessarily refer to the CMS's principles; rather, they pointed to the specificities of medical mission work, particularly in British India, China and the Middle East. Not only the CMS medical missions, but also medical missions of the ABCFM, the London Missionary Society (LMS), the SPG, the Christian Missions in Many Lands (CMML) and the German-based Sudan Pionier Mission (SPM), to name but a few, were started as small outpatient dispensaries, followed by an inpatient department in rented buildings and, after several years, a purpose-built structure.[5]

This step-by-step establishment pattern is the main subject of this chapter. As a quote from an anonymous author described as 'a friend of Iran' suggests, it was necessary to obtain trust and friendship to build a hospital: 'A purpose-built hospital was constructed when the true foundations had been laid in the hearts of the people whose friendship . . . had [been] won through the uphill years before.'[6] The chapter highlights the importance of opening dispensaries and undertaking medical itineration tours in this regard. Additionally, it shows that dispensaries and itineration tours were complementary to the work of the central hospitals: 'the Medical Missionary must not be content with a central hospital, but by branch dispensaries or itineration must try to reach the outlying populations', was stated in a report in 1891.[7] These practices provided social settings for interaction and, through interaction, for perception and sensation between the missionaries and the local people. They allowed a more profound means of communicating with people. They also widened the area under a medical mission's influence, providing missionaries with opportunities to engage with people from the cities themselves and the surrounding villages and other towns further afield. The last part of the chapter analyses rented buildings as emotional set-ups for integrating local people into the mission stations since they were supposedly familiar to the patients.

Much that has been written about activities of mission doctors and nurses do not pay any explicit attention to mission dispensaries and medical itineration tours, viewing them at best ancillary to the development of medical missions. A few studies have recognised the preliminary nature of these two practices but without any further clarification. For example, in her research concerning North American mission hospitals in China, Michelle Renshaw discerns that 'dispensaries always preceded the building of mission hospitals'. Renshaw states that many patients could 'be catered for at little cost and the missionaries could start work as soon as he or she had acquired sufficient Chinese language' through dispensaries. She further asserts that dispensaries 'provided a way to break down barriers because it was easier to persuade potential patients to visit a physician than to enter a foreign hospital'.[8] John R. Stanley makes a similar observation regarding Dr Charles Roys' (American Presbyterian mission) decision to open a dispensary within the city walls in Wiexian (China), stating that his aim was 'to extend the medical facilities to a wider area'.[9] Concerning medical itineration tours, David Hardiman notes their importance in winning the trust of the Adivasis of western India. According to Hardiman, people's 'suspicions' could only be broken down gradually and 'one of the best ways to do this was to take medicine to people in their own villages, where they could accept or reject treatment on their own terms'.[10] Likewise, Samir Boulos states that the visits of SPM missionaries to villages 'promoted the "al-Jarmaniyya" [the hospital] in Aswan and helped gain the trust of local communities'.[11] While scattered, these accounts show that dispensaries and itineration tours played a role in establishing contacts with a more significant number of people and thus preparing the ground for or reinforcing the hospital work.

Even less has been said about rented buildings. Hardiman has made a general observation: '[u]ntil the later years of the nineteenth century, most medical missionaries practiced from their own houses or in rented buildings that had not been built with this purpose in mind and which were often poorly suited to the task.' He continues, 'as biomedical work grew in sophistication, the emphasis gradually shifted towards the purpose-built hospitals.'[12] Hardiman is correct; the construction of purpose-built structures became a subject matter from the later years of the nineteenth century. Still, his statement is incomplete because it disregards that many mission hospitals were established in rented buildings until the 1920s. Some even operated in these structures for more than ten years.

This chapter expands and reshapes these existing observations. First, it highlights medical missionaries undertook many itineration tours and opened a significant number of dispensaries, often in strategic areas such as on a caravan route. Second, they established various dispensaries: permanent, temporary, semi-weekly, bi-weekly, dispensary horses and dispensary boats. Third, providing medical care and preaching the Gospel was sometimes closely allied with other activities such as interacting with patients' family members. The missionaries hoped to attract and engage the people by employing these strategies, thereby increasing their number, and generating a community. Overall, the chapter integrates these practices more fully into the story of the establishment of medical missions.

'A Way through All Obstacles'

Before examining dispensaries, medical itineration tours and rented buildings, it is essential to register the influence of specific practical reasons on the development or otherwise of medical missions more generally. While I aim to illustrate that it was necessary to build trust to construct the hospitals, it would be a mistake to suggest that no other factors delayed the construction of a purpose-built structure. Some missionaries even stated that the work could only be strengthened by constructing a hospital.[13] Missionaries in Kerman tried to build a hospital soon after their arrival but failed.[14] Thus, the first part of this chapter maps some of the difficulties and obstacles missionaries faced.

Missionary societies, in general, had limited resources, both of people and funds and, as a result, medical missions were expanded slowly.[15] The importance of gaining trust and friendship may have partly arisen due to the lack of resources. Writing in the context of Danish missionaries in South India, Karen Vallgårda argues that owing to the scarcity of funds and people, missionaries 'had to rely on persuasion rather than force' to make any impact.[16] Archival sources discussing the CMS medical work in Persia and north-western British India also point to missionaries' lack of resources. As stated in the Introduction, in the 1870s and 1880s the CMS had not yet fully engaged with medical mission work. During that time, some medical missions were opened temporarily without any financial help from the Society. For example, the Medical Committee sanctioned the opening of the Isfahan medical mission in 1879 merely 'as an experiment for three years'.[17] Even after this trial period, it only made an annual grant-in-aid towards its expenses.[18] It was not until 1891 that the Medical Missionary Auxiliary Committee (MMA) was formed to bear all the cost of the Society's medical missions without any grant from the General Fund,[19] and not until 1900 that the Committee accepted the responsibility of providing all new buildings required by the missions.[20] And yet, the missionaries continued to raise money themselves both at home (in Britain) and on the ground (in the mission field) to build a hospital because the Committee was rarely in a financial position to grant sufficient funds to them: 'the Medical Committee to their great regret cannot, in the present state of their funds, make him [Dr Lankester] any definite grant' was stated in an appeal for funds to build the Peshawar hospital.[21] Similarly, missionaries raised most of the funds locally in Kerman, Yazd and Isfahan.[22]

The shortage of workers also hindered the development of medical missions. It is important to note that, with the professionalisation of medicine in Britain from the mid-nineteenth century onwards, the title medical missionary was increasingly reserved only for qualified medical doctors.[23] An 'efficient' medical mission required 'no less than two qualified medical men (and of course in Mohammedan countries lady doctors, in addition, are essential if the women are to be reached), and two nurses', as Dr Albert Cook, the famous missionary doctor of the CMS in Mengo (Uganda), put it in 1902.[24] This requirement was rarely satisfied (even after the Society passed some rules in 1899 to make an annual grant covering the actual cost of the medical education of suitable applicants[25]) due partly to the limited number of interested candidates, partly to the financial difficulties of the Society, and partly to missionaries' illness. As a result, some medical missions were closed down either temporarily or permanently.

The Kerman medical mission is a case in point, where no full-time medical missionary was available between its commencement in 1901 and 1903. Credit for the founding of the Kerman medical mission is due to Dr A. Hume-Griffith, who arrived in the city with his wife, M. E. Hume-Griffith, in 1901. Hume-Griffith's stay in Kerman was short-lived; he had to leave in December 1902 on account of his wife's health and exchanged the station with Dr George Day, who was a medical missionary in Yazd and arrived in Kerman in January 1902, only to resign his post and leave Persia in July 1902 for medical reasons.[26] After Day, the Kerman medical mission remained without a qualified missionary doctor until October 1903. During this time, Miss Mary Bird, who had previously worked in Isfahan and Yazd, oversaw the mission. Moreover, Dr John Orlando Summerhayes, a CMS medical missionary in Quetta, took charge of the medical work for a few months, from December 1902 until April 1903. A full-time medical mission began in autumn 1903 when Dr Winfred Westlake and Dr George Dodson joined the staff.[27] Another example is the Quetta medical mission, which Dr S. W. Sutton started in 1886. Sutton had to postpone the construction of the inpatient department and close the hospital for two years after falling ill with enteric fever. Writing about the progress of the Quetta hospital in 1924, Dr Henry Tristram Holland stated, 'what an example of the harm done to the work by having only one doctor in a station!'[28]

Returning to Cook's statement, he singled out the importance of 'lady doctors' for 'Mohammedan' countries. He was echoing the idea of 'women's work for women'. As will be explained in Chapter Four, women initially contributed to the furthering of mission cause mainly as male missionaries' wives and daughters (unpaid assistants). They became a crucial part of the missionary enterprise in the second half of the nineteenth century because of their access to the zenana – the separate (segregated) quarters for women in some houses in India and the Middle East. The missionary societies were as restricted in employing female medical missionaries despite this. Female medical professionals themselves were against recruiting women without adequate qualifications. Acquiring accreditation was a hard-won battle for female doctors in Britain, and they feared that a failure in treatment could undermine their reputation.[29] Yet, as the number of qualified female doctors was small, many missionary societies continued to employ unqualified women without permitting them to establish a medical mission.[30] As stated above, one such female missionary was Mary Bird, who had the sole charge of the Kerman medical mission in 1902 without being allowed to develop the work. In 1899, the Dera Ghazi Khan hospital had two 'lady workers', but neither was qualified to take up the charge of the hospital. Appealing for a female doctor, Dr Andrew Jukes stated in 1899, 'surely a hospital which last year had 114 women in-patients and 4900 out-patients who paid over 13,000 visits is an agency that should have the superintendence of a qualified lady'.[31] Female missionaries who wished to take charge of a medical mission had to acquire a medical degree, which would postpone the construction of a building, as is evident from the case of the Multan hospital. This hospital was started by Miss Annie Wilhelmina Eger of the Society for the Promotion of Female Education in China, India and the East (FES) in 1885. It was handed over to the CMS in 1899. Having had only rudimentary medical knowledge, Eger left Multan in 1891 for three years to obtain a medical degree. The medical mission was subsequently closed because of the unavailability of a female doctor to continue the work.[32]

The opposition of local people also caused complications and delays. As explained at the beginning of the Introduction, Elmslie had to leave Kashmir during the winter seasons upon the order of the Maharajah. Another example is the Kerman hospital. The construction of this hospital was postponed due to general anti-foreign feelings that existed in the country during the First World War. The missionaries reported that they experienced active 'opposition' during this time to the extent that they had not experienced for many years. In autumn 1915 they closed the hospitals, and the Kerman hospital's construction was ceased. Dodson went to Bombay and was engaged in the Royal Army Corps war in the Colaba War Hospital, and Westlake went to work at the CMS women's hospital in Multan.[33] The hospital remained closed for two years. Dodson and Westlake resumed their work in November 1917 after British troops occupied the cities. However, the nature of the relationship between missionaries and local people was diverse and plural. Furthermore, the opposition of local people was only partly related to sanctions against conversion.[34] Indeed, the underlying reasons varied depending on the context and did not always fit within a threat/resistance formula. For example, according to Philippe Bourmand, the CMS medical mission in Nablus was closed down 'twice' and 'threatened some more times' between 1891 and 1901. The medical missionaries 'treated it as the manifestation of a general confrontation between defensive Christianity and aggressive Islam'. But it 'sometimes originated from unexpected quarters'.[35] Bourmand refers to the decision of the newly appointed medical missionary, Dr Gaskoin Wright, to make redundant the assistant-pharmacist, Šukrī El-Karey. This decision upset 'the bonds of trust' between mission and Šukrī's father who was ready 'to take any step to force Dr Wright out, and the whole CMS if the need arose'.[36] On another occasion, Wright's annual letter, in which he had described 'all Orientals' as 'liars', reached the Protestant congregation of Palestine, who 'petitioned against Wright's remark'.[37]

Because of the difficulties discussed above, the growth of many medical missions was slow. The missionaries partly relied on the British authorities' support to advance their goals and wishes.[38] Another factor that could influence the growth of a medical mission was the missionaries' relationship with local chiefs. As their opposition could hinder missionaries' goals, their support could be beneficial; some were even active participants within the mission fields, cultivating relationships with missionaries to pursue their modernising motives. One such ruler was Zill al-Sultān, the governor of Isfahan (1874–1907), whose 'tacit goodwill' facilitated the transfer of the Isfahan mission from Julfā to Isfahan.[39] Moreover, the missionaries benefited from the support of a wealthy Parsee merchant in Yazd, Mr Mehriban Goodarz, who granted missionaries a caravanserai in 1898 and the land for a men's hospital.[40] Similarly, the Sultan of Oman allowed missionaries to establish a hospital and financially contributed to their causes.[41] The relationship between local chiefs and missionaries was not steady, however, and could oscillate between support, promotion and toleration.[42]

Notwithstanding the financial, practical and socio-political limitations and difficulties, missionaries opened dispensaries and undertook itineration tours. Bourmand explains in detail how missionaries succeeded at handling local mobilisation and creating a 'private, nearly extraterritorial space for their hospital'.[43] But he does not mention that the importance of itineration was brought up as early as 1894 in the Palestine conference.[44] These initiatives could play a role in the development of medical missions. The following two parts of this chapter discuss the importance of these initiatives.

Medical Itineration Tours

The missionaries regularly undertook medical itineration tours, bringing the Christian message to new people. David Livingston popularised itineration as a missionary strategy in the first half of the nineteenth century. While Livingston pursued itineration as opposed to the overwhelming focus of most missionaries around the world on institution building, by the second half of the nineteenth century itineration was regarded as complementary to institution building.[45]

There are accounts of itineration tours in the published reports as early as the 1830s.[46] According to these reports, undertaking itineration became more popular from the 1850s onwards and was taken up by medical missionaries. The title 'itinerating missionary' was increasingly utilised, which implies that itineration gained ground.[47] Itineration was even a reason why recruiting two medical missionaries for each station was essential; with the presence of two doctors, one was always available to undertake regular itineration without leaving the hospital unattended.[48] On medical itineration, the missionaries carried a medical chest, which consisted of surgical instruments and 'a good assortment of the most useful and powerful drugs', a table and a few chairs. They also sometimes borrowed a bed from the villagers.

Besides being a helpful strategy for finding new grounds to advocate the Christian message or finding the best place to start a permanent medical mission,[49] itineration was a means for opening up the region to medical mission work. '[A]s itineration has opened the country, Missionaries should be established in other centres to shepherd inquires and converts' was stated in the minutes of the Persia-Baghdad missionary conference on 6 July 1894.[50] In other words, as Cook put it in 1902, 'as pioneer work it [itineration] is invaluable, softening and disarming prejudice'.[51] Furthermore, the missionaries hoped to make the medical missions 'more widely known' by undertaking itineration and visiting remote villages that were 'cut off from the main hospital.[52] It is essential to discuss the importance of itineration tours by considering these three correlated factors.

The missionaries sometimes visited as many as six or seven villages during a short itineration tour of two weeks or even one day, which illustrates that they aimed to see as many people as possible in a short time (Figure 1.1). More exactly, itinerating was an emotional practice for cultivating relations. Dr Cecil Lankester of the Peshawar medical mission undertook one such itineration tour in March 1902. During a '[f]ortnight's Itineration' Lankester and his wife, Cécile Florence Archibald, visited six villages, including Charsadda, Otmanzai, Tangi and Umurzai. They stayed for five days at Charsadda village; in each of the other five villages they only stopped for one or two days.[53] Dr Theodore Pennell's 'six weeks itineration' in a district of British Afghanistan in 1894 is another example.[54] Pennell undertook a similar itineration tour in the Bannu district in 1896, during which he visited at least five villages on one day.[55] Likewise, Dr and Mrs Dodson of

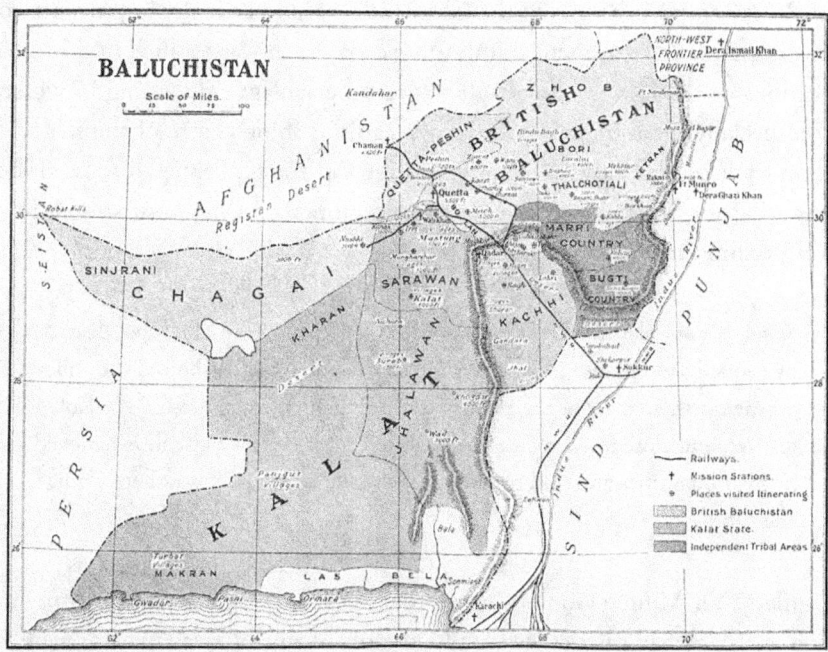

Figure 1.1 Map of Baluchistan showing the places where missionaries visited while itinerating.
CMS Review, 1908, p. 650–1, Church Missionary Society Archive, Cadbury Research Library, Special Collections, University of Birmingham.

the Kerman mission visited 'fourteen villages, besides Seyyedabad, a town of 15,000 inhabitants' in August 1907.[56] Dr Henry White's five-day itineration in Yazd district in 1901 and Neve's twelve-day itineration in Kashmir district in 1899 are also telling. White visited around fifteen villages altogether, and Neve visited seven large villages as well as Islamabad (Anantnag) and Achibal, seeing a total of 1,000 patients.[57]

Moreover, missionaries settled for a few days at villages that were on caravan routes or at populous districts as if visiting many villages in one go was not enough. Take the example of Kerman, where missionaries carried out periodic tours almost every year between 1903 and 1914. A village they frequently visited was Khebis (now Shahdād),[58] a centre of commerce where merchants from other regions in Persia – such as Mashhad and Sīstān – would gather, especially for buying and selling of dates and henna.[59]

At Peshawar, paying visits to the Charsadda was of particular importance to missionaries, the 'commercial importance' of which was testified in the publications of the CMS.[60] Kalabagh was another village, itinerating in which was specially mentioned because it was 'a flourishing centre of the salt and alum trade on the Indus'.[61] Another village was Karak; Pennell discussed the importance of this village as a centre of commerce in the most straightforward fashion in 1905:

> Karak is not only important because it is the market town of all that district, but equally so because it is a great salt mart. The hills that bound the valley on the north are part of the extensive salt range that runs through the Kohat district, and close to Karak are large salt quarries, from which salt is removed in great quantities and sold to traders, who take it for sale to southern Punjab and Sindh.[62]

Similarly, Dr Minnie Gomery stated that 'there is splendid scope for itineration' in Islamabad district, especially in a place called 'Bavan' where 'there is a celebrated shrine, which is the meeting place of large numbers of pilgrims, especially in the Spring season'.[63] The missionaries' deep interest in visiting these villages highlights their concern to construct relations with people from various regions and not just the inhabitants of a specific territory. Miss E. M. Fox, who accompanied the Lankesters on their 1902 itineration tour, reported separately about their time in two parts. In the first part of her report, Fox indicated the instrumental role of the tour in earning people's trust: 'though perhaps not very much result could be expected from a fortnight's camping, yet most certainly good was done, at least, in softening the hearts of the people, and breaking down prejudice.'[64]

Itineration was also a means by which missionaries promoted their work. While itinerating, they encouraged people to bring their sick to the medical mission for extended treatment.[65] Miss J. Biggs of the Yazd hospital made an unequivocal comment on this in 1903 when she wrote, 'again, connected with this village work, one sees the necessity of an itinerating doctor – one who could give himself up entirely to the village work, treating some and sending others into the hospitals.'[66] Writing about her visit to Sanej, a village near Yazd, in 1905, Dr Lucy Molony stated,

We saw 280 patients while we were there, and several of them have been told to come into the hospital for an operation, so we hope to see them again and bring them under further teaching. In this way we hope to get hold of many whom we could not reach otherwise.[67]

Likewise, in 1910, Westlake mentioned a patient called Sharbaun who came to the Kerman hospital after Westlake had visited her village.[68] To take three cases from north-western British India, Dr William Adams reported about an itineration tour in Punjab in 1897: 'several cases could not be treated properly, and these we advised to come into Bannu. Afterwards, some followed us and were cured in Bannu.'[69] In the same year, Pennell wrote, 'you will find a miniature representation of our itineration, for the Bannu Medical Mission, has become a household word in many of these distant homes, and most of our in-patients have first had a journey of from 10 to 150 miles.'[70] Singling out a case, he referred to a man from the Khattak tribe and wrote, 'in whose lands . . . I had often been itinerating'.[71]

At least two examples demonstrate that the missionaries took upon themselves to do activities other than providing treatment and thought about the material arrangements to facilitate doing emotions. In reporting about a 'five day Medical itineration' in Morri country (Muree), Holland mentioned a visit from the 'Nawab of Murris (the head of the tribe)', who had written to Holland before the tour requesting a meeting. Besides conversing with the Nawab, Holland invited him to observe an operation. The operation was a 'series one-lateral lithology', and the Nawab and six or seven Morris, some sat on the floor and some on a bedstead, watched the operation from a 'gallery'. Holland reported that they were critical and even provided suggestions during the surgery.[72] Similarly, Dr Arthur Browne of the Amritsar medical mission invited an 'old Mullah of the village', who had interrupted their preaching and written a letter of opposition, to come and sit by him for a whole day without interfering. Browne reported that the mullah 'withdrew his letter and testified to the work the hitherto despised Christians were doing'.[73]

Studies of missionaries commonly portray an itinerating missionary outside a tent under the shadow of a tree, surrounded by local people. The cases of the Nawab and the old mullah demand revisiting this picture. One wonderfully detailed and rare illustration of diverse forms of itinerating camps is a report published in 1891 entitled 'Itinerating Medical Work'. This account discussed the 'why' and 'how' of undertaking itineration tours by using Kashmir as a case study:

> Hand in hand have medicine and the Gospel visited the remotest parts of Kashmir territories. Even in the quick mosques of sequestered mountain villages, and at the holy springs reverenced by Hindus, have the messages of Divine love, and the ministry of loving care and medical science, been brought to the sick and the ignorant. The rock has been our pulpit; the overarching boughs or groined roof, the shaded lawn our consulting room and church, the turf our operating table, mosques our inquiry rooms, and heathen pilgrim-house our in-patient wards.[74]

This account renders how missionaries carried out itineration tours. Among other things, it shows that missionaries could pitch an itineration camp in diverse places, including a mosque. A sketch, drawn by Arthur Neve, accompanied the report, illustrating this point (Figure 1.2). In his sketch, Neve wrote that they faced no opposition in administrating medicine and preaching the Gospel in a mosque, the reality of which cannot be known with any accuracy. Significantly, missionaries' goal was to enact a tradition in the Muslim world, where hospitals had sometimes been linked to mosques, such as the Princess Turan Malik hospital in Divariği. This hospital was built as part of a complex with a mosque,[75] reflecting an emir's piety, power and care for his people.[76] Missionaries sought to attend to the patients' memory, hoping that, in this way, they would succeed in gaining their trust.

Moreover, there were wandering Ayurvedic physicians in western India and moving hospitals and itinerant apothecaries in Persia.[77] Some patients might have been able to understand itinerating medical missionaries in such terms.[78] Meanwhile, there were internal differences in emotional patterns of itineration according to gender. Eliza Kent states that 'Itinerancy in Colonial India was associated with two groups of Indian women, neither of whom garnered much social status: working women from lower castes who were engaged in trade and wandering religious women who were often associated with prostitution'.[79] Therefore, the missionaries' medical itineration activities could evoke contradictory feelings. Preaching the Gospel and treating patients was also sometimes combined with giving lantern slide performances, which

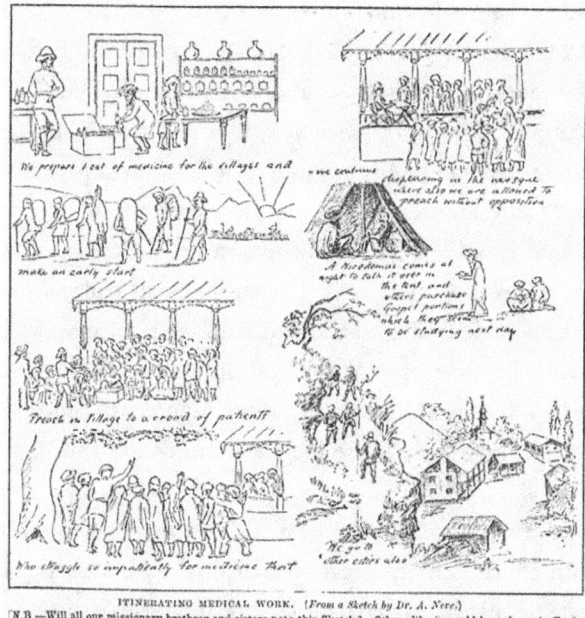

Figure 1.2 Itinerating Medical Work.
The Church Missionary Gleaner 18 (1991): p. 135, Church Missionary Society Archive, Cadbury Research Library, Special Collections, University of Birmingham.

could alter the emotional charges of itineration. Lantern slide performances became popular in Britain in the second half of the nineteenth century. They served the interrelated purposes of 'moving' and 'arousing' interest and garnering financial support.[80] They might have been given by medical missionaries while itinerating to arouse interest through showing, for example, before and after visual techniques, illustrating the transformed life of a relatable convert, a child or a community from 'primitive' to 'civilised', thus evoking 'wishes of belonging'.[81] It is unclear whether the medical missionaries moved people by giving such performances; instead, they might have confused them.

Medical Dispensary

Dispensaries in Britain originated in the first half of the eighteenth century. They increased in number and scale in the second half of the eighteenth century. By the mid-nineteenth century they were one of Britain's primary forms of medical provision until their eventual decline in the early twentieth century. Dispensaries were chiefly urban structures. They were initially established by medical practitioners and dissenting physicians and were run by subscribers and governors who were granted the right to recommend patients. While some had beds, they mainly accepted outpatients and treated medical cases.[82] Dispensaries sometimes damaged the work of such hospitals as The Middlesex Hospital's lying-in service, which 'faced competition' from the Westminster dispensary.[83] Dispensaries also played a crucial role in the evolution of medical education in Britain. For example, in Scotland, dispensary work became part of medical students' standard curriculum.[84] Furthermore, some general infirmaries of the nineteenth century grew out of a successful dispensary such as the North Staffordshire Infirmary at Etruria, Stoke-on-Trent.[85]

The dispensary was transferred from Britain to the United States in the late eighteenth century. By the second half of the nineteenth century, New York and Philadelphia had twenty-nine and thirty-three dispensaries respectively. Similar to dispensaries in Britain, dispensaries in the US were mainly supported by private contributions and often relied on the voluntary services of local physicians. According to Charles Rosenberg, dispensaries had a 'shaky financial condition' in the US. As a result, they often lent 'a portion of their building to commercial tenants'. Besides treating relatively minor ailments, such as bronchitis or colds, they performed an essential public health role by providing vaccination.[86] Some also offered home visiting when a patient was too ill to attend the dispensary. Moreover, they developed ties with other urban charities, such as the Association for Improving the Condition of the Poor (AICP). In this sense, dispensary physicians were '*de facto* social workers'.[87] In the late nineteenth century a change occurred when specialist dispensaries were founded to treat particular ailments.

Nevertheless, to consider dispensaries as primarily urban institutions or to argue that they damaged the work of hospitals is to ignore part of the story. There were exceptions. For example, Bamburgh Castle Dispensary, established in Northumberland in 1772, was not an urban institution; it was situated in a 'remote, coastal location'. Unlike most dispensaries in Britain, the Bamburgh dispensary was 'entirely funded by the Lord Crewe Trust, and administered by Dr Sharp'.[88] Moreover, the picture changes if we examine dispensaries in Britain and the US alongside mission dispensaries. Dispensaries were established in British India in large numbers from the first half of the nineteenth century. As Mark Harrison states, 'the establishment of charitable dispensaries from the 1830s was one of the earliest attempts to provide Western medical care for the Indian people.' Harrison's focus is on government and not on mission dispensaries. He shows that they performed 'useful public health functions acting as local centres for vaccination against smallpox', and were supported initially by 'Indian philanthropists' and, by the 1860s, by 'government, commercial organisations and subscriptions from Europeans'.[89] Mridula Ramanna and Seema Alvi have examined these dispensaries in more detail. Ramanna names Bombay Native Dispensary, which was opened in 1834, as 'the first institution of importance to provide Western medicine to Indians'.[90] Alavi further highlights dispensaries' role as training schools; they 'spearheaded the campaign to disseminate scientific knowledge about Western medical science in Indian society'.[91] Yet, these dispensaries differed on various accounts from dispensaries in Britain and the US. Firstly, they were often established in towns and villages. Moreover, as Alavi states, they 'worked as collaborative institutions where the strained between the two systems of medicine (traditional and Western) were deftly negotiated'.[92]

The first mission dispensaries were also established in the first half of the nineteenth century. In China, dispensaries were established in Sino-Western in 1820, Canton in 1828 and Guangzhou in 1854.[93] In the Middle East they were established in Mosul in 1853.[94] The number and scale of mission dispensaries increased in the second half of the nineteenth century, for the China Medical Missionary Association (CMMA) recorded 241 dispensaries in 1906.[95] Mission dispensaries were not urban structures either; they were founded predominantly in villages while some were temporary. Some mission dispensaries grew out of itineration camps such as the Karak dispensary, an outpost of the Bannu medical mission. As I explained, the missionaries itinerated in Karak in 1895 and 1899. In 1905 they decided to open a permanent outpatient station in this village.[96] Others were established by women, some of whom were not qualified doctors or nurses, or were run by 'native' assistants. The public health function, performed by government dispensaries, was sometimes realised in mission dispensaries. They were also, especially early nineteenth-century mission dispensaries, centres for understanding a region's traditional medicine, as was the case with the Canton dispensary. Additionally, mission dispensaries were complementary to the growth of mission hospitals. They were used to acquire people's trust in Western medical science. The ones that preceded the construction of purpose-built structures 'prepared the ground' for a permanent hospital. The latter point is no more evident than in the Isfahan medical mission.

From the 1890s onwards the missionaries opened several dispensaries in Isfahan proper and the surrounding villages, but these were closed by the local authorities. In 1893 a dispensary was opened in Najafābād – a village eighteen miles from Isfahan – which was closed after a few months. Between 1894 and 1897 no fewer than four dispensaries were opened in Isfahan itself. These dispensaries were established successively in the Jūbbāreh, Bīdābād, Dār Dāsht and Shamsābād districts of the city.[97] According to Heidi Walcher, they were opened because the new secretary of the Persia mission, William St Clair Tisdall (appointed in 1892), was concerned with more 'direct' or 'aggressive' action to occupy Isfahan itself.[98] Nevertheless, it is crucial that this action was pursued primarily through dispensary – and not through, for example, educational work. Perhaps missionaries thought dispensaries would not stand out as a threat because they were modest pursuits. The fact that it was possible to open five dispensaries in rapid succession reveals the nature of this practice for the missionaries: it was a magnet that could easily be moved from one place to another.

Recalling the establishment history of the Isfahan medical mission in 1922, Carr made a statement indicating that a dispensary was more than just a small-scale institution. Carr opened a 'bi-weekly' dispensary in his house in the Shamsābād without facing, according to him, much opposition. When Carr was on furlough in 1899 this dispensary was closed, and Dr Emmeline Stuart opened 'a Saturday Morning dispensary for women' instead.[99] According to Dr Donald Carr, the successful operation of these dispensaries was a sign that 'the medical mission had entered on a new phase'; that is, the time had come to transfer the work from Julfā to Isfahan:

> Kindness again won its way. As we got more among the people, they found that we were not all that we had been painted, and opposition and hatred

soon became markedly less. By 1903 matters had so far advanced that it was felt the time had come to attempt to bring the hospital into town.[100]

This quote implies a link between dispensaries and establishing contact with people. Temporary dispensaries were also opened before the foundation of medical missions in Yazd and Kerman.[101] There are no clear indications as to whether these dispensaries facilitated the foundation of permanent medical missions. In both cases, missionaries expressed positive support for the commencement of a permanent medical mission after the 'successful' opening of a dispensary. For example, Carr opened a dispensary while visiting Kerman in May 1897 to attend to Reverend Henry Carless, who had typhoid fever. In a letter dated 13 April 1898, Carr argued that opening a medical mission in Kerman would be desirable: 'in writing about Kirman [sic], I would emphasise our most earnest plea for a medical missionary for that place.'[102] As I explained in the Introduction, the need for a medical mission in Kashmir was also announced after Mrs Clark opened a temporary dispensary. In addition to short-term, bi-weekly and bi-monthly dispensaries, missionaries had 'dispensary horses' and 'dispensary boats'. For example, in a letter dated July 1904, Reverend Charles Harvey Stileman referred to Carr's 'two dispensary horses', which were funded by the Society.[103]

After the construction of the hospitals, missionaries continued to open branch dispensaries in surrounding villages. These dispensaries, as a note on 'general medical mission policy' stated, were considered as a part of a whole: 'the central and branch hospitals and dispensaries should be so located that the whole may be compact, rather than widely scattered.'[104] In Yazd, missionaries opened branch dispensaries in Khorumshah and Mohammedabad villages. According to White, Khorumshah was five miles from Yazd and Mohammedabad ten miles. Missionaries visited Khorumshah every Wednesday and Mohammedabad every Saturday.[105] The annual report of the medical mission in 1904 noted that Mohammedabad was 'in the centre of a great agricultural district',[106] which recalls missionaries' concerns to reach more people. An example in north-western British India was the Amritsar hospital. It had five outpatient dispensaries at Jandiala, Boorala, Beas, Sultanwind and Ram Dass and was considered 'the largest of any CMS medical mission' in 1900.[107] In 1905, the number of branch dispensaries was recorded as six.

While dispensaries did not have admission register books (or if they did, they have not survived), the missionaries' published reports can provide some insights into the patients' demographic, or at least they can illustrate how missionaries portrayed these figures. Take the example of dispensaries opened in Julfā and Isfahan; Stileman reported that 'no less than 7231 patients' attended the dispensary in Julfā for women between January and November 1894.[108] Likewise, Bird recorded an attendance of 537 during the five weeks that the Bīdābād dispensary was open.[109] In another report, Bird wrote, 'such crowd came that we were obliged to have the doors locked after a certain hour.'[110] In the case of Dār Dāsht, Carr stated in 1904 that 'so anxious were the women to avail themselves of this help, that many, being forbidden by the Mullahs to go, used to climb over the roofs of neighbouring houses in order to gain an entrance'.[111] Another example is the testimony made by Cecil Lankester regarding the temporary dispensary at Nathia Gali: 'the dispensary at the latter place fully justified its existence, attracting patients from all the neighbouring – and many from the distant – hill villages.'[112] In short, the missionaries viewed a dispensary as a means to reach the people and publicise their work, or as Carr put it in 1905, 'to extend the area of operations'.[113]

'It Seems to Him Like Home'

Working in rented buildings was also crucial for evoking people's interest. Apart from the Yazd and Peshawar hospitals, which were established in caravanserais (Figure 1.3), missionaries converted houses to hospitals with wards, an outpatient department and an operating room. They sometimes rented adjacent buildings to increase the number of beds or to form a separate women's hospital. In Yazd, the caravanserai's stables and two neighbouring houses were incorporated into the complex to form a women's hospital with twelve beds.[114] In Kerman, a house was first altered to provide accommodation for both men and women until the missionaries acquired two adjacent houses to increase the number of beds in the men's hospital and form a separate women's hospital (Figure 1.4). Missionaries initially used two caravanserais in Peshawar. They added another caravanserai after a few years (Figure 1.5).

The idea of converting existing structures, especially houses, into hospitals was common in Britain. In particular, many eighteenth-century voluntary

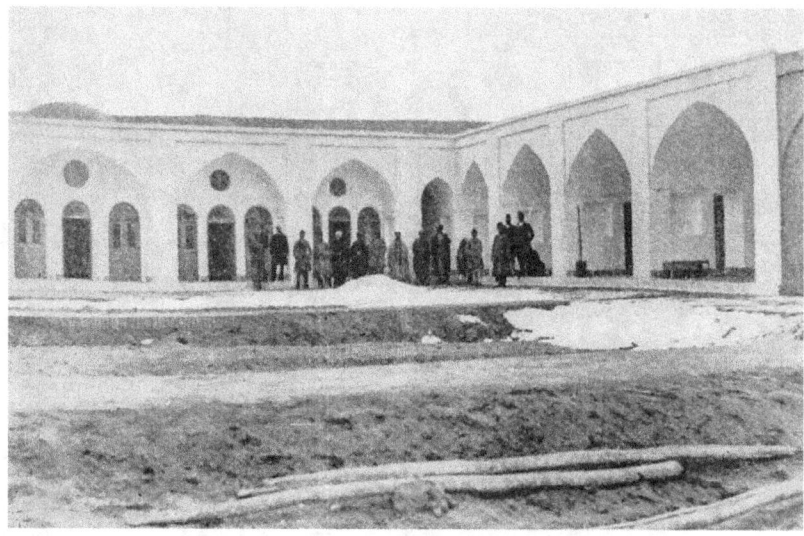

Figure 1.3 The caravanserai that was converted to the hospital in Yazd.
CMS/M/EL2/5, p. 132, Church Missionary Society Archive, Cadbury Research Library, Special Collections, University of Birmingham.

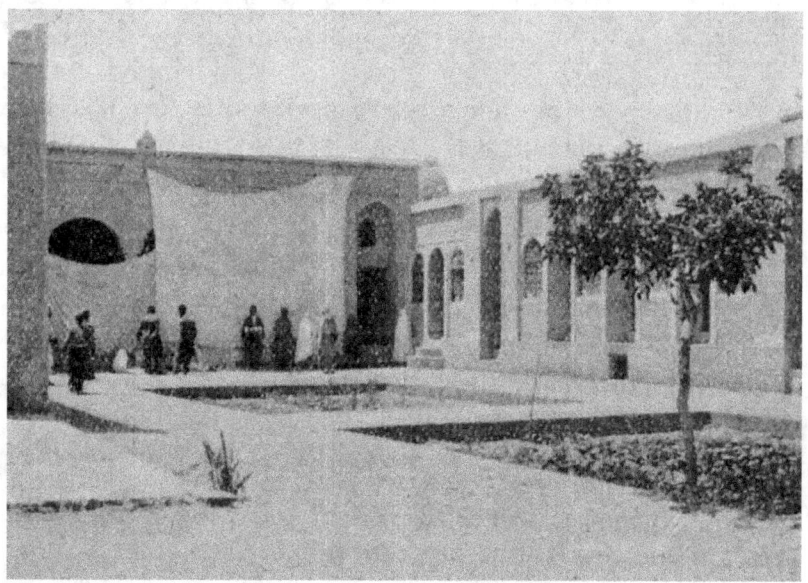

Figure 1.4 The house that was converted to the hospital in Kerman.
CMS/M/EL 2/18, p. 141, Church Missionary Society Archive, Cadbury Research Library, Special Collections, University of Birmingham.

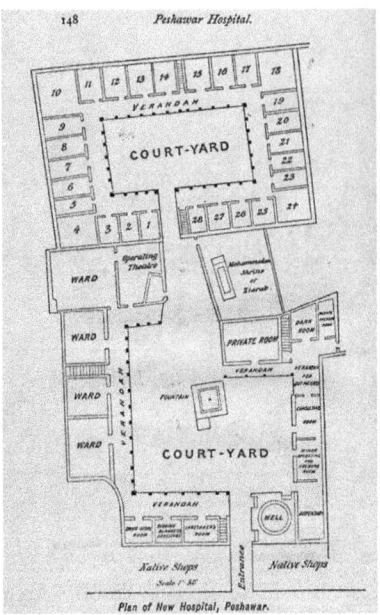

Figure 1.5 The caravanserais that were converted to the hospital in Peshawar. CMS/M/EL2/2, p. 148, Church Missionary Society Archive, Cadbury Research Library, Special Collections, University of Birmingham.

hospitals were established in converted houses, such as the Westminster Public Infirmary, established in 1720, and the Winchester Hospital, opened in 1736. These hospitals were enlarged later by adding new buildings.[115] Examples of converted local buildings to hospitals could also be found across the British Empire, and the missionaries may have patterned themselves after these models. Whilst commencing medical missions in rented buildings was more financially sound in the absence of sufficient support from the CMS, it must also be borne in mind that rented structures were familiar to the patients. The missionaries might not have used local premises merely out of necessity. As a report of the Peshawar medical mission shows, it was beneficial to use local premises during the 'preliminary stage':

> Our present hospital is admirably suited to the taste of the Pathan; with its simple native style, it seems to him like home, and for this reason, has been all that we could desire during the preliminary stage of the work, whilst the reputation of the Medical Mission was being established. Now, however, that the

fame of the hospital has spread far and wide, we are being driven by a variety of considerations to the conclusion that we must leave our native premises.[116]

Lankester repeated this viewpoint at least twice: once in his letter to the Society on 6 January 1903: '[w]hen the work at Peshawar was first started, it was thought best, instead of erecting new buildings, to hire native premises in the city, adapting them as far as possible to the requirements of a Medical Mission.'[117] And another time at his speech in 1899, when he elaborated more, making it as clear as possible that financial deficiency was not the reason:

> From what I know of the intention of the Parent Committee I had reason to believe that if I had asked for 30000 rupees (£2000) for building a fine new hospital, it would probably have been granted; but it seemed better to hire a native building in the middle of the city of Peshawar, a building that people would come to naturally, and not seen too grand. [. . .] we obtained two large native caravanserais, a place where for years past those frontier people had been accustomed to go and put up for the night, and stay, and bring their families; right in the heart of the city, within a hundred yards of the place where all the great caravans come in from Afghanistan.[118]

Lankester's wife echoed his husband's view in 1906, stating that the three caravanserais were 'admirably suited at first to our needs when the number of patients was small, and we wished to allay suspicion by treating them in familiar surroundings'.[119] Also, consider Marie Elizabeth Hayes's statement concerning the SPG hospital at Rewari, which was an adapted 'Indian house': '[a]n Indian house has its advantages, at all events to the Indian mind, which we want to upset as little as possible in such matters.'[120]

These statements demand rethinking how missionaries perceived rented premises. Some missionaries found working in rented buildings beneficial in obtaining people's trust because they thought local structures were familiar to the patients. Missionaries may have hoped to illustrate this point by publishing images of hospitals, showing patients gathered in the courtyards at the fountains (Figure 1.6), yet understanding how patients perceived converted structures requires an examination of their past experiences, education, social class and so on. They had culturally and historically specific

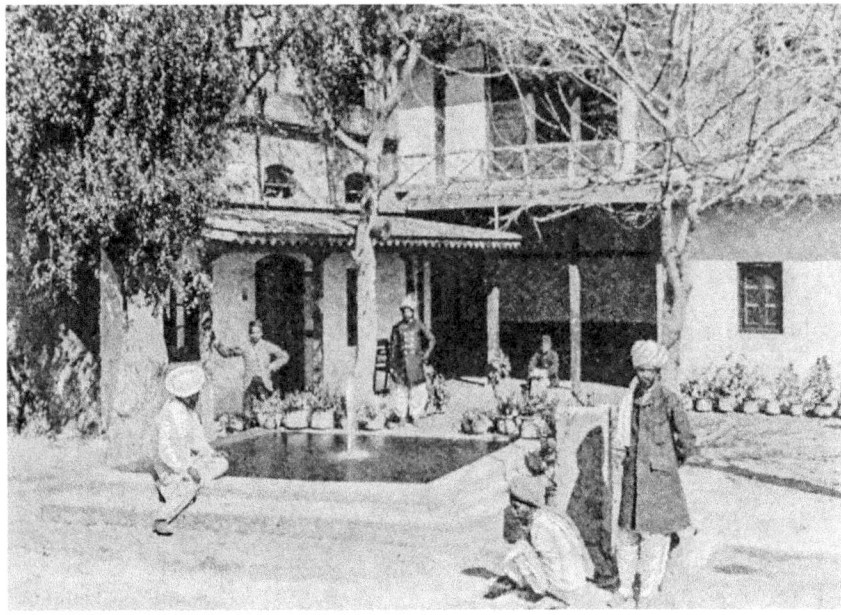

Figure 1.6 Patients gathered around the fountain in front of the doctor's private room and veranda, Peshawar hospital.
CMS/M/EL2/2, p. 138, Church Missionary Society Archive, Cadbury Research Library, Special Collection, University of Birmingham.

preconceptions of what a hospital should look like and these factors would influence their encounter with buildings.[121] Emotional content of converted houses was different from converted caravanserais as some Islamic hospitals were also established in converted houses, such as the Arghun bīmarestān in Aleppo, which was converted from a house by the Mamluk governor, Arghun al-Kamili.[122] In other words, receiving treatment in a converted house may have conformed to patients' expectations and preconceptions, which may not have been the case concerning a caravanserai. Meanwhile, the converted caravanserais in Peshawar had a 'Mohammedan Shrine or Ziarab' (see Figure 1.4) similar to Islamic hospitals such as the bīmarestān al-Qaimari in Damascus.[123] Even if this Shrine or Ziarab was not accessible through the hospital (although the hospital's plan suggests otherwise), given its location in the middle of the hospital and that it might have had a distinctive architectural feature such as a dome, it could influence patients' feelings. It could even fulfil missionaries' desires and make the hospital appear familiar to the patients.

Conclusion

This chapter's discussion has pointed to dispensaries and itinerating activities' central role in developing medical missions. They were more than just small-scale medical activities carried out in addition to or instead of hospital work. They occupied a more important place than previously acknowledged in studies on missionaries and their medicine. They were sites for engaging people and thus laying the foundation of hospital work.

Various factors contributed to the development or otherwise of a medical mission, including lack of resources and staff. But had missionaries not opened dispensaries and undertaken itineration tours regularly and strategically, the number of patients aware of the medical activities of the missionaries would have been considerably lower, meaning that purpose-built structures would not have been built. More precisely, even if a mission had enough doctors, it relied on dispensaries and itinerating activities to help them gain trust to build the hospitals. They visited as many as six or seven villages during a short itineration tour of two weeks, staying at most places for only one or two days. Indeed, itineration camps were practices for accumulating interest. Missionaries mainly visited villages that were on caravan routes, hoping to reach out to people within a larger radius. Itineration tours' performative nature becomes clearer when realising that they were set up at familiar places. Although not to the same extent as itineration tours, dispensaries were also opened to expand the area of operation.

The last part of the chapter discussed the importance of rented buildings for gaining people's trust. Working in rented premises was inevitable given the difficulties missionaries faced, yet this should not diminish the vital role of these buildings in establishing ground. Working in rented buildings was beneficial for another reason. The missionaries were involved in the construction of the hospitals, and working in local premises helped them learn about local ways of construction. Evidence suggests that they drew on the architecture of rented buildings when designing the hospitals. This point will be discussed in the following three chapters.

Notes

1. H. Lankester, 'Medical Missions in Theory', *Mercy and Truth* 4, no. 33 (February 1900): 39.
2. Urania Latham, *Children of Persia* (Edinburgh and London: Oliphant, Anderson and Ferrier, 1911), 90. I am thankful to my friend, James Grannell, for finding this book for me.
3. 'Seventy-Seventh Anniversary of the Church Missionary Society', *Church Missionary Intelligencer*, 1 (1876): 327.
4. Emily Turner, 'The Church Missionary Society and Architecture in the Mission Field: Evangelical Anglican Perspectives on Church Building Abroad. C. 1850–1900', *Architectural History* 58 (2015): 200; Nigel Yates, *Buildings, Faith and Worship: The Liturgical Arrangement of Anglican Churches, 1600–1900* (Oxford: Oxford University Press, 2000), 129.
5. It could take between one and up to twenty years to start the construction of the hospitals. For example, the Isfahan medical mission opened in 1879 and the construction of the purpose-built structures began in 1904. In Quetta, the hospital was built after four years. The Margaret Williamson Hospital in Shanghai was founded in 1884 and the new hospital was opened in 1885. See *Report of the Margaret Williamson Hospital, Shanghai, China* (Women's Co-operating Foreign Mission Boards, 1922), 3–4, Islandora Repository, Women in medicine and history of homeopathy, Drexel University, http://hdl.handle.net/1860/lca:2091; The Sudan-Pionier Mission's hospital in Egypt began with a clinic in 1908 and the hospital was opened in 1913 See Samir Boulos, *European Evangelicals in Egypt (1900–1956): Cultural Entanglements and Missionary Spaces* (Leiden and Boston: Brill, 2016), 181 Mrs Winter began by a box of medicine and then opened a dispensary before establishing the SPG's St Stephen Hospital in Delhi. See Herbert Moore, *Here and There with the SPG in India* (Westminster, 1905), 38.
6. A friend of Iran, *Dawdson: the Doctor: G. E. Dodson of Iran* (London: The Highway Press, 1940), 35.
7. 'Itinerating Medical Work: Why we do it, and how', *The Church Missionary Gleaner* 18, no. 213 (1891): 135.
8. Michelle Renshaw, 'Family-Centred Care in American Hospitals in Late-Qing China', in Graham Mooney and Jonathan Reinarz (eds), *Permeable Walls: Historical Perspectives on Hospital and Asylum Visiting* (Amsterdam and New York: Rodopi, 2009), 57.

9. John R. Stanley, 'Professionalising the Rural Medical Mission in Weixian, 1890–1925', in David Hardiman (ed.), *Healing Bodies, Saving Souls: Medical Missions in Asia and Africa* (Amsterdam: Rodopi, 2006), 123.
10. David Hardiman, 'Christian Therapy: Medical Missionaries and the Adivasis of Western India, 1880–1930,' in *Healing Bodies, Saving Souls* (see note 9), 154.
11. Boulos, *European Evangelicals in Egypt (1900–1956)*, 178.
12. Hardiman, 'Introduction', in *Healing Bodies, Saving Souls* (see note 9), 16–17.
13. For example, Dr Gaskoin Wright of the Nablus medical mission stated that '[a]s long as we have not got a hospital of our own with a firman, these troubles will continue.' See Gaskoin Wright, 'Tribulation – Because of the Word', *Mercy and Truth* 2, no. 20 (1898): 185.
14. For instance, see Dr G. E. Dodson, 6 September 1904, CMS/M/C 2/1 4 no. 34.
15. David Hardiman, 'The Mission Hospital, 1880–1960', in Mark Harrison, Margaret Jones and Helen Sweet (eds), *From Western Medicine to Global Medicine: the Hospital Beyond the West* (New Delhi: Orient BlackSwan, 2009), 204–5.
16. Karen Vallgårda, 'Were Christian Missionaries Colonizers?', *Interventions: International Journal of Postcolonial Studies* 18, no. 6 (2016): 874. Likewise, according to Jennings, a vital element that 'limited the type and range of services that could be offered' was financial constraints. Michael Jennings, '"Healing of Bodies, Salvation of Souls": Missionary Medicine in Colonial Tanganyika, 1870s–1939', *Journal of Religion in Africa* 38, no. 1 (2008): 44.
17. 'Selections from the Proceedings of Committee', *The Church Missionary Intelligencer and Record* 7 new series (March 1882): 188–9.
18. Ibid.
19. 'The CMS Medical Mission Auxiliary – What is it?', *Mercy and Truth* 1, no. 2 (February 1897): 28.
20. 'Things to be Noted', *Mercy and Truth* 4, no. 41 (May 1900): 98.
21. 'Things to be Noted', *Mercy and Truth* 8, no. 89 (December 1904): 353.
22. The CMS Medical Committee sanctioned plans for the Yazd new men's hospital on 6 April 1906. However, it declined to grant any funds and the missionaries had to postpone the construction of the hospital until 1907. 'Things to be Noted', *Mercy and Truth* 10, no. 117 (1906): 258. At Isfahan, a sum of £1,000 was contributed by 'friends in New Zealand through Bishop Stuart . . .' and £1,665 was raised at home. 'The Annual Meeting', *Preaching and Healing, 1903–1904* (1904): 16–17.

23. According to Hardiman, '[i]n this way, medically qualified missionaries distanced themselves from untrained missionary practitioners'. Hardiman, 'The Mission Hospital', 202.
24. Albert Cook, 'Medical Itineration: A Plea for Effective Support of Medical Mission Work throughout the Heathen and Mohammedan World', *Mercy and Truth* 6, no. 66 (June 1902): 175.
25. Vaughan, *Curing their Ills*, 64; see also 'Things to be Noted', *Mercy and Truth* 10, no. 115 (July 1906): 194; 'Things to be Noted', *Mercy and Truth* 3, no. 27 (March 1899): 49.
26. Griffith was accepted as a medical missionary on 6 February 1900. See 'Things to be Noted', *Mercy and Truth* 4, no. 39 (March 1900): 50.
27. For Westlake, see Winifred A. Westlake, 'From Julfa to Kirman', *Mercy and Truth* 8, no. 88 (1904): 116. For Dodson, see 'Things to Be Noted', *Mercy and Truth* 7, no. 80 (August 1903): 224.
28. H. T. Holland, 'Progress of the Quetta Medical Mission', *The Mission Hospital* 28, no. 322 (November 1924): 286.
29. Hilary Ingram, 'A Little Learning *is* a dangerous thing: British overseas medical missions and the politics of professionalism, c. 1880–1910', in Jonathan Reinarz and Rebecca Wynter (eds), *Complaints, Controversies and Grievances in Medicine: Historical and Social Science Perspectives* (London and New York: Routledge, 2015), 76.
30. The unqualified female workers themselves were not willing to take the title of medical missionry. See Ingram, 'A Little Learning', 75–90; see also 'Medical Mission Auxiliary Annual Meeting, May 5, 1898', *Mercy and Truth* 2, no. 18 (June 1898): 138. While not allowed to establish a medical mission, non-qualified missionaries played a role in the transmission of medical ideas to and from Britain. See Ryan Jonson, 'Colonial Mission and Imperial Tropical Medicine: Livingston College, London, 1893–1914', *Social History of Medicine* 23, no. 3 (2010): 549–66.
31. A. Jukes, 'With Dr. Jukes since 1879', *Mercy and Truth* 3, no. 26 (February 1899): 35.
32. S. W. W. W. 'Multan Medical Mission', *The Mission Hospital* 26, no 293 (1922): 105–12.
33. 'Moslem Lands', *Mercy and Truth* 21, no. 247 (October–November 1917): 179.
34. Hans-Lukas Kieser, 'Mission as Factor of Change in Turkey (nineteenth to first half of twentieth century)', *Islam and Christian-Muslim Relations 13*, no. 4 (2002): 392.

35. Philippe Bourmaud, 'Public Space and Private Spheres: The Foundations of St Luke's Hospital of Nablus by the CMS, 1891–1901', in Heleen Murre-van den Berg (ed.), *New Faith in Ancient Land: Western Missions in the Middle East in the Nineteenth and Early Twentieth Centuries* (Leiden and Boston: Brill, 2006), 133.
36. Ibid., 143–4.
37. Ibid.
38. Relying on state sources was not possible everywhere. Femi J. Kolapo, *Christian Missionary Engagement in Central Nigeria, 1875–1891: The Church Missionary Society's All-African Mission on the Upper Niger* (Basingstoke: Palgrave Macmillan, 2019), 137; Heidi Walcher, *In the Shadow of the Kind: Zill Al-Sultan and Isfahan under the Qajars* (London: Bloomsbury Academic, 2008), 241; Jeffrey Cox, *Imperial Fault Lines: Christianity and Colonial Power in India, 1818–1940* (Stanford: Stanford University Press, 2002), 32; Bourmaud, 'Public Space and Private Spheres', 149.
39. Walcher, *In the Shadow of the King*.
40. Missionaries wrote about Mr Mehriban Goodarz on several occassions and even published two pictures of him and his family. See 'Things to be Noted', *Mercy and Truth* 10, no. 117 (1906): 257–8; Dr White, 'Why We Need a New Hospital at Yezd', *Mercy and Truth* 11, no. 122 (1907): 51.
41. Eleanor Abdella Doumato, 'An "Extra Legible Illustration" of the Christian Faith: medicine, medical ethics and missionaries in the Arabian Gulf', *Islam and Christian-Muslim Relations* 13, no. 4 (2002): 388.
42. Walcher, *In the Shadow of the King*, 206.
43. Bourmaud, 'Public Space and Private Spheres', 133.
44. 'Palestine: Precis Book: 22 Nov 1892–8 Sep 1902', CMS/B/OMS/G3 P P4, no. 402, CRL.
45. Andrew C. Ross, *David Livingston: Mission and Empire* (London and New York: Bloomsbury), 56; Jeffrey Cox, *The British Missionary Enterprise since 1700* (New York and London: Routledge, 2008), 152.
46. 'North-India – Foreign Intelligence', *Church Missionary Record* 11, no. 6 (June 1840): 133; 'Australasia – Foreign Intelligence', *Church Missionary Record* 3, no. 4 (April 1932): 80.
47. 'Itinerating Missionary Labour in Bengal', *The Church Missionary Intelligencer* IV, no. 12 (1853): 278–88; 'Itinerating Missionary Work in the Kandian Country', *The Church Missionary Gleaner* 12 (1862): 79–81.
48. Miss J. Biggs, 'First Impressions', *Mercy and Truth* 7, no. 81 (September 1903): 268; 'Memorandum of Interview of Dr. Elliott with Dr. Minie Gomery', 24

March 1905, CMS/M/C 2/1 4, no. 73, CRL; In Palestine conference, held between 6–11 November 1892, request was made for additional works to enable medical itineration to be carried out. See 'Palestine: Precis Book: 22 Nov 1892–8 Sep 1902', no. 402, CRL; A similar statement was made in the conference held in Jerusalem between 3–10 May 1897, 'Palestine: Precis Book: 22 Nov 1892–8 Sep 1902', no. 80–5, CRL.

49. For example, Dr A. Lankester and Dr H. A. Browne were instructed to itinerate in the Peshawar valley in 1897 and report about the best centre for the permanent Medical Mission. See 'Things to be Noted', *Mercy and Truth* 1, no. 9 (September 1897): 193.
50. 'Minutes of Persia-Baghdad Missionary Conference, 6 July 1894', CMS/M/C 1/1 1882-1914, CRL.
51. Cook, 'Medical Itineration', 175.
52. 'News from Beyond the Dead Sea', *Mercy and Truth* 1, no. 9 (1897): 211.
53. Cecil Lankester, 'A Fortnight's Itineration', *Mercy and Truth* 6, no. 68 (August 1902): 236–9.
54. T. L. Pennell, 'Six Weeks Itineration in a New District', *Medical Mission Quarterly*, no. 12 (1895): 82.
55. T. L. Pennell, 'Itinerating in the Bannu District', *Medical Mission Quarterly*, no. 13 (Jan 1896): 16.
56. 'Persia Mission', *Mercy and Truth* 12, no. 142 (October 1908): 316–17; Dr T. L. Pennell, 'An Itineration in the Kurram Valley', *The Church Missionary Intelligencer* XXI new series (1896): 32–4.
57. A. Neve, 'The Story of a few days' district work', *Mercy and Truth* 3, no. 32 (August 1899): 199. A note in 1900 mentioned that 'during a summer itineration in the villages near Yezd, 2570 patients were treated by the doctor and his assistants . . .' See 'The Mission Field', *The Church Missionary Intelligencer* 51 (1900): 211.
58. Mary Bird, 'Village Work Amongst Women in Persia', *Mercy and Truth* 18, no. 209 (May 1914): 140.
59. Iraj Afshar, Narges Pedram and Asghar Mahdavi, *Kerman dar asnād-e Amīnozarb: sālhaye 1280–1351 ghamari* [Kerman according to Amin Alzarb's documents between 1289 and 1351 AH] (Tehran: Soraya, 1385/2006), 339–58.
60. A. Lankester and A. H. Browne, 'Proposed Peshawar Medical Mission', *The Church Missionary Intelligencer* 22 (October 1897): 757.
61. Theodore L. Pannell, 'The Afghan Medical Mission', *Mercy and Truth* 1, no. 5 (May 1897): 105.

62. Dr Pennell, 'More News from the Khattak Hills', *Mercy and Truth* 9, no. 104 (August 1905): 237.
63. 'Memorandum of Interview of Dr Elliott with Dr Minnie Gomery', 24 March 1905, CMS/M/C 2/1 4, no. 73, CRL.
64. Miss E. M. Fox, 'Camping in the Peshawar Valley', *Mercy and Truth* 6, no. 67 (July 1902): 203.
65. Hardiman, 'Christian Therapy: Medical Missionaries', 149.
66. Miss J. Biggs, 'First Impressions', 268.
67. Lucy Molony, 'Itinerating in the Persian Mountains', *Mercy and Truth* 9, no. 108 (December 1905): 365.
68. 'Items: Home and Foreign', *Mercy and Truth* 15, no. 169 (January 1911): 9.
69. Adams, 'Itinerating Medical Work in the Punjab', 116.
70. Theodore L. Pannell, 'The Afghan Medical Mission', *Mercy and Truth* 1, no. 5 (May 1897): 104.
71. T. L. Pennell, 'The Afghan – How can we reach them?', *Mercy and Truth* 1, no. 1 (January 1897): 10.
72. H. T. Holland, 'A Five Days' Medical Itineration', *Mercy and Truth* 8, no. 92 (Aug 1904): 236.
73. Arthur H. Browne, 'An Itineration from Amritsar', *Mercy and Truth* 17, no. 194 (February 1913): 54.
74. 'Itinerating Medical Work. Why we do it, and how', *The Church Missionary Gleaner* (September 1891): 135.
75. Patricia Baker, 'Medieval Islamic Hospitals: Structural Design and Social Perceptions', in Patricia A. Baker, Han Nijdam, and Karine van't Land (eds), *Medicine and Space: Body, Surroundings and Borders in Antiquity and the Middle Ages* (Leiden and Boston: Brill, 2012), 261.
76. Ahmed Rageb, *The Medieval Islamic Hospital: Medicine, Religion, and Charity* (Cambridge: Cambridge University Press, 2015), 46.
77. Hardiman, 'Christian Therapy', 154; Houari Touati, *Islam and Travel in the Middle Ages* (Chicago and London: The University Press of Chicago, 2010); Cyril Elgood, *A Medical History of Persia and the Eastern Caliphate from the Earliest times until the year A. D. 1932* (Cambridge: Cambridge University Press, 1951), 174; Shireen Mahdavi, 'Everyday Life in Late Qajar Iran', *Iranian Studies* 45, no. 3 (2012): 366.
78. Hardiman makes this point regarding Ayurvedic Physician. See Hardiman, 'Christian Therapy', 154.
79. Eliza F. Kent, *Converting Women: Gender and Protestant Christianity in Colonial South India* (Oxford: Oxford University Press, 2004), 154.

80. Ludwig Vogl-Bienek and Richard Crangle (eds), *Screen Culture and the Social Question 1880–1914* (London: Studies in Early Cinema, John Libbey Publishing, 2014), 114.
81. Jane Lydon, *Imperial Emotions: the Politics of Empathy across the British Empire* (Cambridge: Cambridge University Press, 2020), 143–63.
82. Alan Withey, 'Medicine and Charity in Eighteenth-century Northumberland: The Early Years of the Bamburgh Castle Dispensary and Surgery, *c.* 1772–1802', *Social History of Medicine* 29, no. 3 (2016): 457.
83. Bronwyn Croxson, 'The Foundation and Evolution of the Middlesex Hospital's Lying-In Service, 1745–86', *Social History of Medicine* 14, no. 1 (2001): 45.
84. Zachary Cope, 'The Influence of the Free Dispensaries upon Medical Education in Britain', *Medical History* 13, no. 1 (January 1969): 36.
85. Harriet Richardson (ed.), *English Hospitals 1660–1948: A Survey of their Architecture and Design* (The Royal Commission on the Historical Monuments of England, 1998), 25.
86. Charles E. Rosenberg, 'Social Class and Medical Care in Nineteenth-Century America: The Rise and Fall of the Dispensary', *Journal of the History of Medicine and Allied Sciences* 29, no. 1 (1974): 32–54.
87. Ibid.,
88. Withey, 'Medicine and Charity in Eighteenth-century Northumberland', 457.
89. Mark Harrison, *Public Health in British India: Anglo-Indian Preventive Medicine, 1859–1914* (Cambridge: Cambridge University Press, 1994), 88–90.
90. Mridula Ramanna, *Western Medicine and Public Health in Colonial Bombay, 1845–1895* (Hyderabad: Orient Longman, 2002), 51.
91. Seema Alavi, *Islam and Healing: Loss and Recovery of an Indi-Muslim Medical Tradition, 1600–1900* (Basingstoke: Palgrave Macmillan, 2008), 174–85.
92. Ibid., 154.
93. Lazich, 'Seeking Souls through the Eyes of the Blind', in *Healing Bodies, Saving Souls* (see note 9), 62–3; Stanley, 'Professionalising the Rural Medical Mission in Weixian, 1890–1925', 117.
94. Rev. W. S. Tyler, *Memoir of Rev. Henry Lobdell, M.D., late Missionary of the American Board at Mosul* (Cornhill: The American Track Society, 1859), 173.
95. Renshaw, '"Family-Centred Care" in American Hospitals in Late-Qing China', 57.
96. Dr Pennell, 'More News from the Khattak Hills', *Mercy and Truth* 9, no. 104 (August 1905): 237–9.
97. Mary Bird, 'A Women's Work among the Women in Julfa', *Mercy and Truth* 2, no. 14 (February 1898): 35.

98. Walcher, *In the Shadow of the King*, 210.
99. 'A Year's Work in Persia', *The Church Missionary Intelligence* 25 (April 1900): 260.
100. Donald W. Carr, 'What God Hath Wrought', *The Mission Hospital* 26, no. 293 (May 1922): 101.
101. 'Medical Missions', *Preaching and Healing, 1900–1901* (1901): 34.
102. 'A Doctor for Kirman', *Mercy and Truth* 2, no. 21 (1898): 213.
103. Rev. C. H. Stilman, the secretary of the Persia Mission, mentioned these two horses in a letter dated July 1904. See C. H. Stillman, 22 July 1904, CMS/G2/PE/0 1903–1904, no. 125, CRL.
104. Dr Lankester and Dr Browne, 'Some Observations on General Medical Mission Policy', *Mercy and Truth* 1, no. 11 (November 1897): 257.
105. 'Items: Home and Foreign', *Mercy and Truth* 8, no. 89 (May 1904): 133.
106. 'Mohammedan Lands', *Preaching and Healing, the Report of the CMS Medical Mission Auxiliary for 1903–1904* (1904): 51.
107. 'Medical Missions', *Preaching and Healing, the Report of the CMS Medical Mission Auxiliary for 1900–1901* (1901): 36–7.
108. C. H. Stillman, 'Medical Mission Work in Persia', *Medical Mission Quarterly*, no 12 (October 1895): 85
109. Mary Bird, 'A Women's Work among the Women in Julfa', *Mercy and Truth* 2, no. 14 (February 1898): 35.
110. 'Persia in 1894: The Women's Dispensary', *The Church Missionary Gleaner* (April 1895): 56.
111. D. W. Carr, 'Progress in Persia', *Mercy and Truth* 9, no. 103 (July 1905): 208.
112. 'Medical Missions', *Preaching and Healing, the Report of the CMS Medical Mission Auxiliary for 1902–1903* (1903): 52.
113. D. W. Carr, 'Progress in Persia', *Mercy and Truth* 9, no. 103 (July 1905): 208.
114. Urania Malcolm (Latham), 'Work among women in Yezd', *Mercy and Truth* 5, no. 54 (1901): 133; Henry White, 'Why we need a new hospital in Yazd', *Mercy and Truth* 11, no. 122 (1907): 49.
115. Christine Stevenson, *Medicine and Magnificence: British Hospital and Asylum Architecture, 1660–1815* (New Haven and London: Yale University Press, 2000), 132–40.
116. 'Peshawar Medical Mission', CMS/M/FL 1 I7, CRL.
117. A. Lankester, 6 January 1903, CMS/M/C 2/1 4, no. 12, CRL.
118. 'Medical Mission Auxiliary Annual Meeting, May 4th, 1899', *Mercy and Truth* 3, no. 30 (June 1899): 141.

119. Mrs A Lankester, 'The New Hospital at Peshawar', *Mercy and Truth* 10, no. 113 (May 1906): 143–4.
120. Annabella Hayes, *At Work: Letters of Marie Elizabeth Hayes, M.B. missionary doctor, Delhi, 1905–8* (London: Marshall Brothers, 1909), 2019.
121. Benno Gammerl, Philipp Nielsen and Margrit Pernau, 'Introduction: Encountering Feelings – Feeling Encounters', in Benno Gammerl, Philipp Nielsen and Margrit Pernau (eds), *Encounters with Emotions: Negotiating Cultural Differences since Early Modernity* (New York and Oxford: Berghahn, 2019), 4.
122. Baker, 'Medieval Islamic Hospitals', 261.
123. Ibid.

2

MISSIONARIES AND THE DEVELOPMENT OF NOVEL HOSPITAL DESIGNS

'It is not a bit like an English hospital.'[1] This was the reaction that the architecture of the CMS hospital for women in Isfahan, Persia, elicited from the newly arrived missionaries in the early twentieth century. The hospital had inpatient, outpatient, isolation and private blocks familiar to the missionaries but the specific design and arrangement of the buildings and the mode of occupation they engender appeared very different. Planned with almost no reference to the prevailing hospital design principles in Britain, the buildings were arranged to form an enclosed compound and were designed to facilitate free movement between the different parts of the hospital (Figure 2.1). Not only the Isfahan hospital but also some of the hospitals in north-western British India were judged in this way: 'at first one feels "How different to an English hospital",' wrote Miss D. Mellowes in 1919 about her first impressions of work in the Multan hospital.[2] Likewise, Miss F. M. Clarke referred to the Peshawar hospital in 1922 as 'this most un-English hospital'.[3] Not all mission hospitals planned differently from conventional models of the period in Britain. In contrast to the Isfahan, Peshawar and Multan hospitals, the hospital of the London Society for Promoting Christianity Amongst the Jews in Safed, for example, was described as 'English-Like'.[4] But they functioned, and some were designed, to gain the trust of the local communities.

This chapter is the first among the three that focus on hospital buildings. They examine various architectural configurations the CMS medical

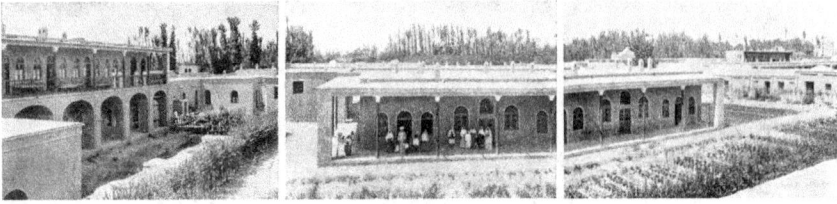

Figure 2.1 Isfahan's new women's hospital.
CMS/M/EL 2/10, p. 366, Church Missionary Society Archive, Cadbury Research Library, Special Collections, University of Birmingham.

missionaries developed to obtain trust and friendship while showing that mission hospitals could not impress upon patients (and visitors) in any simple way. The focus of this chapter is mainly on the design characteristics of the master plan of the hospitals and the general wards, and the following two chapters examine specialised buildings constructed for a whole family and female patients. Meanwhile, they go beyond a mere focus on the layout and appearance to consider smell, taste, touch and sound.

These three chapters also raise questions concerning the internationalisation of hospital architectural forms in the late nineteenth and early twentieth centuries. Hospital architecture in Britain had undergone a radical transformation by the second half of the nineteenth century, when most new and rebuilt hospitals conformed to one basic design known as the pavilion plan.[5] Ideas about the pavilion approach to hospital design originated in France in the late eighteenth century, and they were honed in Britain in the nineteenth century. The advocates of pavilion design were concerned with the high mortality rate in hospitals, seeing it a result of bad air, or miasma, accumulated in dark and stagnant spaces. Their main aim was to limit the spread of hospital infection by allowing air – and natural light – to permeate every part of the hospital. By the late nineteenth century examples of pavilion plan hospitals could be found across Europe and in Asia, Africa, Australia and North America.[6] According to Cor Wagenaar, the pavilion plan was the 'the first revolution' in the history of hospital architecture: 'a victory of science, philosophy and technology'.[7]

In a pavilion hospital each ward was housed in a separate block or pavilion. A pavilion ward was rectangular and had windows facing each other along its length to ensure cross-ventilation. Each pavilion had its own sanitary facilities – baths, sinks and water closets – that were placed usually at the end of the ward, sometimes in detached towers connected to the ward by a small, enclosed passage.[8] As historians have shown, there was a variety of pavilion plan hospitals. For example, in the tropics, the plan was modified to include verandas, and the standard size of the ward was increased in response to climatic conditions.[9] In the United States, one of the most celebrated examples was the Johns Hopkins Hospital (1877–85), in which sanitary towers were designed to the east of the pavilion wards rather than at the end 'to avoid blocking the southern exposure'.[10] However, the key principles – particularly ensuring cross-ventilation – remained the same everywhere.

After 1900 discoveries in bacteriology rendered unnecessary the issue of cross-ventilation, emphasising the importance of hygiene to disease prevention instead. As a result, the pavilion plan design slowly declined, giving way to more compact ward tower (or multi-levelled) buildings in the 1920s and 1930s, in which the movement and interaction of goods and people were increasingly controlled to reduce contamination.[11] The curative value of fresh air and sunlight was still deemed necessary, particularly in the contexts of tuberculosis institutions, where the focus was on remaining outside in all weather conditions, and maternity facilities.[12] As Jeanne Kisacky states in the context of the United States, 'if aseptic barriers and controlled circulation paths become as common in modern hospital design as open windows and fresh air corridors had once been, to portray the shift as complete in the 1920s is to give a false impression.'[13] Securing fresh air became less concerning only in the 1940s and 1950s.

The historiography of hospital architecture in the late nineteenth and early twentieth centuries is predominantly about the pavilion plan. Scholars such as Jeremy Taylor and Kisacky further argue that this type of hospital planning became an international standard by the late nineteenth century.[14] This understanding is perhaps to be expected. After all, Florence Nightingale's *Notes on Hospitals* (1863) partly popularised the pavilion plan; it has a chapter on how to construct a pavilion plan hospital in India.[15] According to Kisasky, 'it became the international bible of late nineteenth-century hospital design'.[16] Moreover, Frederic J. Mouat and H. Saxon Snell's *Hospital Construction and Management* (1867), F. Oppert's *Hospitals, Infirmaries, and Dispensaries* (1883) and Henry C. Burdett's four-volume *Hospitals and Asylums of the World* (1891) showcased examples of pavilion plan hospitals in British India, Australia and Persia.[17] These texts provided models to be copied and recommendations to be followed, and have constituted some of the primary sources in Taylor's, Kisacky's and other scholarship concerning the history of hospital architecture worldwide.[18]

However, there are some stark omissions in these texts. By relying on them, scholars have provided only a partial picture of hospital architecture in a global context. These books exclude hospitals built in China, along with hospitals constructed in Africa and South America, those built by non-British empires and those by North Americans in the colonised world. Moreover, they were published when missionary medicine was still in its infancy. Thus, examples provided in these three books were state or military hospitals.[19] By the turn of the century, medical missions had become one of the main providers of Western biomedical services in colonial territories, if not the only one in some regions. An examination of all these hospitals is required for addressing the extent to which the pavilion plan became an international standard.[20] Protestant mission hospitals are a particularly vital lens through which we can write a history of hospital architecture in a global context. Although the secular and mission medicine in colonies shared characteristics in terms of the ways in which diseases and healing were perceived, it was the missionaries that engaged in major spending on medical facilities at the local level. In many British colonies, indigenous people encountered Western biomedical services for the first time in mission, rather than state or military hospitals. Michael Jennings' statement that the 'first hospitals in Tanganyika, the first clinics and doctors, were missionary' is true for some countries in Africa, some parts of the Middle East as well as for China and India.[21]

This chapter and the following two demonstrate that focusing on Protestant mission hospitals challenges the assumption that the pavilion plan became an international standard. They show that the CMS missionaries disregarded scientific and sanitary approaches embodied in the pavilion plan to provide a space that could feel familiar. The CMS medical missionaries made and remade prevailing approaches to hospital architecture and invented new hospital designs by disregarding some of the medical concerns of the time.

The Punjab Model

It is best to start with a discussion about the architecture of the Kashmir hospital, the first mission hospital of the CMS. The first purpose-built hospital in Kashmir was constructed in 1875 (Figure 2.2). It consisted of 'three buildings occupying three sides of a square', and was designed by Dr Theodore Maxwell with the help of Reverend Robert Clark who, according to Maxwell, 'had great experience in building'.[22] These structures were pulled down and replaced by a hospital built 'on the pavilion plan system', consisting of 'seven blocks, separated from one another', between 1886 and 1895 (Figure 2.3).[23] The construction of the hospital took around ten years due to the limited financial support from the Society.[24] Each year the missionaries raised a specific amount of money, and the 'substantial and suitable brick two-storeyed pavilions' were completed year by year.[25] Two blocks were for women, four were for men, one was for paying patients, and one was for outpatients.[26]

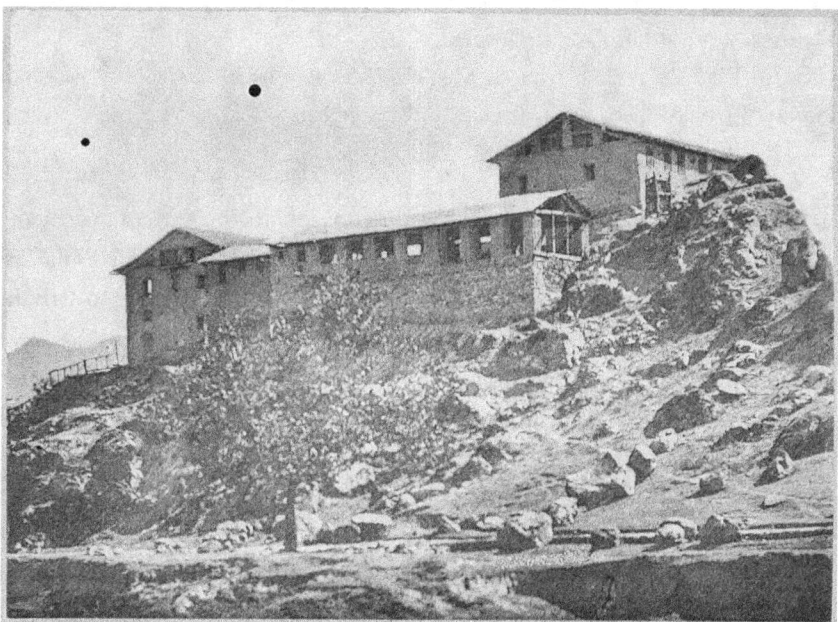

Figure 2.2 The first purpose-built structures in Kashmir.
CMS/ACC 181 Z1, Church Missionary Society Archive, Cadbury Research Library, Special Collections, University of Birmingham.

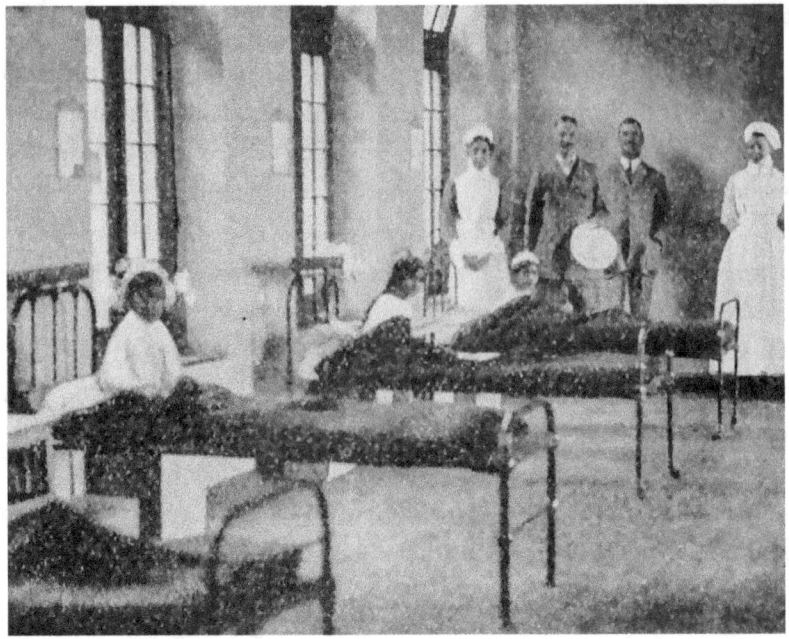

Figure 2.3 A ward in Kashmir hospital.
CMS/M/EL 2/24 p. 282, Church Missionary Society Archive, Cadbury Research Library, Special Collections, University of Birmingham.

The design of mission hospitals was often left to the care of the medical missionaries themselves.[27] They sometimes consulted other missionaries, sought help from military engineers or brought their ideas back to Britain for professional help. But, on the whole, the archival materials offer relatively little help in understanding how they designed the hospitals. They could have drawn on new and approved design criteria that were disseminated through journals and books.[28] If it was not possible for them to avail themselves of copies of relevant publications,[29] many of them studied and practised medicine in pavilion plan hospitals before joining the mission field,[30] and could model their design after these hospitals. Arthur Neve, for example, had worked as a house physician in the Royal Infirmary, Edinburgh,[31] which was considered as one of the best pavilion plan hospitals.[32] As stated by G. A. Bremner and Louis P. Nelson, the transfer of European architecture overseas in the nineteenth and twentieth centuries, among other things, had to do with memory and architectural literature – journals, magazines and pattern books.[33] Additionally, there were missionary examples and publications: almost seven years after the construction of the Kashmir hospital was started, in 1892, the London Society for Promoting Christianity amongst the Jews proposed a scheme for a hospital in Jerusalem, drawn by Arthur Beresford Pite, an English architect. After his initial design was rejected, Pite proposed a second design, built and completed in 1900. Both schemes were designed according to pavilion principles.[34] The final design consisted of four pavilions radiating outwards from a central building.[35] Mark Crinson and Samuel Albert have examined the design of this hospital. They are concerned with Pite's attachment to the London Society (he served on the Society's general committee) discussing how the project allowed him to follow 'devoutly evangelical beliefs', rather than his experience in hospital architecture.[36] Pite had designed at least two hospitals in England before the 'hospital for Jews'[37] and, according to a statement published in the *Jews Missionary Intelligence*, had visited about twenty different hospitals before designing the hospital in Jerusalem.[38] As this and the Kashmir medical missions were among the first in the Middle East and British India, they could have served as models for other medical missions built in subsequent years, especially as their design was disseminated in missionary journals and meetings. The design of the 'hospital for Jews' was published in *The Builder*.[39] Moreover, the plan of a proposed pavilion plan hospital for West Africa was published in *Mercy and Truth* in 1899.[40] However, many mission hospitals built in British India, Persia, Palestine and Egypt did not live up to the principles of the pavilion plan. The 'hospital for Jews' acted as a model insofar as it was one of the first buildings in the 'Orientalist' style, but not for being one of the first pavilion plan mission hospitals.[41] Albert compares the layout and style of the hospital to other 'national' hospitals in Jerusalem, for example the French Hospital and the German Hospital. He states that it contrasted them all markedly, arguing that 'it was actively representative of the (medical) modernity Britain was attempting to bring to the Holy Land'.[42] But the hospital contrasted British mission hospitals too, including the CMS hospitals in Nablus and Gaza.

The CMS often opposed episcopal oversight and hence was less disciplined and establishmentarian, allowing individual missionaries to follow their stance on architecture.[43] Nevertheless, the SPG, which had a corporate structure and highly regulated the recruitment of its applicants,[44] also constructed hospitals with various layouts.[45] We need to see beyond the organisational structure of individual missionary societies and consider how they were united for the common purpose of gaining trust and affection to explain their approach to hospital design. We can gain a picture of the diversity of medical missions of various Protestant missionary societies from the second volume of James S. Dennis's, a member of American Presbyterian Mission in Beirut, three-volume study, *Christian Missions and Social Progress: A Sociological Study of Foreign Missions* (1899) and A. R. Cavalier's *In Northern India* (1899).[46] As these volumes show, a more common design was the single (sometimes U-shaped) pavilion. The missionaries also developed hospitals with irregular designs in addition to one-block, two-storey structures.

In north-western British India, the CMS missionaries designed hospitals with diverse layouts. In 1903 Neve toured the medical missions in north-western British India as the secretary of the Punjab Medical Sub-Conference.[47] After the tour, he prepared a memorandum in which he discussed architecture.[48] Although he had designed a pavilion plan hospital in Kashmir, he appraised the design of two hospitals, neither of which were modelled on the pavilion plan. The first was the Dera Ismail Khan hospital, which was built to the design of Dr W. B. Heywood and was opened on 6 February 1902.[49] According to the memorandum, the hospital was 'the newest and best' and the wards were 'well-planned built and fitted'.[50] The buildings were built around three sides of a square (Figure 2.4). In particular, Neve admired the design of the largest and newest ward (Figure 2.5). It measured 61 feet long, 20 feet broad and 18 feet high and was 'lighted by fourteen windows, and ha[d] six large doors, two on each side and one at each end', while a covered veranda ran along three sides of the building.[51] While Neve declared in the memorandum that the ward was 'unnecessarily wide and lofty for any other station',[52] he echoed a different opinion in a published report and referred to the ward as 'a first class of what a ward in a hot country should be'.[53]

The second ward was the new 'eye block' at the Bannu hospital. Neve regarded this ward 'more suitable to adapt as the standard pattern' and called it the Punjab model: 'It might be adopted as a Punjab model.'[54]

DEVELOPMENT OF NOVEL HOSPITAL DESIGNS | 75

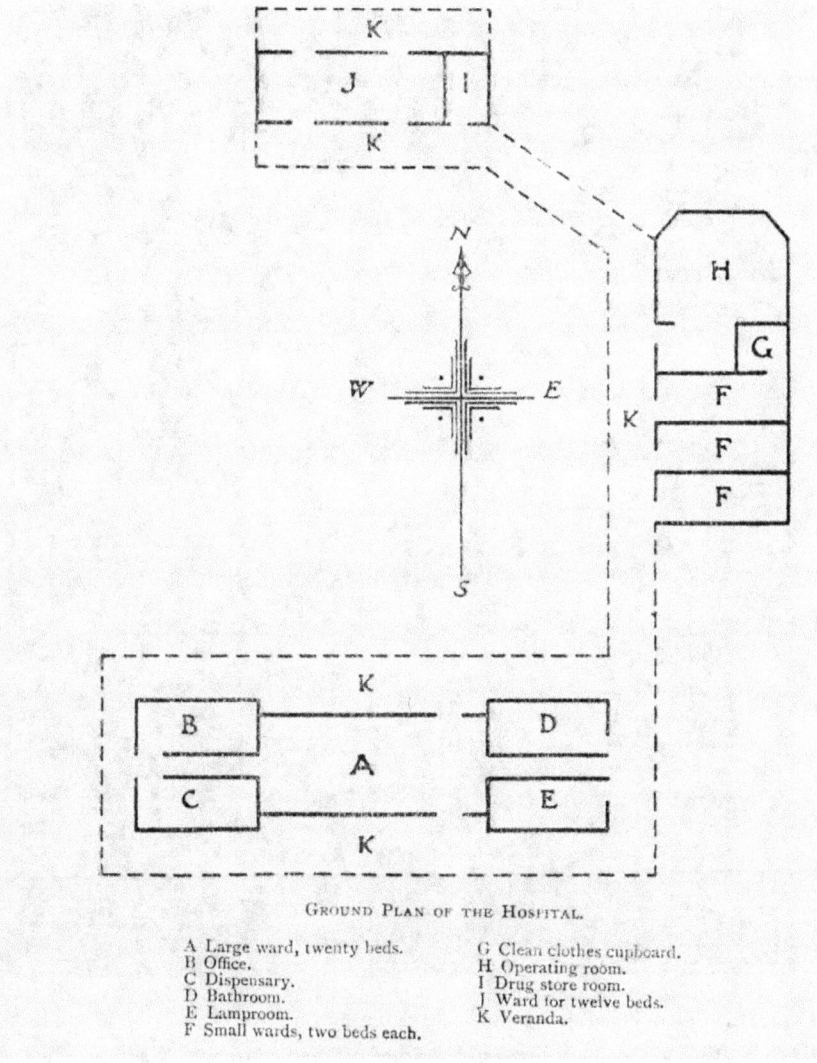

Figure 2.4 Ground plan of Dera Ismail Khan hospital.
CMS/M/EL 2/7 p. 82, Church Missionary Society Archive, Cadbury Research Library, Special Collections, University of Birmingham.

The Bannu hospital was commenced in 1894 by Dr Theodore Pennell and the Society sanctioned the construction of the new eye block in 1901.[55] It was completed a year later and was opened on 3 October 1902.[56] It had two wards that were smaller than the ward at the Dera Ismail Khan

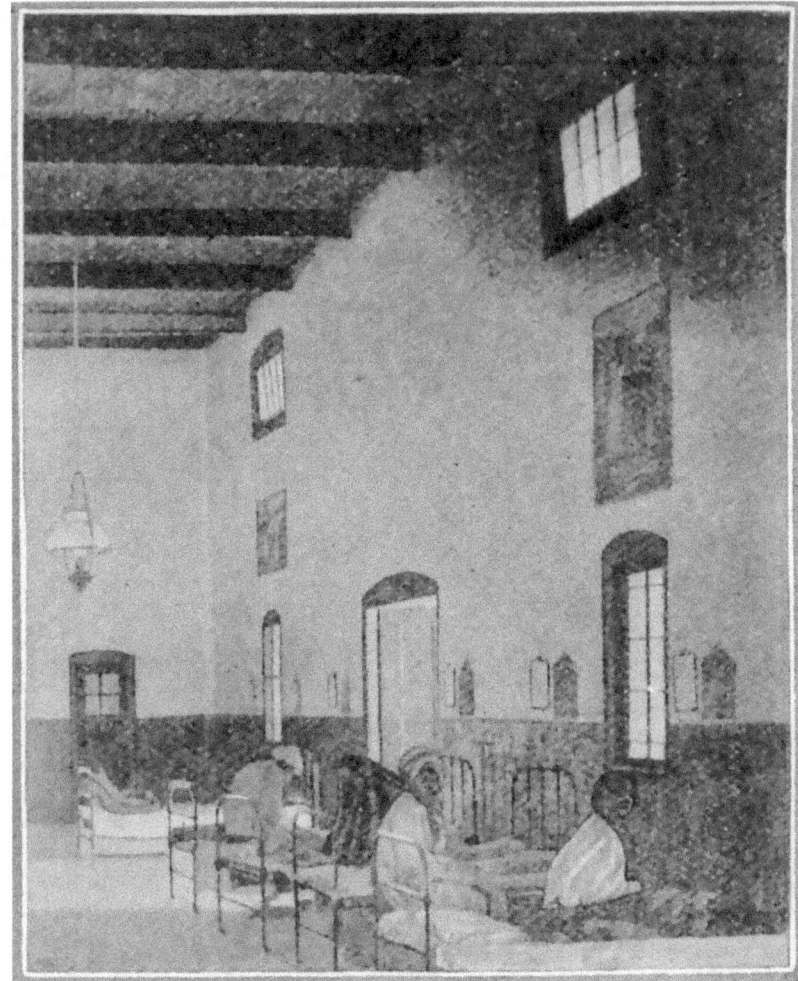

Figure 2.5 Dera Ismail Khan medical mission.
CMS/M/EL 2/7 p. 80, Church Missionary Society Archive, Cadbury Research Library, Special Collections, University of Birmingham.

hospital. They measured 30 feet by 16 feet and were lit by windows at the top of the walls on opposite sides, with four opposing doors – two on each side. Like the new ward at Dera Ismail Khan, a veranda ran around three sides of the block (Figure 2.6). Together, these wards provided accommodation for twenty patients, bringing the hospital's total capacity up to fifty beds.

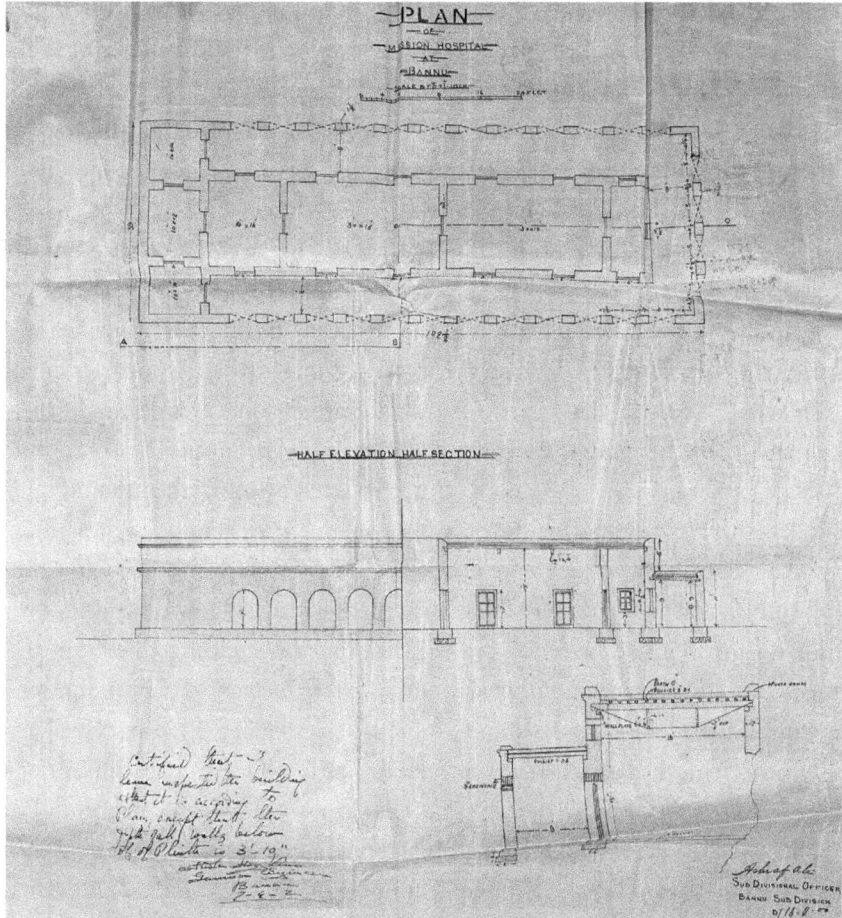

Figure 2.6 Plan of the eye ward at the Bannu hospital.
CMS/M/FL 1/I 2/3, Church Missionary Society Archive, Cadbury Research Library, Special Collections, University of Birmingham.

In opting for the eye block, Neve might have been familiar with the debates on the health benefits of the so-called block plan or smaller rooms over older pavilion plan wards. The rationale was that smaller rooms were less crowded and noisy, and thus more comfortable and easier to manage.[57] But neither the new ward at Dera Ismail Khan nor the eye block at Bannu were cross-ventilated. If the hot climatic condition of the region was the deciding factor, the missionaries could have followed Nightingale's advice. There were also available models of pavilion plan hospitals constructed in hot and dry areas in Burdett's book.[58] Nightingale recommended adding verandas but advised against minimising the size or number of windows. Her advice that 'each ward should [be] so arranged as to prevent the patient going out or holding communication with persons outside'[59] was not realised either; both blocks had several points of entry and exit.

The missionaries drew on 'standard plans' that were developed by the Public Work Department of the Government of India (PWD).[60] The initial 'frame' of these standard plans was that of a pucka bungalow, transformed in a hospital to admit air and light to the upper volume.[61] The missionaries might have opted for these plans due to the lack of professional architectural expertise.[62] As Bremner states regarding churches built in South Asia, they were mostly 'rather generic and "incorrect" in character, owing to the input of military engineers'.[63] Examining how the missionaries went about designing these two hospitals and who they were in contact with is important and could reveal new information about the PWD planning conventions, previously unknown 'experts', missionaries' view of and contribution to tropical architecture and medicine, and their relationship with military engineers.[64] But if we turn our attention to the missionaries' aim to build trust and affection, other considerations begin to surface. We start to see that the PWD planning conventions could have conformed to the expectations of, for example, a small group of wealthy Indian elites who inhabited houses designed after these conventions. The hospitals would make a different impression on these Indian elites than on the Indian servants who worked in these houses.[65] Indeed, while there are some merits in examining these buildings as 'symbol[s] of Britain's commercial and military might',[66] there are also limitations. A focus on building trust and affection, and emotions more broadly, demands turning our attention to the patients and avoiding generalisations about their feelings towards these buildings. The new ward at the Dera Ismail Khan hospital and the 'eye-ward' at Bannu (Figure 2.7) could not affect patients in any unequivocal and straightforward way. They could fit into their surroundings without the overtones of a public building or appear familiar, a fact that might have even influenced missionaries' decision to opt for the PWD conventions.

Even if the hospitals did not adhere to the principles of the pavilion plan, they still had beds in neat rows, a factor that has made some historians such

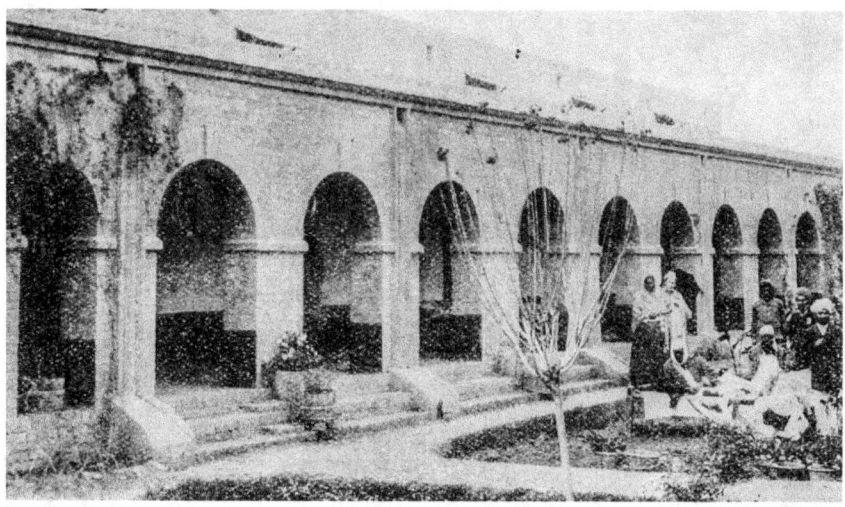

Figure 2.7 The eye ward at the Bannu hospital.
CMS/M/EL 2/11 p. 201, Church Missionary Society Archive, Cadbury Research Library, Special Collections, University of Birmingham.

as David Hardiman argue that mission hospitals imposed 'forms of discipline and ritual on their patients'; that they 'were designed to demonstrate Christian order and cleanliness'.[67] Similarly, in his book on the global production of the bungalow, Antony D. King provides an image of the CMS hospital in Ranaghat, Bengal, which was a bungalow, stating that the building was 'Indian' but the institution it contained was 'European'.[68] However, in some parts of the Islamic world, wards with beds in neat rows might not have appeared as new to the patients. Although information is limited, a painting of Abulcasis (Abū al-Qāsim) (936–1013), an Islamic Spanish physician, in the hospital at Cordoba (Figure 2.8) and a description of the al-Mansūrī hospital in Cairo by Evliya Çelebi, a seventeenth-century Ottoman traveller, indicate that there were also rows of beds in the Islamic hospitals. Elebi wrote that patients 'were provided with bed-clothes and were placed in beds with silk sheets'.[69]

Broadly speaking, the spatial arrangements of the buildings were not contextualised so much based on functional design and discipline as autonomy for patients. Apart from preaching routines and changing clothes, no strict regulations were laid down, dictating 'appropriate' behaviour. Even the

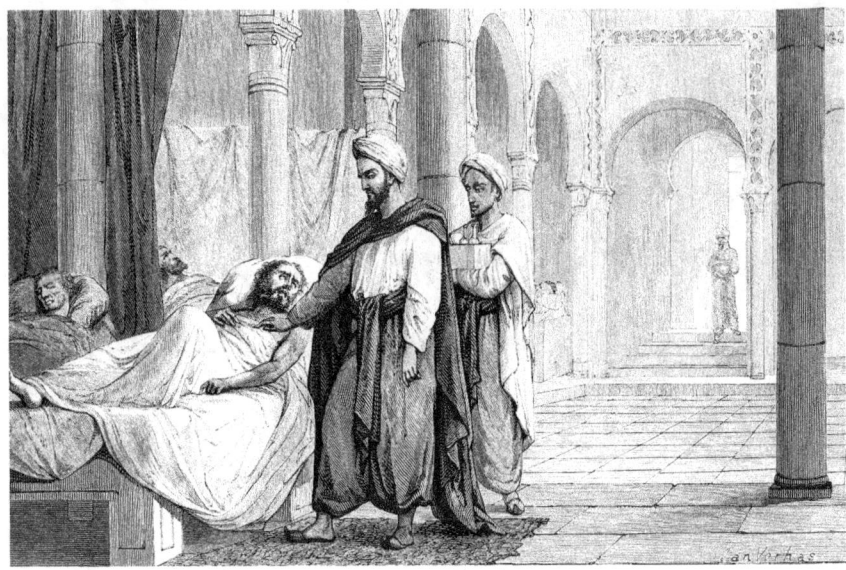

Figure 2.8 Abulcasis (936–1013), Islamic Spanish physician in the hospital at Cordoba, Spain. He attends a patient, while an assistant carries a box of medicine. H401/0289, Sheila Terry / Science Photo Library.

former was not consistently enforced. This accommodating approach also led to the development of new hospital designs. The Peshawar hospital, which opened three years after the Bannu hospital, provides a clear perspective. Not only the master plan of the hospital but also the internal spatial arrangement of the individual buildings represents distinct designs.

The Four-part Garden

The construction of the Peshawar hospital began in 1904. Dr Arthur Lankester and a local builder named Miran Baksh planned the hospital. Miran Baksh was, according to Lankester, 'a Moslem from Sialkot, who had built many of the better class of Indian houses in his own town'. After preparing the sketch plans, Lankester and Miran Baksh prepared the 'detailed plans drawn to scale' under the 'close supervision and help of experienced engineer officers of the Military Works Department'.[70] Lankester and Miran Baksh also superintended the construction of the buildings.[71] The hospital was opened in February 1906, although some buildings were added later.

As mentioned at the beginning of the chapter, the Peshawar hospital was perceived as not being 'English'. In part, the specific condition of the site dictated this dissimilarity. Located 'about 200 yards' from the 'City Gate', the land was a terraced plot. The missionaries decided to build the hospital 'in stages' to take 'the fullest advantage' of the 'natural features of the site'. Moreover, the site was surmounted by a mausoleum of considerable size or 'Said Khan's Tower', which was built by 'a former ruler of Peshawar' (Figure 2.9).[72] The outpatient block consisted of a large waiting room, consulting room, operation room, a room for women outpatients and a dispensary. The inpatient block was a two-storey U-shaped structure consisting of an operating theatre, offices and wards. A staircase on the left corner provided access to the upper floor. The lower and upper floors of the connecting wing contained a large ward for sixteen beds. The lower floor of the right wing housed the operating theatre and offices. Each floor of the left wing had eight four-bed wards.

The hospital contained modern requirements for the care of the sick. Particularly noticeable are two operating rooms. As Lankester explained, the outpatient operating room was for patients who did not 'call for elaborate aseptic precautions', while the inpatient operating room was preserved for

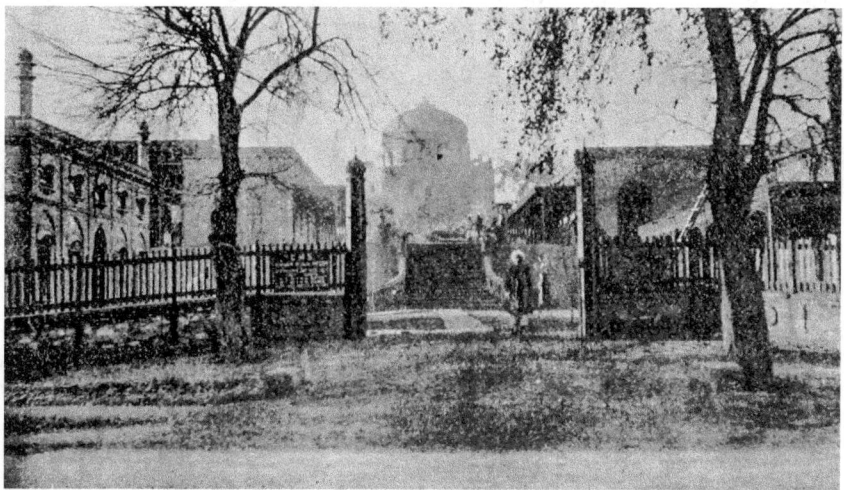

Figure 2.9 Peshawar hospital, view from the main entrance.
CMS/M/EL 2/11, p. 396, Church Missionary Society Archive, Cadbury Research Library, Special Collections, University of Birmingham.

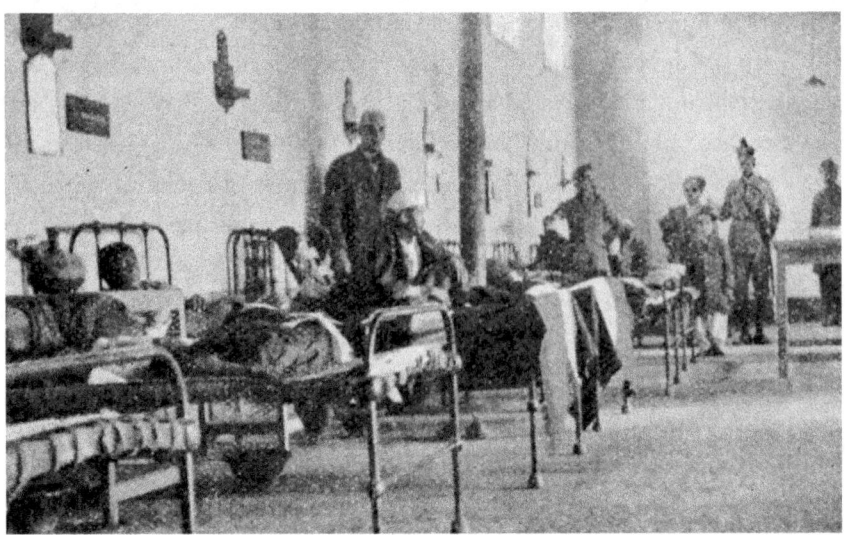

Figure 2.10 Inside of one of the large wards at Peshawar.
CMS/M/EL 2/28, p. 261, Church Missionary Society Archive, Cadbury Research Library, Special Collections, University of Birmingham.

'septic cases' and 'out-patients who come in their own dirty clothes'.[73] This arrangement alludes to contemporary concerns with germ theory and aseptic surgery, which required the thorough disinfection of every instrument, object, person and material.[74] Lankester viewed the advantage of having a septic operating room 'very great indeed'. Moreover, the interior of the large wards represents the general effect of a pavilion plan ward with neat rows of beds, but they were not cross-ventilated (Figure 2.10).

Notwithstanding these, as early as 1903, when the missionaries had just started thinking about architecture, Dr Cecil Lankester expressed his doubt whether 'a hospital at all on Kashmir lines would be suitable in Peshawar, while there has I think been evidence of appreciation of the more "desi" [Indian] style of the present place'.[75] Cecil Lankester neither judged the design of the Kashmir hospital as inadequate nor did he condemn the transfer of ideas regarding hospital design from Britain to British India. Instead, he meant that the pavilion plan was not suitable for Peshawar. This statement demonstrates that issues other than climatic restrictions and site availability were involved. The missionaries were concerned with the feelings of the people, such that the Peshawar hospital retained 'those features of the oriental simplicity which patients find so attractive in the latter [rented caravanserais]'.[76] The buildings of the hospital were not only built on two different slopes but also were arranged in a way to give a 'truly oriental character to the whole'.[77] The desire of the missionaries to attract the patients determined the site's layout, which correlated with the layout of the four-part cross-axial Islamic gardens, a powerful landscape design technique in various parts of the Islamic world, including north-western British India. It consisted of axial, sometimes intersecting, walkway(s) and water canals.[78] While the Peshawar hospital's site did not have water streams for the main axes or pools of various shapes at focal points, it was divided into four sections with a central pathway connecting the large gateway of the hospital to the historic tomb, along which was planted 'an avenue of trees'.[79] In this way, the tomb was visible from the gateway and acted as a central building.

We might compare the style of the Peshawar hospital buildings to that of the Peshawar's All Saints' Memorial Church, constructed in 1882–3. Like this church, the outpatient block was built in Indo-Saracenic style, decorated with details and ornamentations associated with the Mughal era, including rhythms of arches worked in carved wood, minarets at the corners and leaf pattern decorations around the edges (Figure 2.11).[80] Indo-Saracenic had varied applications in British India depending on its practitioners.[81] It was used in All Saints' Memorial Church to make Christianity responsive to converts' needs and thus

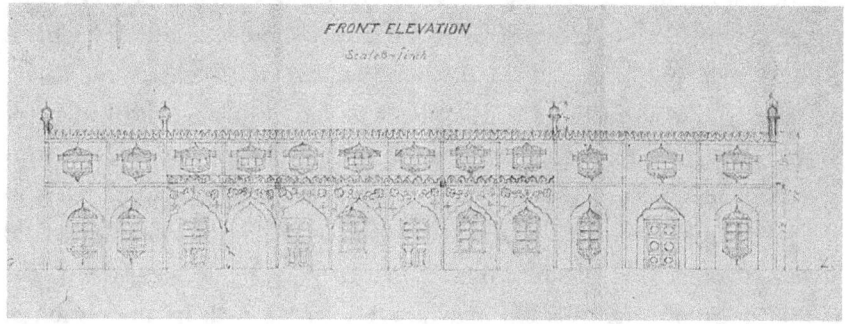

Figure 2.11 The outpatient block, Peshawar hospital.
CMS/M/FL1/I 7, Church Missionary Society Archive, Cadbury Research Library, Special Collections, University of Birmingham.

accessible and relevant,[82] under the influence Henry Venn's mission strategy. Venn, the secretary of the organisation, shifted the focus of the CMS in the 1840s and put in place a mission strategy that advocated the integration of local cultural traditions as the best method of missionary work. Venn's ideas influenced the CMS's stance on building, although more in theory than in practice. Nonetheless, the architecture of All Saints' Memorial Church was not received 'very positively' in missionary circles.[83] Moreover, Venn's ideals, which held sway after his retirement and death,[84] were eventually jettisoned in 1901. From this time on, the CMS envisaged a 'territorial' approach with reduced local independence.[85] Thus, the Peshawar hospital was most likely designed without Venn's principles in mind; Lankester intended to provoke the interest of the people. '[A]s this block of building faces an important thoroughfare, it was necessary to make them as attractive as possible which is being done in a very inexpensive style,' he stated in 1905.[86] He highlighted the minarets writing that 'the towers will be higher than as showing in the plan. They are to be built inexpensively of native materials.'[87] Similar construction details were incorporated into the façade of the inpatient block, although the minarets were omitted.

Whether patients could access the various and contradictory emotional registers of Islamic gardens or ornamentations depended on multiple factors. As patients visited the hospital from various locations (according to the missionaries' reports), their spatial sensibilities, and thus the frameworks through which they could experience and express emotions, had developed via diverse, sometimes overlapping, media – poetry, sounds and scents. Moreover, the hospital might not have been grasped as 'unfamiliar' even if missionaries had opted for the Gothic Revival style. As Preeti Chopra has argued, the Gothic Revival style was 'accepted' in Bombay because 'the ecclesiastical flavor' of this style 'may not have been evident to most Indians who had never visited Oxbridge'. Thus, they would grasp the meaning of this style 'in terms of experiences or concepts familiar or relevant to them'.[88] Chopra refers to the involvement of local builders as a reason as to why the Gothic Revival style was accepted in Bombay, arguing that they were 'intermediaries'.[89] The participation of Miran Bakhsh may have influenced patients' impression of the Peshawar hospital. Still, he could not access the local people's diverse emotional styles. However, these are not the matter because even if patients' records were available, the material environment of the hospital could evoke very different emotions once its interpretation changed over time.[90] The garden, for example, could trigger 'mystical longing' as well as 'more mundane emotions' linked to the economic significance of gardens.[91] At the same time, incorporating the garden into a hospital could disrupt the link between people and gardens and thus no longer evoke certain emotions. What is significant is that the missionaries' strategy was to provide a 'familiar' environment, so much so that the hospital was not merely a variant of hospital buildings in Britain. Besides outpatient and inpatient blocks, the hospital consisted of a structure called the 'James serai', which was designed similarly to a caravanserai where patients could stay with their family and friends. The James serai, the architecture of which shall be explored in the next chapter, was a novel hospital design. If missionaries designed the outpatient and inpatient blocks by copying and adapting metropolitan forms to local structures, they developed the James serai by disregarding these forms.

Persian Courtyard House

As the Peshawar hospital was being built, the Isfahan hospital for men had just been completed. A hospital for women was constructed next to the men's hospital in 1908. The two hospitals were separated by a wall. Dr Donald Carr designed the plan of the men's hospital, and Carr and Dr Emmeline Stuart jointly designed the women's hospital.[92] The involvement of female missionaries in the design and construction process of the hospitals is an important point that has not been considered by historians of gender and mission and will be taken up in Chapter Four. It is not clear who drew the plan of the men's hospital to scale. Mr J. MacIntyre, an engineer of the Indo-European Telegraphs, drew the plan of the women's hospital to scale. According to Carr, MacIntyre had been in the country for 'thirty years' and thus 'thoroughly' understood 'all the details of building'.[93] Due to strategic reasons, related to 'opposition by the Mullahs', Sheikh-ul-Aragin, 'a large landowner and an experienced builder', was initially recruited to oversee the construction of the buildings.[94] The missionaries withdrew this decision accusing the Sheikh of dishonesty.[95] Carr's 'fears that there is a tendency on the part of the Sheikh man not to do the work well and also to increase the charges in various directions' reflect racial prejudice. Meanwhile, the possibility remains that the missionaries had upset their 'bonds of trust' with the Sheikh.[96]

The hospital was designed without reference to the principles of pavilion plan hospitals. The main inpatient block in both the men's and women's sections of the Isfahan hospital was U-shaped (Figure 2.12). It was located in the middle of the site, surrounded by all the other buildings: the outpatient block, private block, storage rooms, cooking and bathrooms. The U-shaped building in the male section opened to the west while the one in the female section opened to the east. The southern and northern wings comprised the wards, and the theatre occupied the connecting wing. Each wing housed several wards, which were not cross-ventilated: each ward contained twelve beds placed along the longer walls, while the windows were located in the shorter walls. There were two windows in each of the shorter walls with a door between the window set. The wards' floor plan is comparable to those

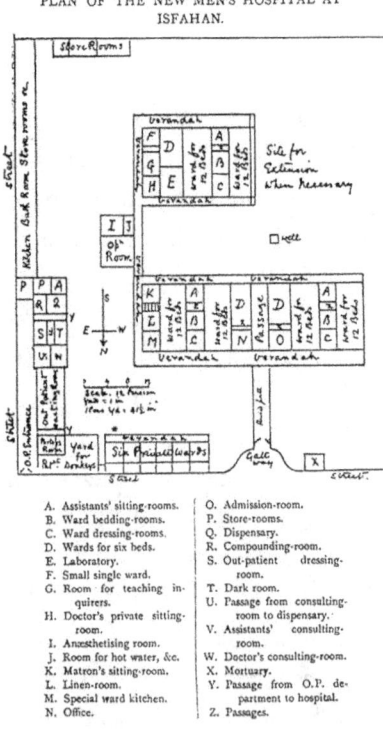

Figure 2.12 Plan of the new men's hospital in Isfahan.
CMS/M/El 2/9, p. 211, Church Missionary Society Archive, Cadbury Research Library, Special Collections, University of Birmingham.

in the Royal Victorian hospital in Belfast (1900–3). But the Royal Victorian hospital was equipped with mechanical ventilation – there were fresh-air ducts that fed air out to the ancillary spaces and the wards.[97] The Isfahan hospital had no mechanical ventilation.

Carr wrote in 1903 that 'I have every reason to believe that a building on the lines of these plans will provide a hospital which will be suited for our work and conditions'.[98] This statement recalls that of Cecil Lankester regarding the Peshawar hospital, signifying there was more at stake than just adaptation to climatic conditions. One of the most noticeable features of the Isfahan hospital is that all the blocks and rooms were accessible directly from the yard. 'There were no covered corridors or halls between several blocks, and you must go into the open air, dry and sunny even in the cold winter, to get from ward to ward,' wrote Dr Catherine Ironside in 1915.[99] During the late nineteenth century, several hospitals in Britain were designed with detached blocks, but in the Isfahan medical mission almost all the rooms were accessible from the outside, even the sanitary facilities. Part of the reason for designing sanitary facilities 'in out-lying parts of hospital compound away from wards' was to achieve efficiency. Carr believed that using a 'water-closet system' was not efficient in the 'East' and doubted 'whether expensive water-closet system when set up would be satisfactory on account of difficulties of choked and leaking drains, etc'. Thus, sanitary facilities were designed in such a way that the 'cesspools' could be 'emptied from the street'.[100] But, the routes from ward to ward and from the wards to the operating room, dispensary and kitchen were also through the yard. Thus, as Miss V. Eardley stated in 1935, 'one lives practically out of doors in hospital'.[101] Eardley was not talking about open-air treatment, as would have been familiar in a tuberculosis hospital in the 1930s. Her focus was on on how all comings and goings took place through the outside.

The Isfahan hospital was not entirely dissimilar to a Persian courtyard house. Firstly, in the Persian courtyard houses, all the rooms were accessible from the outside.[102] Moreover, as far as materials and structure were concerned, the buildings depended predominantly on the regional architecture of Isfahan. For instance, the wooden columns and carved flat wooden ceilings of the hospital's verandas (Figure 2.13) copied similar timber structures used in the area since the seventeenth century. They were not only a feature

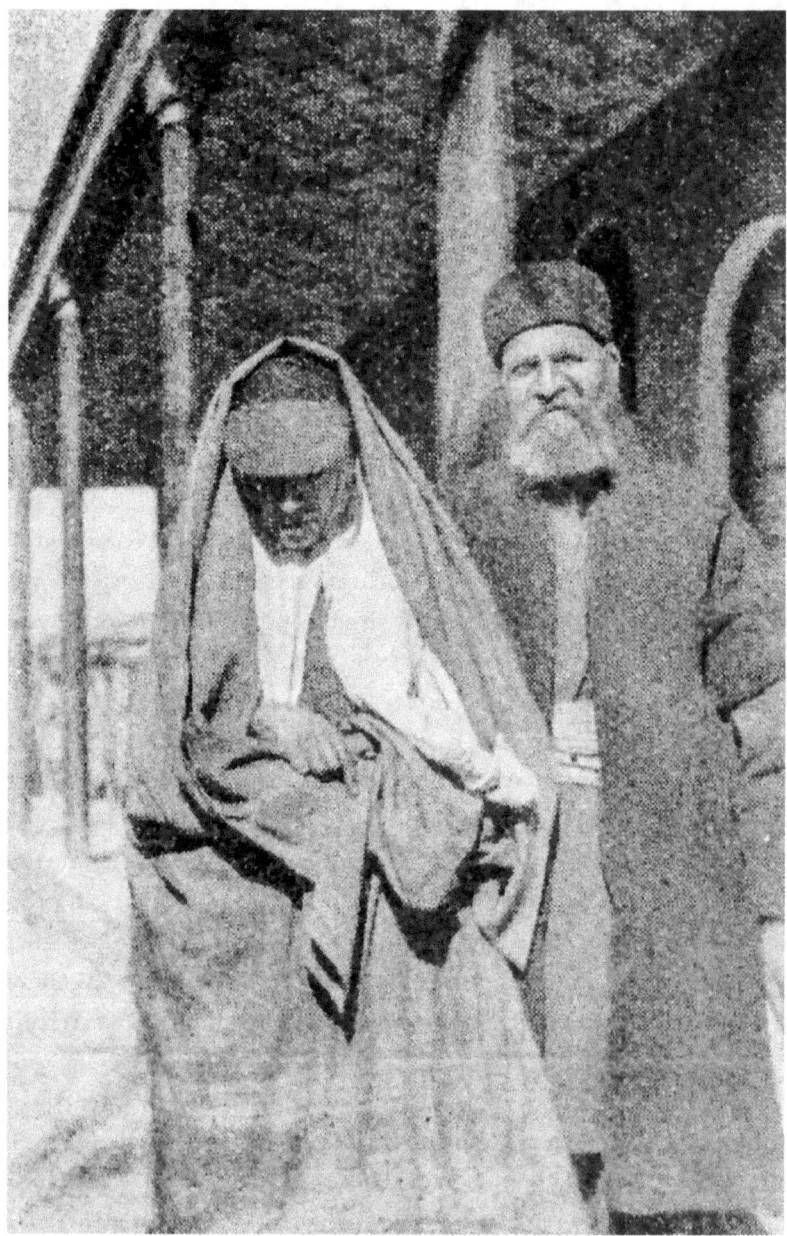

Figure 2.13 Old villager and his daughter, Isfahan hospital. The carved flat wooden ceiling of the veranda is visible.
CMS/M/EL 2/35, p. 62, Church Missionary Society Archive, Cadbury Research Library, Special Collections, University of Birmingham.

DEVELOPMENT OF NOVEL HOSPITAL DESIGNS | 89

of some of the most important buildings of the city (as they still are) but were also commonly used in the construction of houses, both in Isfahan and in the surrounding villages, such as Abyāne.[103] Another, more implicit, indication of the attention paid to the habits of the patients in their daily lives outside the hospital is the similarity between two photographs of women's wards. The first is of a ward in Julfā women's hospital, where the hospital was converted from a house (Figure 2.14), and the second is of the new purpose-built hospital in Isfahan (Figure 2.15). The second echoes the first in the rectangular shape, the arrangement of the beds and the window openings. Familiarity seems to have been more important than an 'up-to-date' hospital design. Rather than being merely a place of healing, the hospital had to be an attractive place to spend time.

A further aspect of the supposedly welcoming nature of the hospitals was that the missionaries permitted the patients to 'play gramophones' or have 'tea parties' in the wards. These mainly happened in private wards for

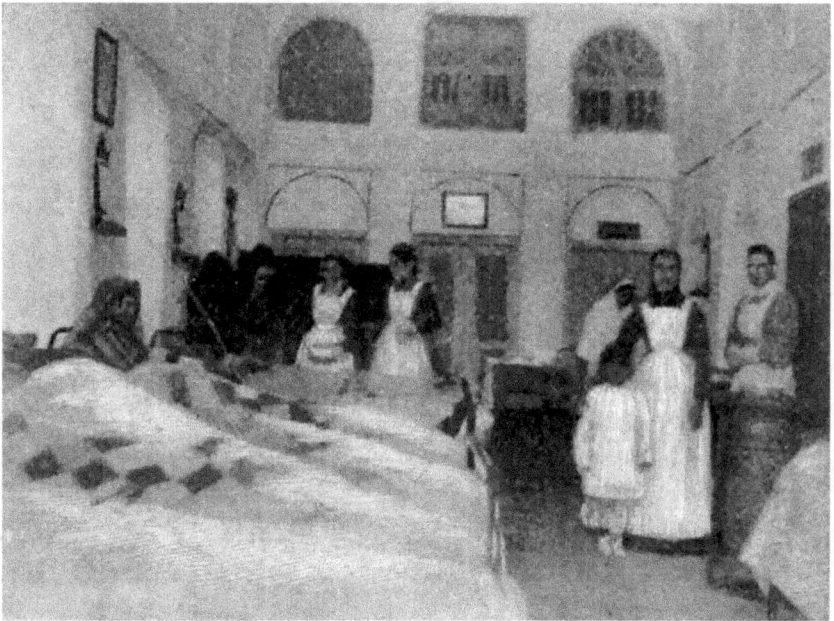

Figure 2.14 A ward in rented buildings, Isfahan women's hospital.
CMS/M/EL 2/3, p. 138, Church Missionary Society Archive, Cadbury Research Library, Special Collections, University of Birmingham.

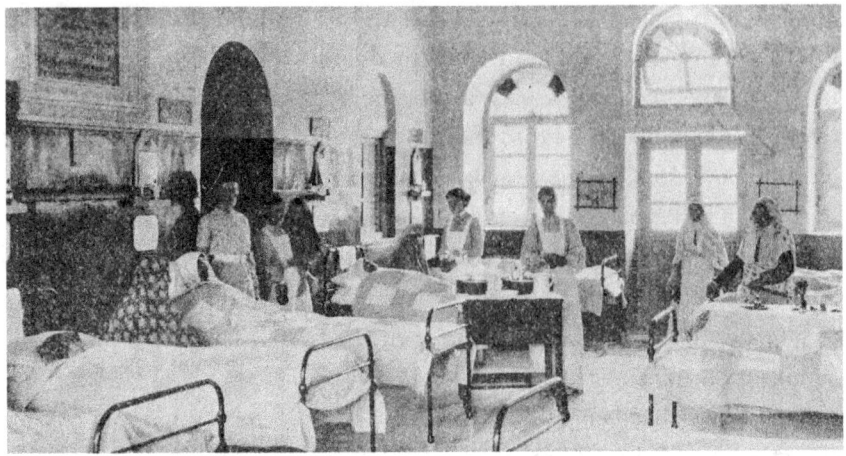

Figure 2.15 A ward in Isfahan new hospital.
CMS/M/EL 2/11, p. 312, Church Missionary Society Archive, Cadbury Research Library, Special Collections, University of Birmingham.

paying patients. We should distinguish between the sound of gramophone and noises produced by staff. While hospitals in Britain, in general, were intended to be calm and quiet zones, staff often interrupted the patients with prayers or readings of rules and regulations. Such noises were considered as 'productive' noises, and it was patients who were discouraged from noise-producing activities such as talking to one another.[104] The missionaries also prayed at patients' bedsides or preached the Gospel, sometimes every day, and even sang hymns in the wards. However, the sound of the gramophones was a noise that patients produced. The private blocks were located some distance from the general wards, and probably the sound of gramophone could not have been heard in all parts of the hospital. Still, it is significant that the missionaries allowed the patients to play gramophone as it meant the respective patients could listen to a preferable noise.

Allowing patients to have tea parties meant creating a familiar smell and taste in the hospitals. Tea was introduced to Persia sometime in the sixteenth century and became the country's 'national beverage' by the twentieth century. It was a popular beverage (and still is) throughout the country, among urbanites and country dwellers alike, and among people of different socio-economical and religious backgrounds.[105] Private patients could also bring their bedding and necessities to the hospital. Patients liked to bring 'carpets [. . .], cushions, curtains, cooking utensils, trays, firewood, and charcoal', transforming the plain, small space 'into a cosy living room', stated Miss Eardley.[106] Eardley' use of the word 'living room' clearly alludes to the missionaries' aim: they hoped to provide an environment that felt – appeared, smelled and tasted – familiar. To my knowledge, no photographs were published of private blocks. This lack of visual evidence makes it difficult to understand how the patients transformed the private wards. It may point to the 'semi-secret' status of these wards. The missionaries were reluctant to photograph these wards, which might be taken as evidence of their 'disordered' state. While the missionaries were happy to settle with it in return for local people's friendship, the general public at home would not have, and since they wished to raise money, the status of these wards had to remain 'semi-secret'.[107]

The missionaries repeated the layout of the Isfahan hospital's inpatient section in the Yazd hospital where Mr MacIntyre was again employed as the 'invaluable architect' (Figure 2.16).[108] Dr Henry White prepared the site plan of the hospital, and the plan of the hospital was drawn jointly by MacIntyre and White.[109] MacIntyre also oversaw the construction of the hospital, which was completed in 1907. Like in Isfahan, the inpatient section consisted of a U-shaped building that opened to the north (Figure 2.17). The two wings of

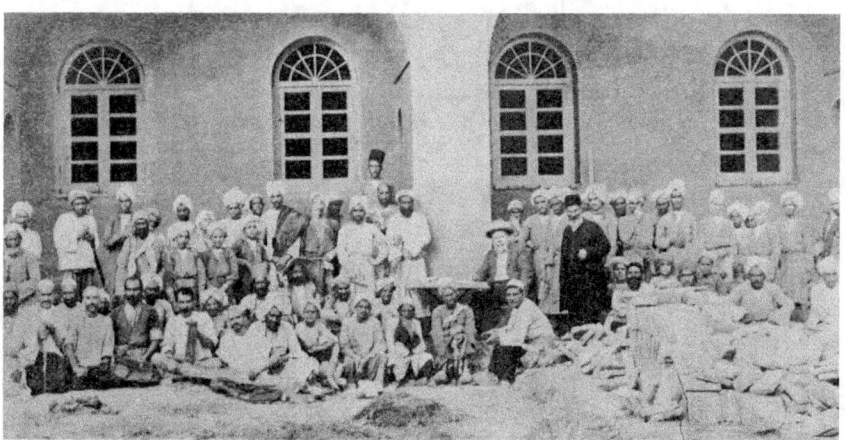

Figure 2.16 The new outpatient department with workmen at Yazd.
CMS/M/EL 2/12, p. 41, Church Missionary Society Archive, Cadbury Research Library, Special Collections, University of Birmingham.

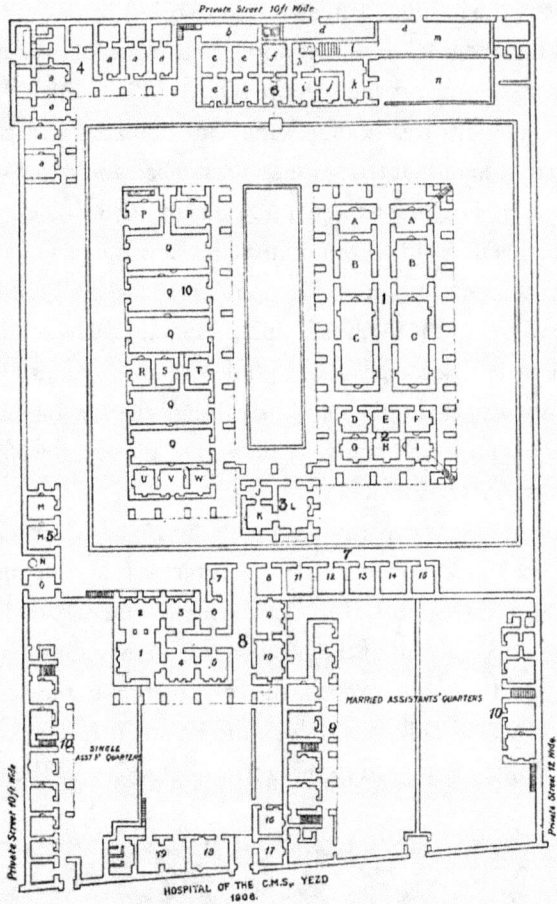

Plan of the Men's Hospital, Yezd.

1. Block of wards for forty-eight pat ents.
2. Dressing-room, assistants' day and night rooms, matron's room, room for women's work (relatives and friends of patients).
3. Operating-theatre, sterilising room, and anæsthetic room.
4. Eight wards fo well-to-do private patients.
5. Isolation wards.
6. Kitchen, well, and storerooms, wash-house, and drying yard.
7. Stores.
8. Out-patient block: Waiting-rooms, doctors' and assistants' consulting-rooms, dressing-room, out-patients' theatre, dispensary, and drug stores, porter's lodge, and receiving-room.
9. Assistants' quarters.
10, 10, 10. Proposed new block and assistants' quarters.

Figure 2.17 Plan of the new hospital at Yazd.
CMS/M/EL 2/12, p. 359, Church Missionary Society Archive, Cadbury Research Library, Special Collections, University of Birmingham.

the U-shaped building contained the wards, accommodating a total of ninety-six patients, and the bottom wing housed the operating theatre. The paths going from wards to the operating theatre, kitchen and bathrooms were by way of the garden: the U-shaped building was located in the middle and was surrounded on the north side by rooms for a kitchen, storeroom, washroom and private wards and on the west side by isolation wards. Both wings were initially planned similar to the ones in the Isfahan hospital, but the design of the eastern wing was modified during the construction for unknown reasons. It consisted of six wards arranged on each side of a central corridor – there was one ward for twelve beds, one for eight beds, and another one for four beds on each side.

In contrast to Isfahan, the rooms at the Yazd hospital were vaulted using a method of arching, which MacIntyre described as 'the method of arching in Persia'.[110] When the missionaries forwarded the plan and details of the new hospital to the CMS Home Office for approval, Mr J. W. Rundall, one of the members of the CMS Committee, criticised the proposed 'constructive details'[111] (Figure 2.18). White went through Rundall's criticism with MacIntyre and, in response, voiced his disagreement with Rundall's opinion: '[i]t is obvious that to those acquainted with buildings in other countries, the Persian method must sound very unsatisfactory. The specification by Mr MacIntyre is in accordance with what is universally adopted in Central Persia.' The Persia Medical sub-conference backed up White's response and called for no alteration.[112] The missionaries in Mosul also proposed a plan like the Isfahan hospital, which was never built. It is interesting that here, again, a different construction method was used, and the façade of the proposed hospital was designed completely different from the façade of the Isfahan hospital (Figure 2.19). It is telling that the missionaries used different construction techniques in all these cities, for these areas shared several construction methods. Thus, developing a model hospital to be utilised whenever required was possible and financially more sound. But using a local construction method was more important to them. The Kerman medical mission, the last hospital built in the period under consideration in this study, was designed entirely differently from both the Isfahan and Yazd medical missions. The missionaries also used a local construction technique specific to Kerman.

94 | EMOTION, MISSION, ARCHITECTURE

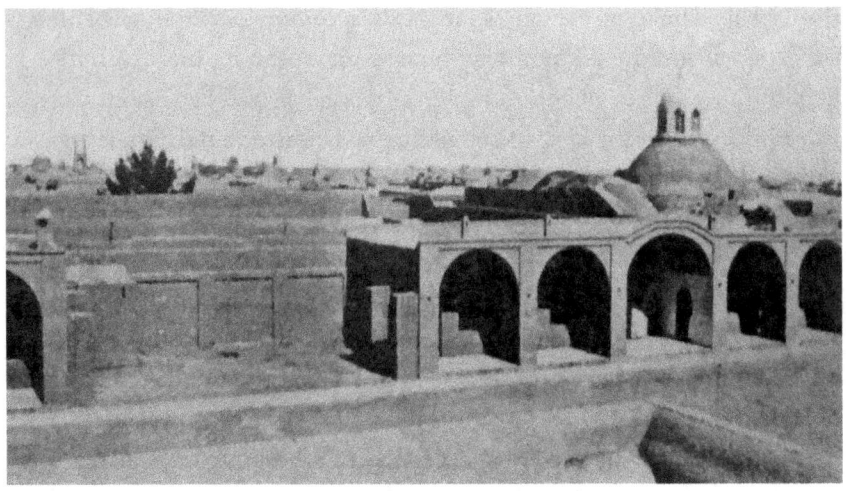

Figure 2.18 Men's hospital in Yazd.
CMS/M/EL 2/37, p. 318, Church Missionary Society Archive, Cadbury Research Library, Special Collections, University of Birmingham.

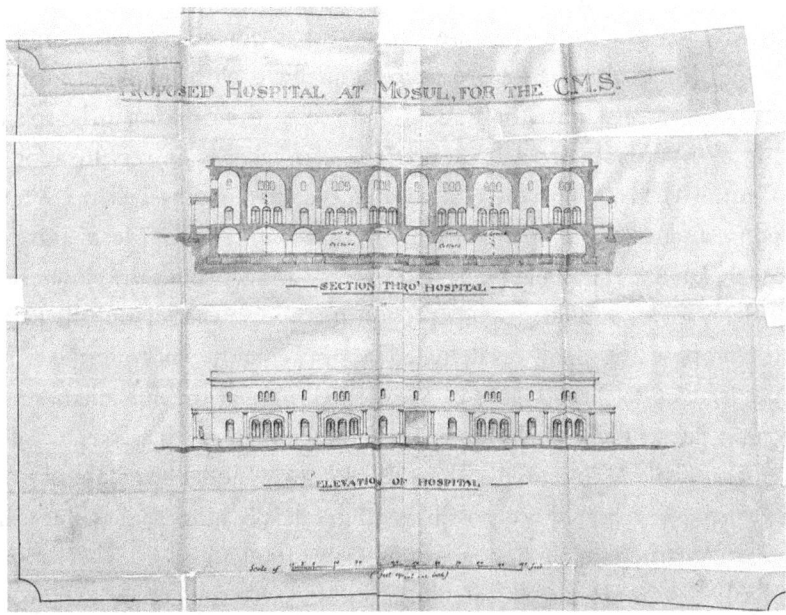

Figure 2.19 Section and elevation of the proposed hospital at Mosul.
CMS/M/FL 1/TA 1, no. 2, Church Missionary Society Archive, Cadbury Research Library, Special Collections, University of Birmingham.

The Kermanī Arch

Dr George Dodson and Dr Winifred Westlake designed the Kerman hospital buildings. They were constructed between 1914 and 1928. After sketching out the plan of the hospital, Dodson brought their ideas back to Britain, and he possibly received some professional help in developing them into a design for a building, although this is not certain.[113]

As in Isfahan, the CMS hospital in Kerman had separate sections for men and women designed side by side. Between the men's and women's sections of the hospital ran a straight narrow blind alley. This narrow blind alley can be taken as the first indication that the hospital's layout was to act as reminiscent of the local people's daily lives (Figure 2.20). The hospital was located outside the north-east walls of the city, on the Seyyedī road. The narrow alley branched off the Seyyedī road and domed at an interval. The gates to the inpatient section in both the men's and women's hospitals were in this domed

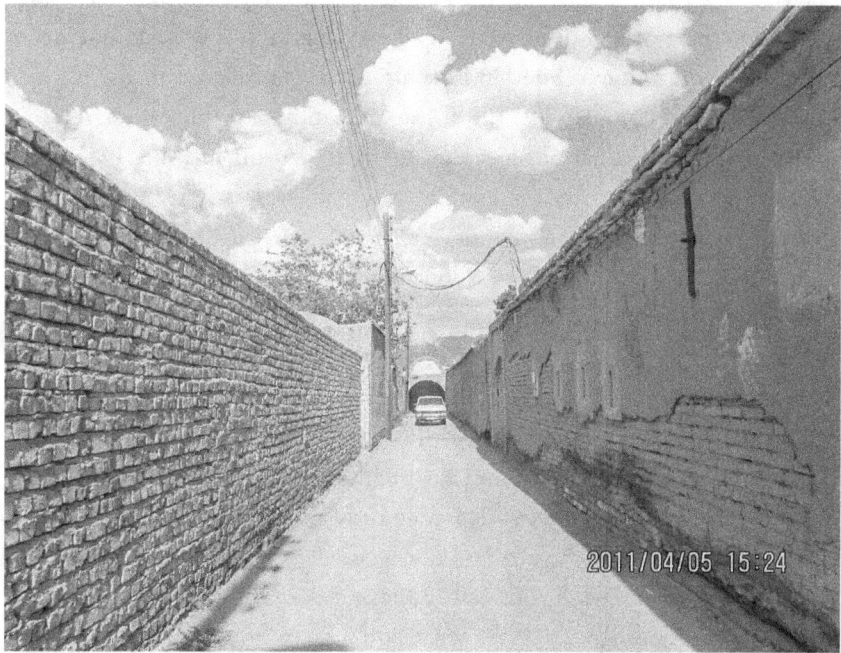

Figure 2.20 The narrow blind alley run between the men's and women's hospitals at Kerman.
Photo by author.

area and thus, to reach the inpatient sections, people had to turn from the Seyyedī road into the alley. This narrow blind alley resembled the blind alleys leading to the entrance of houses in traditional cities in Persia, including Kerman. According to Masoud Kheirabadi, blind alleys (known as *bunbasts* in Farsi) formed 'the most common lanes seen in plans of traditional Iranian cities'.[114] The Kerman hospital was built before the 1920s–30s, when drastic changes had not yet reshaped the appearance of the city.[115] The form of the city had remained relatively the same since the Safavid period.[116] Although every patient and even urban dwellers of Kerman individually might have felt differently,[117] having been part of the daily lives of many patients, blind alleys could allow specific experiences and evoke certain emotions.[118] The missionaries, most likely, hoped to transfer emotions associated with blind alleys into the context of medical mission.

While it was built when pavilion plan was on the decline, the Kerman hospital was modelled after pavilion plan institutions. It consisted of long, one-storey pavilions that stood apart amid a garden (Figure 2.21). Each pavilion hosted one ward, and the space between the pavilions was enough for the free circulation of air. While Dodson himself never referred to the Kerman hospital as a pavilion plan institution, an indication of pavilion design can be found in his sister's description of the buildings. Writing in 1933, Dr Eleanor Dodson declared that 'the [men's and women's] hospitals are on the block system';[119] the block system was another name for the pavilion plan.[120] In particular, the plan of the men's section can be compared to the Royal Herbert Hospital, Woolwich. Like the Herbert hospital, each pavilion was reached through a spine corridor. Additionally, the floor plan of the ward blocks is comparable to the floor plan of the large ward in the Dera Ismail Khan hospital (Figure 2.22). Eleanor worked in north-western British India and her brother might have learned about the architecture of the Dera Ismail Khan hospital through her and have adapted it for Kerman. As was the case in Dera Ismail Khan, cross-ventilation was not secured in Kerman: the wards were dark; they were designed with four opposing doors (two in the north wall and two in the south) with a veranda shading them from both the north and south sides. There are no windows, and there is no evidence of a mechanical ventilation system. As I will explain below, this was not purely, or possibly at all, a response to the heat outside.

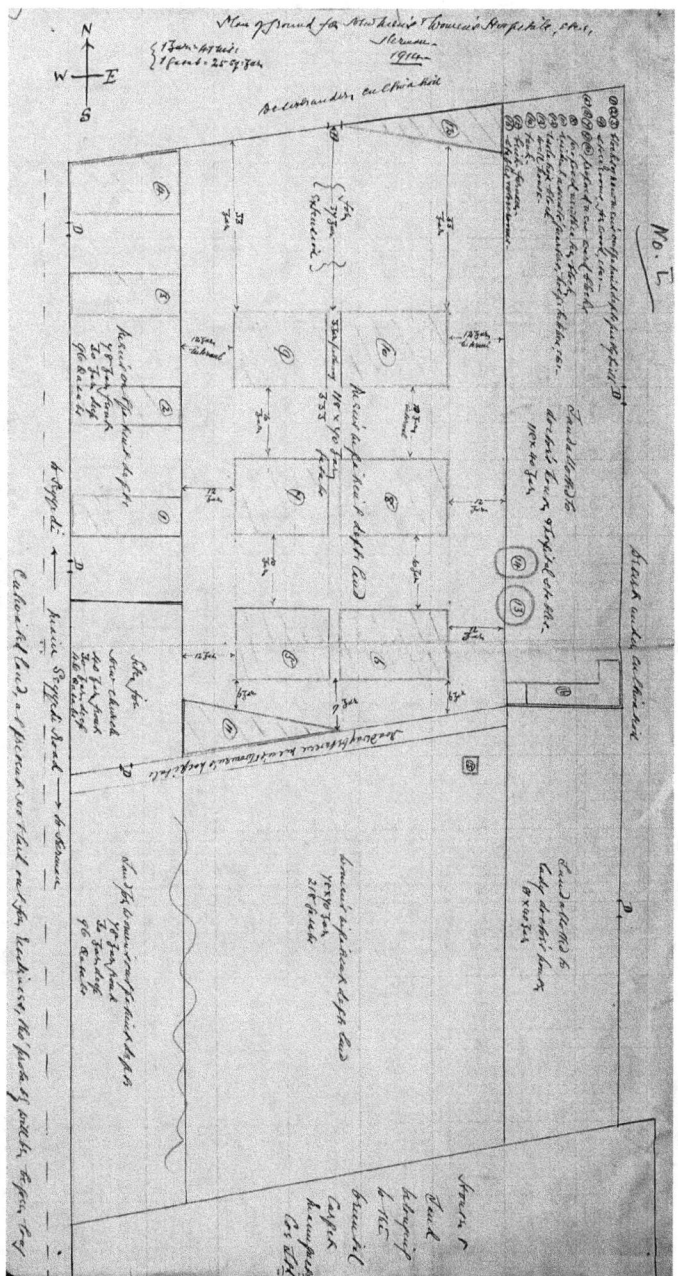

Figure 2.21 Sketch plan of the men's hospital in Kerman.
CMS/M/FL 1/PE 2 [no.9], Church Missionary Society Archive, Cadbury Research Library, Special Collections, University of Birmingham.

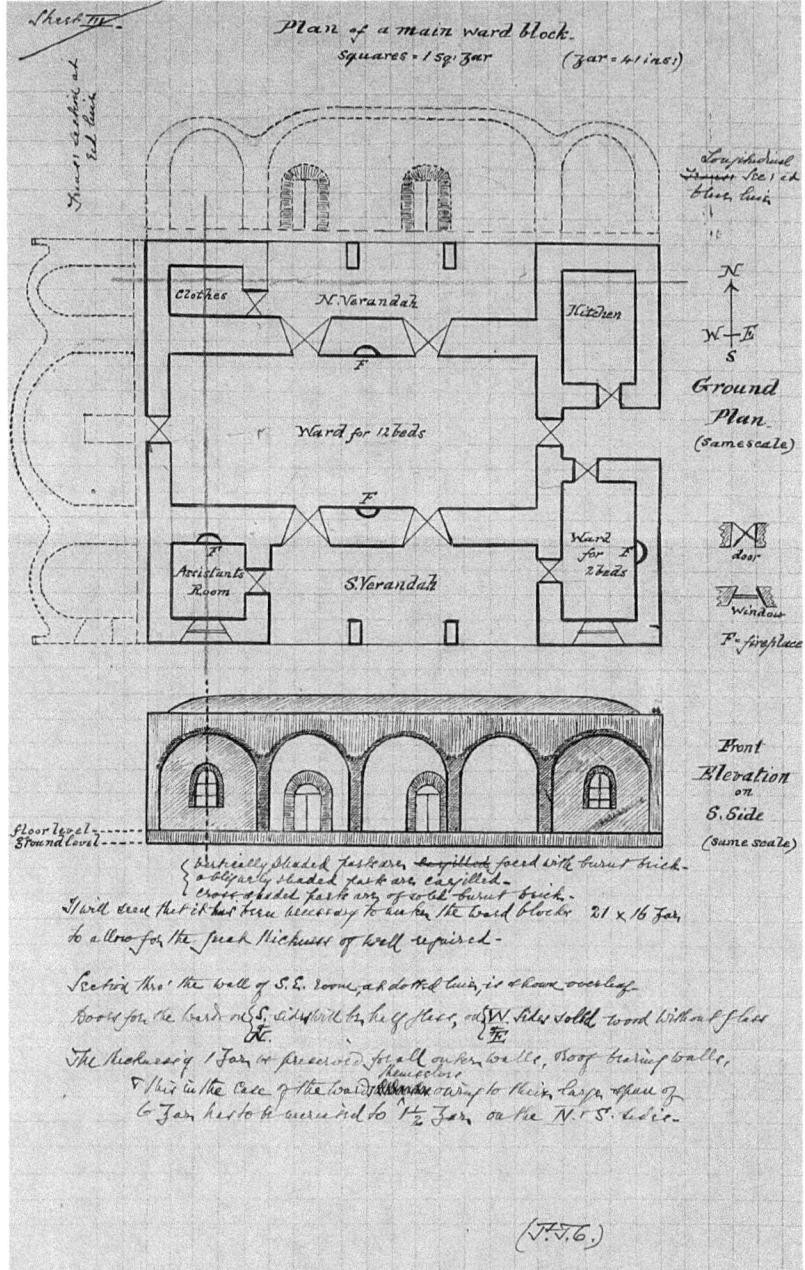

Figure 2.22 Floor plan of one of the wards in Kerman hospital.
CMS/M/FL 1/PE 2 [no. 4], Church Missionary Society Archive, Cadbury Research Library, Special Collections, University of Birmingham.

As one of Dodson's letters indicates, the primary building material was brick produced on the site. As the foundations were dug, the soil was taken and mixed with lime and straw to make mud and mould bricks. Some of the bricks were laid out to bake in the sun, while others were fired in kilns for the covering of walls and columns.[121] Moreover, the ceilings mainly were vaulted using a round vault known as the Kermanī (Figure 2.23), local to the region, and found primarily in domestic buildings. This may represent the missionaries' effort to use a locally sourced construction technique and incorporate one that was related closely to the people's daily lives. Like other types of vaults in Persia (namely the knife-shaped and the Roman), the Kermanī vault is constructed using square bricks; the bricks measure approximately 25 x 25 x 5 cm. Except in the ribs, which strengthen the vault approximately every 50 cm, the bricks are laid with the largest face forming the internal surface of the vault; they are only connected along their side, that is, along the depth of the brick. It is not a method of vaulting suitable for large spans. As mentioned above,

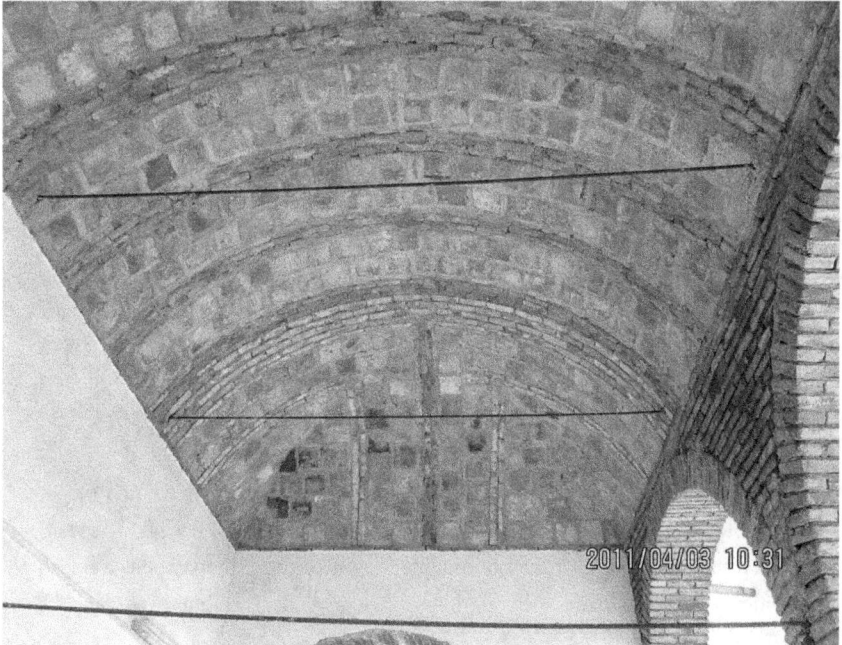

Figure 2.23 The men's hospital in Kerman. Note the Kermanī arch. Photo by author.

the Kermanī vault is mainly found in houses. The largest room in a courtyard house in Kerman was usually approximately 10.5 m wide, while the general wards in the Kerman hospital are 15.6 m wide, that is, almost twice as wide as the standard domestic room.[122] The vault at the Kerman hospital spans this distance while being carried on the longer walls – the walls in which the doors are placed. I would suggest that this is partly why the wards have so few doors and window openings – it makes the arching roof more stable. Combined, these show that using the Kermanī arch was very important, to the extent that the missionaries sacrificed much of the principle of cross-ventilation.

The archives of the CMS contain a children's game that incorporates the fictional story of thirteen-year-old Mariam, a patient in the Kerman hospital (Figure 2.24). Written by missionaries sometime after 1935, the story begins with a description of Mariam's home and her condition:

> 'Zahra, come here! I'm going to hospital', [. . .]. The speaker was thirteen-year-old Mariam, a little crippled carpet weaver in a hill village in Iran. [. . .]. Her home was a one-roomed mud hut beside which was a smaller, lower room, dark and damp. Here, damp, bad air, hard work and poor food had made Mariam a cripple. [. . .] Mariam was at last going to the Christian hospital in Kerman to have her crooked knees and arms straightened. [. . .].

The importance that the missionaries gave to the hospital's architecture as a means for gaining trust becomes apparent in the description of Mariam's arrival there:

> Next morning, as the donkey on which Mariam was seated reached the other side of the town, Mariam could see low buildings with humped roofs and surrounded by a high wall, standing at the edge of the desert. [. . .] Bright green trees showed above the walls and, behind the hospital, the dog-tooth hills showed clear-cut against the brilliant blue sky. [. . .] It all seemed bright and welcoming to Mariam. [. . .] Inside the ward it was bare enough. The walls were brick, and though many doors opened on to the veranda there were no windows. It was cool and rather dark – a refuge from the burning sun outside.[123]

On the surface, Mariam's story underlines the colonising approach of the missionaries to the built environment.[124] It makes a comparison between her

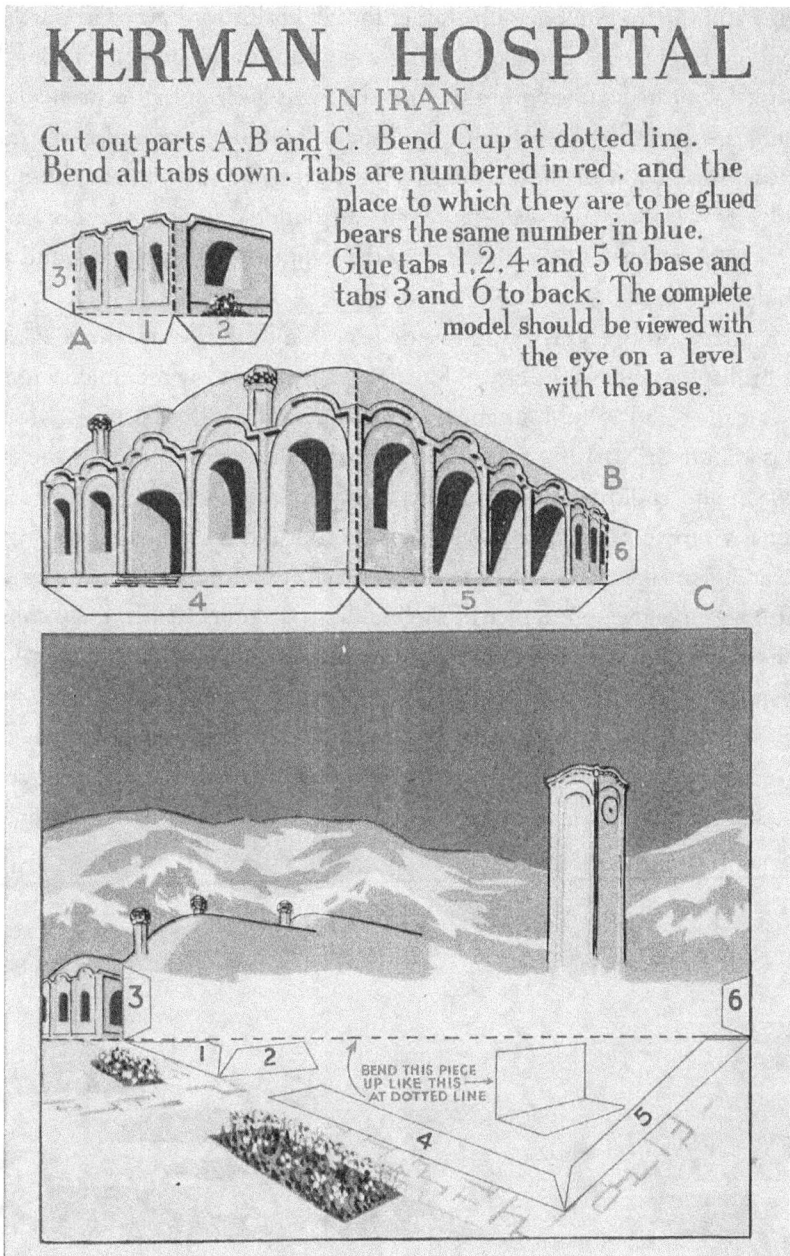

Figure 2.24 Kerman hospital game.
CMS/H/H5/E2, Church Missionary Society Archive, Cadbury Research Library, Special Collections, University of Birmingham.

home and the hospital, demonstrating that ill health was caused as much as anything by the dark and damp living conditions of the home, whereas the hospital appeared to bring health. But the word 'welcoming' is particularly significant, as it directly refers to the issue of building trust and friendship. Its use, together with the particular reference in the story to the 'humped roofs' visible above the wall, represents an outlook among the missionaries, which drew a connection between the familiarity of the setting and the building of trust.

Mariam's story also refers to 'the dog-tooth hills showed clear-cut against the brilliant blue sky'. The city of Kerman is surrounded by mountains; to the east are the Kūh Payeh Mountains, and on the north are the Darmānū Mountains (Figure 2.25). These peaks formed the broader landscape of the medical mission and could provoke unanticipated reactions. Although patients' (as well as visitors') experience was defined by conditions other than just sight, including smell, touch and taste, it is crucial to consider that patients did not merely see the appearance of the buildings. In other words, these conditions should not disqualify the importance of sight, but rather, discussions regarding sight should go beyond a mere focus on the visual appearance or the 'doctor's gaze' to consider the wider landscape. The missionaries may not have read much out of the mountains than they were an essential source of water.[125] At the very least, however, the Kūh Payeh and Darmānū mountains

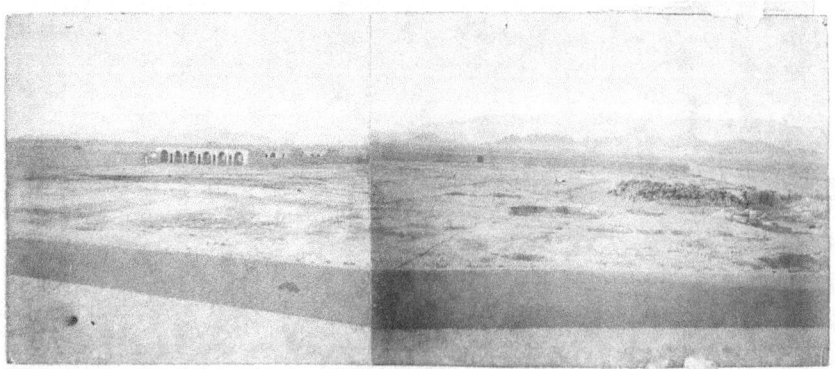

Figure 2.25 Kerman hospital site. Note the mountains.
CMS/M/FL 2/ PE 2 [photo 3], Church Missionary Society Archive, Cadbury Research Library, Special Collections, University of Birmingham.

may have helped the patients to find their way to the hospital. It is also possible that the name of the hospital and the mountains became interchangeable. At Isfahan, the dome of Soltānī theological and clerical school was visible from the hospital (see Figure 2.1). It could distract the patients' gaze from the church built between the hospitals. Some patients might have employed gazing at this dome as a coping strategy in their encounter with the church.

Like Isfahan, the patients were permitted to make and drink tea and even smoke in the hospital. It remained relevant in the 1910s to compromise on the idea of 'absolute cleanliness'. Its importance to obtaining the trust of the people was made explicit in a 1912 article entitled 'Principles and Practice of Medical Missions'. The unknown author of this article emphasised that adapting local conditions had a particular application for the work of a medical mission:

> There are many points to be considered in the planning of a hospital, for local conditions have to be taken into account, and it is not possible always to reproduce in the Mission field exactly the same conditions to which we are accustomed in a hospital at home. This is true in all branches of missionary work to some extent, . . . but it is still more true in the working of a hospital.[126]

The author then went on to single out one case: 'it may be necessary at the outset to conform to the ways of each country so far as this is consistent with hygienic rules, and even these must not always be pressed too rigidly.'[127] Integration of local architectural elements and techniques without confining to contemporary hospital design principles distinguishes the medical missionaries' approach to architecture.

Conclusion

What is clear, then, is that missionaries employed a wide range of construction methods in north-western British India and Persia and different types of hospital plans and ward designs. The missionaries neither used nor suggested or developed a standard design for hospitals. Meanwhile, most of the hospitals were adapted to local conditions. Among a variety of factors that influenced the architecture of the hospitals – local climate, availability of materials or condition of the sites – the needs and requirements of the patients was one of the main factors. As I have explained, the missionaries accommodated the needs and requirements of the people to earn their trust.

The missionaries adapted local architectural traditions in a different way than their counterparts. They used local elements that permeated people's daily lives without enforcing contemporary hospital design principles in the West. By the second half of the nineteenth century, hospital architecture had been revolutionised in Britain; the pavilion plan hospital had become the basic design in response to concerns with bad air or miasma. The pavilion plan remained popular throughout the early twentieth century, with various examples being built across Europe and in North America, Asia and Africa. While the Kashmir medical mission, the first medical mission of the CMS, adhered to pavilion plan hospital guidelines, it was not widely utilised thereafter. Instead, the missionaries drew on what was familiar to the patients regarding buildings' layout and appearance and construction methods, considering matters such as ventilation and cleanliness less critical than familiarity.

The case of Peshawar showed that even the individual buildings of a medical mission were sometimes designed differently to accommodate the needs of various local communities. The importance of adapting local conditions was as relevant in the 1910s when the Kerman hospital was built. The point that I wish to emphasise in drawing this analysis to a conclusion is that gaining trust required toleration and an ability to accommodate the needs and requirements of locals, rather than forcing ideas upon them. I argue that when considering the issue of gaining trust, a case should be made for finding alternative terms of reference to those typically used in studying missionary medicine. The missionaries referred to the medical missions as attractive agencies. This phrase captures the aim of medical missions very directly.

Notes

1. Catherine Ironside, 'In the Women's Hospital, Ispahan', *Mercy and Truth* 19, no. 228 (1915): 390. For a discussion on how 'the idea of "England" was taken for granted as signifying Britain', see G. A. Bremner, 'The expansion of England? Rethinking Scotland's place in the architectural history of the wider British world', *Journal of Art Historiography*, no. 18 (2018), DOI: https://arthistoriography.files.wordpress.com/2018/05/bremner.pdf
2. 'The Foreign Field', *Mercy and Truth* 23, no. 264 (1919): 226.

3. F. M. Clarke, 'In a Frontier Hospital', *The Mission Hospital* 26, no. 291 (1922): 59.
4. Quoted in Yaron Perry, 'Anglo-Judeo Confrontation: Jewish Antagonism towards the English Medical Mission in Nineteenth-Century Palestine', in Barbara Haider-Wilson and Dominique Trimbur (eds), *Europe and Palestine 1799–1948: Religion – Politics – Society* (Wien: Austrian Academy of Science Press, 2010), 311.
5. Jeremy Taylor, *The Architect and the Pavilion Hospital: Dialogue and Design Creativity in England 1890–1914* (London and New York: Leicester University Press, 1997).
6. Jeremy Taylor, *Hospital and Asylum Architecture in England 1840–1914: Building for Health Care* (London and New York: Mansell Publishing Limited, 1991); see also Hilary Marland, 'The Changing role of the hospital, 1800–1900', in Deborah Brunton (ed.), *Medicine Transformed: Health, Disease, and Society in Europe, 1800–1930* (Manchester: Manchester University Press, 2004), 31–60.
7. Cor Wagenaar, 'Five Revolutions: A Short History of Hospital Architecture', in Cor Wagenaar (ed.), *The Architecture of Hospitals* (Rotterdam: NAi Publishers, 2006), 26.
8. Harriet Richardson (ed.), *English Hospitals, 1660–1948: A Survey of their Architecture and Design* (London: Royal Commission of the Historical Monuments of England, 1998), 8.
9. Jiat-Hwee Chang, 'Tropicalising Technologies of Environment and Government: The Singapore General Hospital and the Circulation of Pavilion Plan Hospitals in the British Empire, 1860–1930', in Michael Guggenheim and Ola Söderström (eds), *Reshaping Cities: How Global Mobility Transforms Architecture and Urban Form* (London and New York: Routledge, 2010), 123–42.
10. Annmarie Adams, *Medicine by Design: The Architect and the Modern Hospital, 1893–1943* (Minneapolis and London: University of Minnesota Press, 2008), 27.
11. Jeanne Kisacky, 'Germs are in the details: Aseptic Design and General Constructors at the Lying-In Hospital of the City of New York, 1897–1901', *Construction History* 28, no. 1 (2013): 83–7.
12. Ken Worpole, *Here Comes the Sun: Architecture and Public Space in Twentieth-century European Culture* (London: Reaktion Books, 2000), 49.
13. Jeanne Kisacky, *Rise of the Modern Hospital: An Architectural History of Health and Healing, 1870–1940* (Pittsburgh: University of Pittsburgh Press, 2017), 243.
14. Taylor, *Hospital and Asylum Architecture*; Kisacky, *Rise of the Modern Hospital*, 23–4.

15. Florence Nightingale, *Notes on Hospitals*, 3rd ed. (London: Longman, 1865), 150–5.
16. Kisacky, *Rise of the Modern Hospital*, 23.
17. The Takhtsingji Hospital was built to the design of Mr W. Emerson. See Frederic J. Mouat and H. Saxon Snell, *Hospital Construction and Management* (London: J. & A. Churchill, 1883), 270–3; the Tehran Hospital was built in 1890–1 to the design of Mr Ernest Turner. See Henry C. Burdett, *Hospitals and Asylums of the World: their Origin, History, Construction, Management, and Legislation*, vol IV, Hospital Construction, with Plans and Bibliography (London: J. & A. Churchill, 1891), 122; and the European Hospital in Bombay was designed by Mr T. Roger Smith, see F. Oppert, *Hospitals, Infirmaries, and Dispensaries: Their Construction, Interior, and Management* (London: J. & A. Churchill, 1883), 179–81.
18. Taylor, *Hospital and Asylum*; Chang, 'Tropicalising Technologies of Environment and Government',123–42.
19. The *Hospitals and Asylums of the World* also included state-aided hospitals and hospitals built by local philanthropists. *Hospital, Infirmaries, and Dispensaries* refers to a Missionary Hospital in Canton but without describing the architecture of the building: Oppert, *Hospitals, Infirmaries, and Dispensaries*, 181.
20. Simon De Nys-Ketels has recently examined the Clinique Reine Elisabeth of Coquihatville in the Belgian Congo. Nevertheless, his focus is also on state hospitals. Hospitals that were built by missionaries in the Belgian Congo need to be considered too if we want to acquire a better picture. See Simon De Nys-Ketels, 'A hospital typology translated: Transnational flows of architectural expertise in the Clinique Reine Elisabeth of Conquilhatville, in the Belgian Congo', *ABE Journal* 19 (2012), URL: http://journals.openedition.org/abe/12715
21. Michael Jennings, 'Healing of Bodies, Salvation of Souls: Missionary Medicine in Colonial Tanganyika, 1870s–1939', *Journal of Religion in Africa* 38, no. 1 (2008): 28; Megan Vaughan states that '[t]hroughout most of the colonial period and throughout most of Africa, Christian missions of one sort or another provided vastly more medical care for African communities than colonial state'. Megan Vaughan, *Curing Their Ills: Colonial Power and African Illness* (Stanford: Stanford University Press, 1991), 56. It was estimated in 1947 that there were 300 mission hospitals in China and 256 hospitals and 250 branch dispensaries in India. See David Hardiman, 'The Mission Hospital, 1880–1960', in Mark Harrison, Margaret Jones and Helen Sweet (eds), *From Western Medicine to Global Medicine: the hospital beyond the West* (Hyderabad: Orient BlackSwan, 2009), 198.

22. T. Maxwell, 'The Opening of the Door in Kashmir, 1873–1876, Part II', *Mercy and Truth* 1, no. 9 (1897): 199–200.
23. A. Neve, 'Medical Mission Auxiliary Annual Meeting, May 5, 1898', *Mercy and Truth* 2, no. 10 (1898): 134.
24. 'The Mission-Field', *The Church Missionary Intelligencer*, no. 22 (1897): 843.
25. A. Neve, 'The Opening of the Door in Kashmir, 1882–1897', *Mercy and Truth* 1, no. 12 (1897): 274.
26. H. E. Rawlence, 'Work in a Kashmir Hospital', *The Church Missionary Gleaner* 36, no. 426 (1909): 88.
27. There were exceptions. For example, plan of the Nablus hospital was drawn up by a 'qualified architect'. 'Palestine Precis Book: 22 Nov 1892-8 Sep 1902', CMS/B/OMS/G 3 P P4, no. 402–29, CRL.
28. Sir Douglas Galton, *Healthy Hospitals: Observations on Some Points Connected with Hospital Construction* (Oxford: Clarendon Press, 1893).
29. Some mission stations were isolated and hence missionaries had little contact with the outside world. For example, Rev. C. H. Stilman wrote in 1904 that 'it is impossible to send from Kerman such plans and estimates for hospital buildings as it is customary to receive in India.' See C. H. Stileman, 7 June 1904, CMS/M/C 2/ 1 4, no. 54, CRL; Emile Turner has highlighted this point in her article on the CMS Church Building Abroad. See Emily Turner, 'The Church Missionary Society and Architecture in the Mission Field: Evangelical Anglican Perspectives on Church Building Abroad. C. 1850–1900', *Architectural History* 58 (2015): 202; For a discussion concerning connection and isolation in global history, see Ronald Wenzlhuemer, *Doing Global History: An Introduction in 6 Concepts* (London and New York: Bloomsbury Academic, 2020), 54–64.
30. For example, Dr W. B. Heywood and P. S. Sturrock finished their medical education at the London hospital. See 'Medical Reinforcements, 1897', *Mercy and Truth* 1, no. 10 (1897): 228–30.
31. Ernest F. Neve, *A Crusader in Kashmir: Being the Life of Dr Arthur Neve, with an Account of the Medical Missionary Work of Two Brothers & Its Later Developments Down to the Present Day* (London: Seeley, 1928), 18.
32. The design of the Royal Infirmary, Edinburgh was published in several books and journals. For example, see Oppert, *Hospitals, Infirmaries, and Dispensaries*, 187–8.
33. G. A. Bremner and Louis P. Nelson, 'Propagating Ideas and Institutions: Religious and Educational Architecture', in G. A. Bremner (ed.), *Architecture and Urbanism in the British Empire* (Oxford: Oxford University Press, 2016), 160.

34. Mark Crinson, *Empire Building: Orientalism and Victorian Architecture* (London and New York: Routledge, 2013), 225.
35. Ibid., 218–26; Samuel D. Albert, 'Egypt and Mandatory Palestine and Iraq', in *Architecture and Urbanism* (see note 33), 434–4.
36. Crinson, *Empire Building*, 221.
37. Taylor, *Hospital and Asylum*, 32 and 234.
38. Yaron Ferry and Efraim Lev, 'The Medical Activities of the London Jews Society in Nineteenth-Century Palestine', *Medical History* 47 (2003): 76.
39. *The Builder* 70 (1896): 404.
40. 'A Memorial to the Late Joseph Sydney Hill, Bishop in West Africa', *Mercy and Truth* 3, no. 27 (1899): 61.
41. Albert, 'Egypt and Mandatory Palestine and Iraq'.
42. Ibid., 434.
43. T. O. Beidelman, 'Alturism and Domesticity: Images of Missionizing Women among the Church Missionary Society in Nineteenth-Century East Africa', in Mary Taylor Huber and Nancy C. Lutkehaus (eds), *Gendered Missions: Women and Men in Missionary Discourse and Practice* (Ann Arbor: University of Michigan Press, 1999), 114.
44. As an 'official' Church of England Association, the SPG had a great deal of influence on Anglican ecclesiastical architecture in Britain's empire during the mid-nineteenth century in such a way that 'can be seen to amount for a form of corporatisation'. See G. A. Bremner, 'The Corporatisation of Global Anglicanism', *ABE Journal* [Online], 2 (2012). DOI: https://doi.org/10.4000/abe.357 For more on corporation, see G. A. Bremner and Diego Caltana, 'Corporations, Corporate Identity, and Imperial Architecture?', *ABE Journal* [Online], 2 (2012), DOI: https://doi.org/10.4000/abe.352
45. For an account of SPG medical work, see C. F. Pascoe, *Two Hundred Years of the SPG: An Historical Account of the Society for the Propagation of the Gospel in Foreign Parts, 1701–1900* (London, 1901), 816a–818. St Catherine Hospital, St Stephen Hospital and St Elizabeth Hospital were the three main hospitals of SPG in India. They were designed differently. See *Here and There with the SPG in India* (Westminster, 1905), 51 and 55.
46. James S. Dennis, *Christian Missions and Social Progress*, vol. 2 (New York: Fleming H. Revell Company, 1899); see also John S. Chandler, *Seventy-five Years in the Madura Mission: A history of the Mission in South India* (Madras, 1912); A. R. Cavalier, *In Northern India: A Story of Mission Work in Zenanas, Hospitals, Schools and Villages* (London: S. W. Partridge, 1899).

47. Consisting of all the qualified medical missionaries of the Punjab mission and a Secretary (appointed by the Parent Committee), the responsibility of the Sub-conference was to review the progress and financial efficiency of medical missions. See 'Rules for Medical Sub-Conferences', 4 April 1899, CMS/M/AP 2/1, CRL.
48. Arthur Neve, 'Memorandum on the CMS Medical Missions of the Punjab & N. W. Frontier,' CMS/M/C 2/1/4, no. 64. CRL.
49. 'Medical Missions', *Preaching and Healing, The Report of the CMS Medical Mission Auxiliary for 1902–1903* (1903): 54.
50. Neve, 'Memorandum on the CMS Medical Missions'.
51. Dr Haywood, 'The New Hospital at Dera Ismail Khan', *Mercy and Truth* 7, no. 75 (1903): 81.
52. Neve, 'Memorandum on the CMS Medical Missions'.
53. Arthur Neve, 'A Visit to Dera Ismail Khan', *Mercy and Truth* 7, no. 78 (1903), 207.
54. Neve, 'Memorandum on the CMS Medical Missions'.
55. 'Medical Missions', *Preaching and Healing: The Report of the CMS Medical Mission Auxiliary for 1901–02* (1902), 46.
56. 'Items: Home and Foreign', *Mercy and Truth* 7, no. 75 (1903), 71.
57. Adams, *Medicine by Design*, 113.
58. Burdett, *Hospitals and Asylums of the World*, 122.
59. Nightingale, *Notes on Hospitals*, 153.
60. For a discussion regarding Public Work planning, see Peter Scriver, 'Empire-Building and Thinking in the Public Works Department of British India', in Peter Scriver and Vikramaditya Prakash (eds), *Colonial Modernities: Building, dwelling and architecture in British India and Ceylon* (London and New York: Routledge, 2007), 69–92.
61. Peter Scriver, 'Rationalization, Standardization, and Control in Design: A Cognitive Historical Study of Architectural Design and Planning in the Public Works Department of British India', PhD diss. (Delft Institute of Technology, 1994), 503–4.
62. As Neve stated in 1912, '[an] English builder or architect was not be [*sic*] of much help' in north-western British India because R. E. Officers were experienced in building and, importantly, because 'senior medical missionaries know by long experience the cheapest and strongest materials and relative advantage of same . . .' See A. Neve, 3 March 1912, no. 62, CMS/M/C2 1/10, CRL.
63. G. A. Bremner, *Imperial Gothic: Religious Architecture and High Anglican Culture in the British Empire* (New Haven: Yale University Press, 2013), 292.

64. For example, see Cathy Keys, 'Designing hospitals for Australian conditions: The Australian Inland Mission's cottage hospital, Adelaide House, 1926', *The Journal of Architecture* 21, no. 1 (2016): 68–89.
65. Miki Desai and Madhavi Desai, 'The origin and indigenisation of the Imperial bungalow in India', *The Architectural Review* (22 June 2016).
66. Ibid.
67. Hardiman, 'The Mission Hospital', 204.
68. Anthony D. King, *The Bungalow: The Production of a Global Culture*, 2nd ed. (New York and Oxford: Oxford University Press), plate 6.
69. Patricia Baker, 'Medieval Islamic Hospitals: Structural Design and Social Perceptions', in Patricia A. Baker, Han Nijdam and Karine van't Land (eds), *Medicine and Space: Body, Surroundings and Borders in Antiquity and the Middle Ages* (Leiden and Boston: Brill, 2012), 255.
70. A. Lankester, 24 August 1904, CMS/M/C 2/ 1–4, no. 135, CRL.
71. Arthur Lankester, *Stepping Stones: A doctor's memories* (London? John Lankester, 2013), 73. 92 LAN, Crowther Mission Studies Library, Church Mission Society, Oxford.
72. A. Lankester, 'More about Peshawar Hospital', *Mercy and Truth* 10, no. 119 (1906): 336. This domed building was converted to the hospital's chapel in the 1910s.
73. Ibid., 337.
74. Kisacky, *Rise of the Modern Hospital*, 107–8.
75. Cecil Lankester, Notes on Dr A. L.'s letters re. Hospital building, CMS/M/FL 1/I 7, CRL.
76. 'A New Hospital for the Peshawar Medical Mission', 1904, CMS/M/FL 1 R1, CRL.
77. Lankester, 'More about Peshawar Hospital', 336.
78. D. Fairchild Ruggles, *Islamic Gardens and Landscapes* (Philadelphia: University of Pennsylvania Press, 2008), 39–40.
79. Ibid.
80. Turner, 'The Church Missionary Society and Architecture', 198–200; The CMS was not alone in this regard. For example, see G. A. Bremner, 'The Architecture of Universities' Mission to Central Africa: Developing a Vernacular Tradition in the Anglican Field, 1861–1909', *Journal of the Society of Architectural Historians* 68 (2009): 514–38.
81. Preeti Chopra, *A Joint Enterprise: Indian Elites and the Making of British Bombay* (Minneapolis: University of Minnesota Press, 2011), 31–72; Thomas R. Metcalf,

An Imperial Vision: Indian Architecture and Britain's Raj (Berkeley: University of California Press, 1989).
82. C. Peter Williams, *The Ideals of the Self-Governing Church: A Study in Victorian Missionary Strategy* (Leiden: Brill, 1990); C. Peter Williams, 'The Church Missionary Society and the Indigenous Church in the Second Half of the Nineteenth Century: The Defence and Destruction of the Venn Ideals', in Dana L. Robert (ed.), *Converting Colonialism: Visions and Realities in Mission History, 1706–1914* (Grand Rapids and Cambridge: William B. Eerdmans, 2008): 86–111.
83. Turner, 'The Church Missionary Society and Architecture', 215.
84. Williams, *The Ideals of the Self-Governing Church*, 52–101.
85. This Memorandum resulted from the 1899 centenary systematic review of all the CMS policy. See Kenneth John Trace Farrimond, 'The Policy of the Church Missionary Society Concerning the Development of Self-Governing Indigenous Churches, 1900–1942' (PhD diss., University of Leeds, 2003), 51–90. See also Williams, *The Ideals of the Self-Governing Church*, 263; Kevin Ward, 'The legacy of Eugene Stock', *International Bulletin of Missionary Research* 23, 2 (1999), 76.
86. A. Lankester, 13 December 1905, CMS/M/C 2/1 4, no. 1, CRL.
87. A. Lankester, 20 December 1905, CMS/M/C 2/1 4, no. 9, CRL.
88. Preeti Chopra, *A Joint Enterprise* 61.
89. Ibid.
90. Margrit Pernau, 'Mapping Emotions, Constructing Feelings: Delhi in the 1840s', *Journal of the Economic and Social History* 58, no. 5 (2015): 646.
91. Ibid., 655.
92. D. W. Carr, 15 December 1903, CMS/M/C 2/1 4, no. 5, CRL.
93. Ibid.
94. D. W. Carr, 3 March 1903, CMS/M/C 2/1 4, no. 46, CRL.
95. D. W. Carr, 30 September 1903, CMS/M/C 2/1 4, no. 118, CRL.
96. For example, missionaries upset the 'bonds of trust which united the mission and El-Karey's family' in Nablus. See Philippe Bourmaud, 'Public Space and Private Spheres: The Foundations of St Luke's Hospital of Nablus by the CMS, 1891–1901', in Heleen Murre-van den Berg (ed.), *New Faith in Ancient Land: Western Missions in the Middle East in the Nineteenth and Early Twentieth Centuries* (Leiden and Boston: Brill, 2006), 133.
97. Taylor, *The Architect and the Pavilion Hospital*, 189.
98. D. W. Carr, 2 May 1903, CMS/M/C 2/1 4, no. 72. CRL.
99. Ironside, 'In the Women's Hospital', 390.

100. Dr Carr, 3 April, 1914, CMS/M/C2 1 10 1912–1914, no. 23, CRL.
101. I. E. Eardley, 'News from Isfahan', *The Mission Hospital* 39, no. 444 (January 1935): 3.
102. Gholamhossein Memarian and Frank Brown, 'The Shared Characteristics of Iranian and Arab Courtyard Houses', in Brian Edwards, et al. (eds), *Courtyard Housing: Past, Present and Future* (Abingdon: Taylor & Francis, 2006), 21–30.
103. Kleiss Wolfram, 'Safavid Palaces', *Ars Orientalis: The Arts of Islam and the East* 23 (1993), 271.
104. Johnathan Reinarz, 'Learning to Use Their Senses: Visitors to Voluntary Hospitals in Eighteenth-Century England', *Journal of Eighteenth-Century Studies* 35, no. 4 (2012): 505–20.
105. Rudi Matthee, *The Pursuit of Pleasure: Drugs and Stimulants in Iranian History, 1500–1900* (Princeton and Oxford: Princeton University Press, 2005), 237–66.
106. Eardley, 'News from Isfahan', 3.
107. Jane Lydon, *Imperial Emotions: The politics of empathy across the British Empire* (Cambridge: Cambrdige University Press, 2019), 54.
108. 'Ask the Lord, And Tell His People', *Mercy and Truth* 12, no. 134 (1908): 42.
109. 'Plan of the proposed new men's hospital, prepared by Mr McIntyre and Dr White', 21 August 1905, 1905, CMS/M/C2 1–4, no. 75, CRL.
110. 'Rough sketch showing method of arching roofs in Persia', CMS/M/FL 1/PE 4, no. 17, CRL.
111. 'Memorandum by Mr J. W. Rundall regarding the design and estimate for the proposed Men's Hospital at Yezd', 23 October 1905, CMS/M/C 2/ 1–4, no. 94, CRL.
112. Medical Sub-Conference, Julfa, 18 January 1906, CMS/M/C2 1–4, no. 15, CRL.
113. 'Report Furnished by Dr. G. E. Dodson Regarding Hospital Building, Kerman', 7 July 1915, Medical precis book 18 September 1914–25 October 1921, CMS/M/C 2/1/11, no. 18, CRL.
114. Masoud Kheirabadi, *Iranian Cities: Formation and Development* (Syracuse: Syracuse University Press, 2000), 30.
115. Heinz Gaube, 'Iranian Cities', in Salma K.Jayyusi, Renata Holod, Attilio Petruccioli and Andre Raymond (eds), *The City in the Islamic World*, vol. 1 (Leiden and Boston: Brill, 2008), 159.
116. Lisa Golombek, 'The "Citadel, Town, Suburbs" Model and Medieval Kerman', in *The City in the Islamic World*, vol. 2 (see note 115), 445–63. This study

was based on a collaborative project between the Iranian Cultural Heritage Organisation, the Royal Ontario Museum of Toronto and the University of Michigan, which was undertaken in 2001.
117. 'These experiences are (and were) very much a product of age, class, status, and gender.' See 'Introduction', *The City in the Islamic World* (see note 115), xv.
118. Margrit Pernau, 'Space and Emotions: Building to Feel', *History Compass* 12, no. 7 (2014): 545.
119. Eleanor Dodson, 'A Holiday Letter from Persia', *The Mission Hospital* 27, no. 424 (May 1933): 102. Eleanor Dodson visited Kerman from Multan in summer 1932 in response to an invitation from her brother.
120. Adams, *Medicine by Design*, 113.
121. G. E. Dodson, 1914, CMS/M/FL 1 PE2, CRL.
122. This information is based on fieldwork in Kerman conducted in 2011 and 2015.
123. 'Kerman Hospital', CMS/H/H5/E2 (Box 6), CRL.
124. For example, see Zoë Crossland, 'Signs of Mission: Material Semeiosis and Nineteenth-Century Tswana Architecture', *Signs and Society* 1, no. 1 (2013): 79–113.
125. Paul Ward English, 'The Origin and Spread of Qanats in the Old World', *Proceedings of the American Philosophical Society* 112, no. 3 (1968): 170.
126. C. F. H. 'Principles and Practice of Medical Missions: Chapter V, In-patients', *Mercy and Truth* 16, no. 185 (1912): 154.
127. Ibid.

3

HOSPITAL VISITORS AND A HOSPITAL FOR A WHOLE FAMILY

When I examined the architecture of the Peshawar hospital in the previous chapter, I mentioned that it consisted of a caravanserai for traveller patients – patients who travelled from other cities – and their family and friends. This chapter, the focus of which is on hospital visiting, returns to this architectural configuration. A focus on visitors and visiting is beneficial to understanding the distinct nature of mission hospitals, as it can reveal much about the relationship between the institutions and the communities they served. In their edited collection on hospital visiting, Graham Mooney and Jonathan Reinarz assert that 'visiting involved the comings and goings not only of relatives and friends, but also of administrators, managers, philanthropists, lay care-givers, priests and ministers, entertainers, and tourists'.[1] Mission hospitals also received visitors from various groups. This chapter identifies these groups, focusing ultimately on patients' visitors, namely family and friends. Protestant missionaries of various denominations allowed family and friends to visit and even live in the hospitals in Persia, British India, China, the Persian Gulf region, Uganda and Nigeria.[2] The chapter examines who family and friends were, what they did and discusses the reasons that counted for their presence. Additionally, it demonstrates that the presence of family members had an architectural manifestation; that is, the missionaries developed a specific building to host a 'whole family' in a hospital. In so doing, the chapter identifies a new hospital type developed at the beginning of the twentieth century.

Mooney and Reinarz find it surprising 'how little has been revealed about the historical evolution of this seemingly universal practice'.³ Reinarz further states that 'the history of hospital visiting has been a strangely neglected theme in the history of medicine'.⁴ More than ten years after the publication of their volume, hospital visiting is still a relatively marginalised topic.⁵ There is an even greater shortage of research on hospital visiting beyond the European and North American contexts. Only a few scholars have explored the specificities of the boundaries between asylums (or hospitals for the insane) and the extra-institutional world in Australasian Colonial World and South Asia.⁶ The only scholar that has examined the topic of visiting mission hospitals is Michelle Renshaw, who recognises that 'it was not uncommon for family members to live with the patients in American-run hospitals' in China. The reasons that Renshaw identifies to account for this include:

> [A] lack of resources to employ staff; Chinese cultural norms concerning the inappropriateness of women nursing men; customary familiar involvement in caring for the sick; and the fact that missionaries were prepared to make concessions to these norms and customs so that Chinese patients would agree to come into hospital to undergo unfamiliar procedures and perhaps even receive a dose of religious instruction.⁷

Besides drawing on Mooney and Reinarz's work, I am guided by Renshaw's observations in this chapter. I identify reasons like hers concerning the presence of family and friends in mission hospitals in Persia and British India. Ultimately, my focus is on the latter reason; I argue that the issue of gaining trust or friendship legitimised the presence of family and friends. Renshaw agrees, although she does not elaborate on this in any detail. She argues that even with enough nursing staff, it was advisable to allow the family and friends to accompany the patients as this practice responded to the 'Chinese custom of family members taking an active role in caring for the sick'.⁸ While missionaries found the presence of family and friends irksome, they allowed them to accompany the patients and stay in the hospitals because this plan would increase the number of people with whom the missionaries came into contact.

None of the essays in Mooney and Reinarz's volume explicitly addresses the built form; how architectural decisions conditioned, and were conditioned by, hospital visiting. There are only passing references to the façade and the internal arrangements of the buildings in various chapters, including Renshaw's.[9] She refers to the design of examination areas in dispensaries and explains how they were partitioned off but remained in full view. Thus, 'patients who were still waiting and any friends and relatives who had accompanied them could see what the doctor was doing'.[10] In another section, Renshaw refers to a 'commodious and very convenient inn' designed in the LMS Robert Memorial Hospital in Hebei to accommodate patients and their family members.[11] This idea of the inn – or a distinct design to accommodate an entire family – is particularly important to this chapter. Renshaw does not analyse the architecture of the LMS Robert Memorial Hospital's inn. It might have consisted of identical rooms where patients could stay with their close associates. This chapter suggests that this design might have originated in north-western British India.

A Visit to the Mission Hospital

Mooney and Reinarz divide visitors into four categories to better understand who they were and what they did: patients' visitors, public visitors, house visitors and official visitors. Patients' visitors include family and friends; public visitors refer to those members of the public who 'were not associated with the direct administration of the hospital or with familial ties to the patients'; house visitors were 'usually involved in the formal management and government of the hospital by way of a donation or subscription'. They also performed 'quality control tasks' and took 'an active interest in patients'. The final category, official visitors, were 'usually salaried inspectors of the state, and were responsible for monitoring and reporting on the performance of, and conditions inside, institutions'.[12] Visitors were subjected to regulations that were highly diverse across time and place. They also fulfilled many roles and were essential to hospitals economically, socially, politically and even morally. Mooney and Reinarz's classification is based on the most crucial function.[13] In this part, I focus on the last three groups, comparing circumstances in mission hospitals vis-à-vis their counterparts in provisional England* before moving on to patients' visitors in the following two sections.

The wider public gained a chance to visit the hospitals on the occasion of their openings. At the opening ceremony of the Peshawar hospital, for example, 'nearly 150 people, English and Indian' were present, among whom was Sir Harold Deane, the Chief Commissioner of the North-West Frontier Province. After Deane declared the hospital open, guests were invited to 'see over the Hospital'.[14] Likewise, '[s]everal English residents and a large number of Hindus and Mohammedans came to the [opening] ceremony' of the new hospital at Dera Ismail Khan. According to Dr W. B. Heywood, '[t]he whole hospital was open to the inception of visitors both before and after the [opening] service'.[15] Throwing an opening ceremony, as was the case with the first voluntary hospitals in England, might have been a strategy for showcasing the benefits of the new hospital.[16] The missionaries might have also used opening ceremonies to demonstrate their legitimacy.[17] In other words, the very act of visiting a mission hospital as part of an opening ceremony was an emotional practice, so much so that if the missionaries were uncertain about the potential affective results of an opening ceremony, they would opt for none: 'in view of past oppositions' no opening ceremony took place at Isfahan because the missionaries' aim was 'to get to work as quietly as possible in the new buildings without attracting more attention than was necessary,' wrote Dr Donald Carr in 1905.[18]

It is unclear whether 'English residents and Hindus and Mohammedans', 'English and Indian' and 'Hindu and Mohammedans' inspected the hospitals simultaneously. People of various religions interacted in shared sacred spaces of popular religion in India,[19] but interaction as part of the opening ceremony of a mission hospital, especially as it involved 'English residents', might have appeared different to them. Even if Hindus and Mohammedans and English residents visited the hospitals together, they may have been from a specific social group and may have shifted their values and modes of expression according to expectations associated with opening ceremonies.

---

* I refer to hospitals in provisional England because there is no work on hospital visiting in Scotland, Wales or Ireland.

Public visitors, exclusive of local people – Hindus and Mohammedans or Indian – visited the hospitals beyond the opening ceremonies. One case is Miss Ella Sykes, the sister of the Consul-General in Kerman, Major Percy Molesworth Sykes. Miss Sykes visited the Kerman hospital in 1904 and provided an 'outsider's view' or an 'amateur view' of the work in *Mercy and Truth*.[20] Moreover, fellow missionaries sometimes visited one or several medical missions on their way to and from Britain, as was the case with Dr Andrew Jukes, who visited the Old-Cairo hospital on his way back to British India in 1901.[21] Another example is Miss Harriet Ellen Finney's visit to the Amritsar hospital in 1905. A CMS missionary in Kandy (Ceylon), Miss Finney accompanied the doctor on 'his usual round of visits' upon his invitation.[22] Additionally, some visits to the CMS hospitals were paid by missionaries of other missionary organisations. Two examples are Miss Wauton and A. R. Cavalier; Wauton visited the Amritsar hospital in June 1903 upon the doctor's request. Wauton was a missionary of the CEZMS Zenana Mission house at Amritsar and called chiefly upon the female patients.[23] Cavalier was the Secretary of the Zenana Bible and Medical Mission (and formerly a CMS missionary in Ceylon and South India) and visited several mission hospitals, including the Peshawar hospital, on his tour of mission stations in Bombay, the Punjab and North-West Provinces in 1897–8.[24]

Financial gain was one of the main reasons why the members of the wider public were allowed inside the walls of the voluntary hospitals beyond the opening ceremonies. As Mooney and Reinarz state, '[h]ospital administrators . . . regarded such visits as ideal fundraising opportunities, some having even contemplated the introduction of admission changes.'[25] Published reports imply that patients were the main focus of public visitors, who played a role in the general rejuvenation of the patients. Wauton, for example, listened 'for a little while to the sorrowful complaints of some of the sufferers', believing that they 'seem all the better for pouring them out'.[26] Nevertheless, the very reports of these visits were meant to secure financial support at home by emphasising the value of a medical mission as an 'evangelistic agency' or by commenting on the 'busy' state of the hospitals. Finney's aim, 'more especially', was to see an old Mohammedan man, who occupied 'a small room containing only one "charpoy" or native bed'. She commented on the old man's 'expression of gratitude, confidence, and deep affection', stating that he was not only 'a believer in Christ, but a Christian of a high and beautiful type'. The rest of her report explained in detail how the old man 'came to be here'.[27] Likewise, the Lieutenant-Governor of Punjab, Sir W. Mackworth Young, visited the Kashmir hospital in 1902 and commented on the hospital's buildings in the visitor book. According to a published note, Young wrote, 'I could not help thinking how the sight of the fine buildings, the pretty substantial church, and the hospital work in full swing, would have gladded the heart of Dr Elmslie.'[28] Young's note was possibly altered to meet the expectations of a home audience.[29]

Drawing on the sociologist Erving Goffman's study of the institutional visit,[30] Mooney and Reinarz state that hospital and asylum visits often resembled 'choreographed theatrical performances'.[31] That is, given the financial implications of many visits, hospital and asylum governors and staff tried to 'convey certain impressions to visitors'. My examination of mission hospital visiting echoes this view. Missionaries opened the entire hospital for inception as part of an opening ceremony. Still, they controlled how hospitals were presented to the public and home visitors beyond the ceremonies. Hospitals were open to the public and home visitors only upon invitation. For example, Miss Sykes visited the Kerman hospital upon the request of Mary Bird. Although she resided in Kerman for some time, she most likely did not repeat her visit.

European explorers, government officials and local chiefs were house visitors to mission hospitals. As already mentioned, house visitors were involved in a hospital's formal management through a donation or subscription. In other words, they played a promotional role. According to Mooney and Reinarz, public visitors monitored the management of healthcare facilities as well as 'various aspects of institutional life and house rule, expenditures, and the compliance of patients and practitioners'.[32] Hospitals' reliance on charity slowly declined from the early twentieth century until 1948, when central taxation and management replaced the old system. Although house visitors to mission hospitals contributed to the institution's management through donation, they did not monitor healthcare facilities or institutional life and rules.

European explorers rarely engaged in hospitals' management, but one exceptional and known case is Isabella Lucy Bird, later Mrs Bishop. Being a clergyman, Bird's father brought her into contact with missionaries. Moreover, one of her cousins was Miss Mary Bird.[33] Isabella Bird also developed an active interest in medical science, which she shared with her husband of eight years, Dr John Bishop. She also received training in nursing for three months at St Mary's Hospital in London in 1887. Bird surveyed medical missions, visiting the Kashmir and Isfahan missions in the late 1880s and around twenty-eight medical missions in China and Japan between 1894 and 1897.[34] Besides writing about medical missions in both her books and private letters, Bird gave a lecture at the Annual Meeting of the London Medical Missionary Association in 1897,[35] followed by another address at the Missionary Loan Exhibitions held at Norwich in April 1898, to a 'packed audience'.[36] In general, she had a favourable opinion of medical mission work and was interested in how missionaries combined medical and evangelistic work. However, according to Gili Adair, Bird represented medical missions in her published travel narratives 'as honourable and well-intentioned, but also, at times, rather naïve individuals, whose failure is suggested as inevitable'.[37]

Bird is also an exceptional case because she was among a few female house visitors. Like their counterparts in England, female house visitors to mission hospitals were excluded from the governing and decision-making rules and processes. There are names of many women in the Islamabad (Anantnag) women hospital's visitor book, but these women were most likely public visitors, not house or official visitors.[38]

As hinted at above, Sir Harold Deane, the Chief Commissioner of the North-West Frontier Province, attended the opening ceremony of the Peshawar hospital, and Lieutenant-Governor of Punjab, Sir W. Mackworth Young, visited the Kashmir medical mission in 1901. Whether they donated towards the fund is not mentioned in the reports. But British government officials were among the main house visitors, whose support, as I mentioned in Chapter One, was beneficial to the advancement or otherwise of medical mission work. Official civil and military supporters of the CMS missions in Punjab and Persia included Herbert Edwardes, Henry and John Lawrence, Robert Montgomery, Donald McLeod, Reynell Taylor, Robert Cust, Arthur Roberts, William Martin, C. B. Saunders and Sir Percy Sykes.[39] For example, Sykes visited the Kerman and Yazd medical missions several times and played a role in missionaries' unsuccessful attempt to acquire land for building a purpose-built structure in Kerman in 1904.[40] Much has been written about

British government officials' relationship with missionaries, yet their role as house visitors has been disregarded.

The role of local chiefs and elites as house visitors has not been discussed either. I explained in Chapter One that local chiefs' or elites' support and contribution towards the fund, for their varied reasons, could also play a role in the success or otherwise of a medical mission. Notably, they sometimes contributed a donation after visiting and inspecting the hospitals. One example is the governor of Yazd, Jalal-ud-Dowlah, a son of Zill al-Sultān, the governor of Isfahan, and a nephew of the Shah of Persia. Jalal-ud-Dowlah paid a visit to the Yazd hospital in 1900 and 1903. During his 1900 visit, according to Dr Henry White, Jalal-ud-Dowlah inspected every part of the hospital (dispensary, operating room and the wards) and 'made a good donation towards the funds'.[41]

It is essential to look beyond people who visited the hospitals physically concerning mission hospitals' house visitors to include the general public at home, or 'friends at home', who visited the hospitals through published reports. These 'emotional scripts', to use Elizabeth Elbourne's term,[42] or 'narrative tropes', to use Stephen Cummins' and Joel Lee's term,[43] sought to evoke feelings in their readers through conversion narratives and through creating and leaving an impression of a hospital's environment. Miss Sykes, for instance, took the reader on a tour of the hospital, describing the building (courtyard, wards, kitchen and dispensary) and commenting on the patients.[44] More telling examples are those reports entitled, 'A Walk Through the Wards of the Women's Hospital, Multan' or 'A Walk Through the Wards of a Mission Hospital'. The author of these reports encouraged the reader to accompany them on a tour of the hospital, going from ward to ward, thus helping them to comprehend the character of medical missions.[45] The same applies to missionary exhibitions, which became popular from the 1880s due to their entertaining nature.[46] The CMS and the LMS were two of the most active missionary organisations in curating exhibitions. The CMS had a 'Medical Mission Court' at one or even two exhibitions per year, displaying models of hospital wards and operating theatres (Figure 3.1) or fitting up part of the court as a hospital ward.[47] By way of these exhibitions, the public at home, especially the lower-middle and artisan classes, visited the hospitals.[48] Medical missions were presented in a court at the Dublin Mission Loan Exhibition

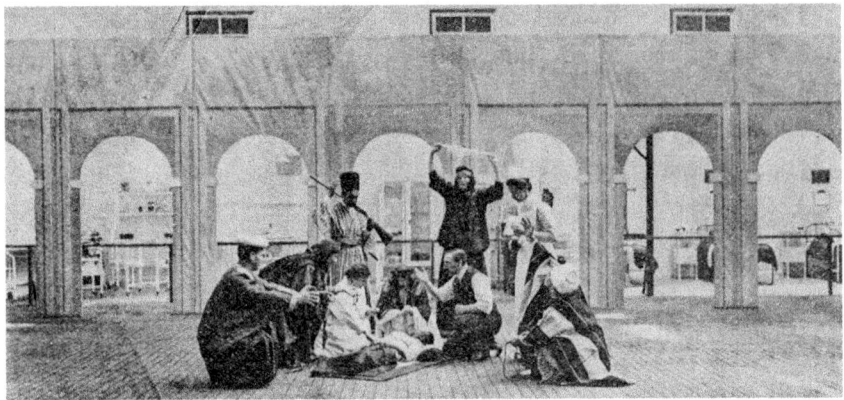

Figure 3.1 Realistic hospital sense.
CMS/M/EL 2/13, p. 272, Church Missionary Society Archive, Cadbury Research Library, Special Collections, University of Birmingham.

in 1899. A note stated, 'several new models of Mission Hospitals help them in picturing the surroundings of our Medical Missions'.[49] Missionaries also displayed models of hospitals at larger exhibitions attended by a more diverse group of people, such as the 1925 British Empire Exhibition at Wembley, where a model of the Peshawar hospital was on display.[50]

There were initially no official visitors to mission hospitals. In the case of the CMS, the Home Committee passed a resolution in 1899, sanctioning the formation of Medical Sub-conferences.[51] Consisting of all the qualified medical missionaries of a mission and a secretary (appointed by the Parent Committee), a Sub-conference could be formed after three medical missionaries of a mission (such as the Persia Mission or the Punjab Mission) had passed their second language examination. While receiving opinions of members by correspondence was sufficient for preparing their report, secretaries occasionally made a tour of medical missions and can be counted as official visitors. The responsibilities of a Sub-conference included reviewing the progress and financial efficiency of medical missions, commenting on the training of 'Native Medical Assistants' and, when asked, reporting on any 'medical or sanitary matters'.[52] Secretaries also commented on the geography of the regions, the patients' demography and medical and surgical cases in their reports. Reinarz states that 'many individuals visited English hospitals to view their technological and architectural features'. These visits partly contributed to standardisation and uniformity among hospitals.[53] The purpose of none of the secretaries' visits was strictly educational and, as I showed in the previous chapter, Dr Arthur Neve's tour of medical missions in north-western British India and his suggestions did not lead to standardisation.

Neve's tour was well documented, and it is worth examining it in more detail. Neve of Kashmir medical mission was the secretary of the Punjab Medical Sub-conference between 1900 and 1919 (his death). He toured medical missions several times during his tenure, in 1903, 1910 and 1915. Reports of his 1903 tour were published in a series of articles in *Mercy and Truth*. He also prepared a Memorandum.[54] Besides writing about the architecture of medical missions, he commented on the topographical location of the hospitals. His reports indicated that the Quetta medical mission was located 'just outside the town' and the Dera Ismail Khan hospital lied 'on the outskirts of cantonment, quite close to the city'. Additionally, Neve remarked on the geography of the regions. For instance, he wrote, 'Sind looks like a veritable desert to the traveller, who strains his eyes to see any sign of fertility or verdure.' In his Memorandum, he also discussed branch dispensaries and itineration, the financial situation of the missions and provided advice on improving hospitals' performance.[55]

If, overall, it seems that mission hospitals' walls were not as permeable, the picture changes when the focus turns to patients' visitors. In general, mission hospitals were open to patients and their families and friends. Close associates were, in fact, a noteworthy feature of a mission hospital. As one missionary put it, medical work brought missionaries into contact with 'a whole family'. Again, this sits in sharp contrast to the situation in nineteenth-century provisional England.

'These are Family and Friends'

Family and friends' access to hospitals in England was increasingly controlled and became subject to strict rules from the mid-nineteenth century onwards. The rules and regulations were not uniformly adopted in every hospital in England; they varied from hospital to hospital, depending on their finances and type. At many well-supported voluntary and specialist hospitals, only a limited number of guests were permitted by medical staff to visit each patient two or three days a week. In contrast, in some of the less well-supported voluntary hospitals, visitors were permitted to stay overnight to offset the expense of hiring night nurses. In children's hospitals, guests could visit on fixed days and when inmates' wounds were being dressed. Mothers were occasionally charged as paying patients to reside in the hospital with their children.[56] Moreover, the opinion of matrons about patients' visitors differed from that of medical staff; the former welcomed guests because they brought clean linen with themselves, whilst the latter were against visitors because they would introduce many prohibited items to the hospitals. From the 1880s onwards, restrictions became even tighter due to deep concerns about the state of hospital hygiene; there were fears that guests might introduce dirt and hence infection.

Medical missionaries were not alone in permitting family and friends to enter the hospitals. For example, as John Chircop shows, relatives regularly, if not daily, visited '[t]wo forgotten lunatic asylums' set in Corfu and Malta. Although these two asylums were built to impose social regulations based on colonial state documents, the picture was more complex. The circulation of bodies and objects was not restricted, and hence Chircop questions the extent to which these institutions functioned as 'state instruments of social control management, from top to bottom, with little if any interference from outside'.[57] The situation was even more complicated with respect to mission hospitals because relatives resided in the hospitals, fed their patients, changed their bedding and kept them company.[58] The number of relatives sometimes exceeded that of the patients.

As mentioned at the beginning of this chapter, Michelle Renshaw identifies the lack of resources to employ nursing staff as one of the reasons for the presence of relatives in North American-run mission hospitals in China. Historians such as John R. Stanley and David Hardiman also identify family members' involvement in nursing their patients. Indeed, nursing their patients is the only reason that has been widely acknowledged. Stanley states, regarding Dr Charles Roy's hospital at Weixian (China), that 'because there were no professional nurses, the relatives or friends of patients were allowed to remain on the premises to provide care, increasing the overcrowding even more'.[59] Similarly, Hardiman writes regarding the CMS hospital at Lusadiya that 'there were no nurses, so that the care of inpatients had to be carried out by relatives or friends'.[60] The CMS accepted its first nurses in the 1890s. According to the figures for 1894, the CMS did not have any nurses, but, by December 1898, there were thirteen, including Miss Emmeline Stuart of the Isfahan hospital and Miss Neve of the Kashmir hospital.[61] The number of nurses increased to nineteen in the following year, thirty-six in 1902[62] and sixty in 1911.[63] Reading these figures against statistics of the number of medical missions, it becomes clear that most missions had no or only one nurse. In 1901 none of the hospitals in British India had nurses among their staff except the Kashmir hospital. The number of nurses does not include missionary wives, who engaged in nursing, even if they were not qualified. For example, Mrs White and Mrs Brown were mentioned in the 1898 report 'Nurses Working in CMS Hospitals', but only on the side and were not included in the statistics.[64] Missionary wives also helped in other activities, such as home visiting and itineration, which means they could nurse patients only occasionally.

Writing about the lack of nursing staff and the presence of family members, Reverend Arthur Russell Blackett compared the Isfahan hospital to a home in 1898: 'Hospital nursing as understood in civilized land is out of the question here. The patient brings his nurse with him, a father, son, wife (one or more), sometimes his whole family. So, the institution is a home as well as a hospital.'[65] Two years earlier, Carr had similarly questioned the status of the institution: 'in many ways it is more like a "hostel" where patients can come and stay for treatment, than a hospital, because we have no system of nursing.'[66] Blackett and Carr's statements refer to the transformed nature of nursing in late nineteenth-century Britain. The modernisation of the hospital and the nursing profession went hand in hand to such an extent that the status of a hospital could be questioned due to the lack of nurses. Nurses maintained strict standards of cleanliness and the good order of the hospital, cared for and assessed the patients and helped during surgery.[67] Without good nursing, the Isfahan hospital was not a hospital in the strict sense. Meanwhile, it is worth asking how urgent was the need for nurses? Dr Pennell asked this same question in 1897:

> Here too, with such cases, do we feel the want of trained nurses most acutely; most patients have either brother or father or wife to attend on them, and he or she will sleep on the floor beside the bed of their sick relation and attend to their wants in a rough but kindly way; but the greasy garments and long unwashed skin of this dilettante nurse send many a misgiving to the heat of

the surgeon, especially when he is seen to have found some very old and dirty rags from his own person round the dressings of an aseptic joint case to make it most softly. Yet to dispense with these willing but uncouth, unwashed, and often blundering helpers is quite impossible, as most of the patients would refuse to stop without their friends to care for and guard them.[68]

Pennell was clear that the hospital would have been less 'untidy with nurses present'. At the same time, he referred to a family member as a 'dilettante nurse', stating that many patients would not have come without their presence. The impression being that they had to choose between a 'tidy' but empty hospital or an 'untidy' but busy one; they made a compromise. Missionaries were not all for close associates and their presence in the hospitals; they tolerated their attendance because patients would not have come otherwise, and, in turn, family members took up the much needed role of nurses. Miss Wauton elaborated on this in 1903:

> In this country the members of a family cannot bear separation from each other, and on this account often refrain from coming to the hospital; but the open door here admits not only the sufferer but the relations also who can stay with them, providing their food, and many thankfully avail themselves of this permission, thereby greatly increasing the number of those who through the Medical Mission come to hear and understand something of Christian truth.[69]

Apart from caring for and feeding their patients, family members introduced many goods to a hospital. Sister F. M. James of the Kerman hospital discussed this in detail in 1938 by recalling the situation ten years earlier. First, she noted how family and friends caused complications; they not only crowded the hospital, but also made it 'untidy': '[they sat] on the floor [. . .], surrounded with pots and pans, cups and saucers, teapots, and last but not least, a samovar [. . .], and a galyun or water pipe.'[70] Then she compared the 'untidy' situation of the Kerman hospital with the 'spick and span condition of an English hospital', stating why the missionaries acquiesced and allowed all these habits to continue. According to her, while this was upsetting at first sight, the missionaries gradually learnt to shut their eyes to some 'innocent things' that went on because patients would not come.[71] Sister James's use of the term 'innocent things' clarifies that attracting people was such an important factor that the missionaries were ready to abandon the idea of absolute 'cleanliness' and 'order'.

Close associates were everywhere: in the hospital compound, waiting-halls and wards, and their number was sometimes more than necessary for nursing. Put categorically, if the patients did not come with their relatives, the number of people missionaries met would have been considerably less. For example, a report on 15 March 1907 declared that there were thirty-eight traveller patients in the Peshawar hospital accompanied by thirty-two relations.[72] Interacting with these extended guests was considered an important part of the missionary work. In this regard, it is helpful to ask who family and friends were? As used in the letters and reports of missionaries, family extended beyond relatives of varying closeness and friends to include neighbours and servants. Thus, allowing them into the hospital meant bringing different age groups and classes. Consider the Yazd hospital: a photograph was published in 1910, illustrating that a Shahzada was in the hospital (Figure 3.2). This

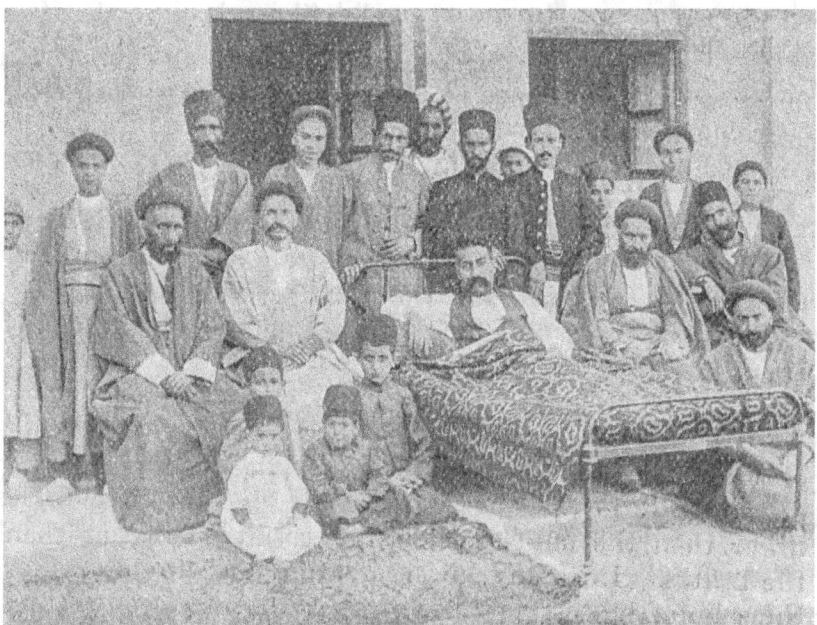

Figure 3.2 A Shahzada with his children, friends and servants in Yazd hospital. CMS/M/EL 2/14, p. 267, Church Missionary Society Archive, Cadbury Research Library, Special Collections, University of Birmingham.

photograph shows the patient surrounded by people, and the description of the photograph explicitly notes that 'the men around the patients were their children, friends, and servants'.[73] Surely, not all these people were engaged in nursing. With their presence, the number of potentially interested people increased. While in the hospital, they saw and learned about the missionaries, and consequently, the chance for earning belief became remarkably greater.

Shahzada refers to the male descendants of the king of Persia. According to Mooney and Reinarz 'any discussion about using the restriction of visiting non-infectious disease hospitals as a tool of infection control by the medical staff is thrown into dispute – if not revealed as grossly hypocritical – when class distinctions are considered'.[74] Conversely, close associates were permitted inside the walls of a mission hospital regardless of a patient's class status. Examples are, in fact, boundless: in 1916, writing about a child who was staying in the Isfahan hospital, Dr Catherine Ironside stated that 'the whole family, who had carefully avoided us before, were brought into touch with us daily and hourly for the two or three weeks that the child was in'.[75] A particularly telling case is a mullah called Maizullah Khan, who was of the Afghan tribe of Khost and stayed in the Bannu hospital for two months until his death. Maizullah Khan's visitors were not his family members or friends but his pupils. Pennell wrote, 'I have no doubt that all these future mullahs were more or less favourably influenced towards Christianity.'[76]

The presence of family members might have decreased the infection rate in mission hospitals. As Renshaw explains, concerning North American mission hospitals in China, the practice of washing every sore indiscriminately with the same sponge in British hospitals in the nineteenth century – which would result in the spread of infection throughout the ward – 'was less likely happen' in mission hospitals because 'all patients had their personal attendants'.[77] However, Pennell's report hints at a divergent story, not least because it stated that a family member used his 'very old and dirty' rag as 'dressing'. In another report, Pennell made mention of a boy who came to the hospital with his father. One hour after changing the boy's clothes and putting him in a bed, missionaries found the boy on the 'cold floor'. The father carried the boy away after learning this was not allowed, which by itself illustrates the importance of making compromises.[78] Some missionaries also claimed that family members hindered their teaching: '[n]o restraint is put upon visits from their friends, and many stay in the wards and help their relatives. We have to be a little watchful, lest Muhammadan mullah should come and try secretly to counteract our teaching,' stated Neve in 1897.[79] These statements, of course, are constructed around ideological and imperial biases, yet family members of different patients possibly exchanged goods with one another, which puts Renshaw's argument under question. A more probable scenario might be that, with family members present, patients did not need to leave their family surroundings. Even if they had to confront missionaries who expressed and practised their emotions in unfamiliar ways, they could be in the comfort of a familiar voice, smell and touch. In short, obtaining the trust of the people was the determining factor. This becomes clearer when realising that the absence of family members was interpreted as a sign of change in people's attitude towards missionaries. Dr Marcus Eustace wrote in 1897:

> I am glad to tell you that I see a distinct improvement in the general conduct of the people towards us. In former years every in-patient brought someone to look after him and obstruct us in our work as much as possible; but now, except in cases of sick children and helpless cases, most of our patients remain contentedly in the hospital without the dear and dirty companion.[80]

Sister James made a similar statement in 1938. Comparing the situation between 'then and now', she stated '[a]t one time patients would not stay in a foreigners' hospital if no friends were with them, but this is not so today. They are more used to us now and know that we do not like to see the hospital untidy and dirty.'[81] Nonetheless, missionaries never restricted patient visitors to once or twice a week. Some missionaries would come to favour the 'homelike' atmosphere of the hospitals. As Dr W. Hamilton Jefferys, a missionary of the American Episcopal Missions's St Luke's hospital in Shanghai observed, mission hospitals in China were 'far more homely and far more human' than North American hospitals.[82] Similarly, Dr Paul Harrison of the Arabian mission stated that 'America would do well to imitate us'.[83] At the Isfahan women's hospital each patient could have a family member with them all the time in 1915. Ironside stated that untidiness was an issue, but that 'the plan brings nearly twice as many within reach of regular Gospel teaching as would otherwise come, and many of the friends are able to learn when the poor patients are too ill to listen'.[84] Her statement recalls those of Pennell's and Miss Wauton's, clarifying the importance of family members. At Kerman, friends could visit from noon until sunset, except for patients on the danger list, who could have a family member all the time. And many hospitals in north-western British India had 'family wards'.

The Serai Hospital

The previous chapter demonstrated that cross-ventilation was not secured in many CMS hospitals. Another noteworthy feature of a pavilion plan hospital was that each ward had one entry and exit point. It was hoped that nursing staff could control the movement of patients and visitors in this way. As Cynthia Imogen Hammond states, the Nightingale Ward 'allowed for continual surveillance and control of the patients'.[85] By contrast, wards in many CMS hospitals had more than one entry and exit point, and this is another element that distinguishes them from a pavilion plan hospital. Preeti Chopra makes a similar observation regarding the Bombay hospital wards. Highlighting how patients were segregated by class and religion, she argues that 'the various social divisions precluded the easy implementation of something like a Nightingale Ward'.[86] But, as I showed in the previous chapter, wards in the Persia Mission's hospitals also had more than one point of entry and exit. Another reason might have been climatic conditions. As Cathy Keys writes, the Australian Inland Mission's cottage hospital was designed with ward doors, and verandas wide enough to allow beds to be taken easily out whenever desired to deal with 'periods of oppressive heat'.[87] Given that patients could stay in the hospitals with their close associates, this layout might have also had to do with facilitating direct interactions between patients and their family members. Indeed, this arrangement might be linked to the debates surrounding building trust; that is, the importance of attracting as many people as possible.

The missionaries even developed a rather novel ward design for housing patients with their close associates in the hospital. It is unclear when and where this idea was developed and whether it was an invention of the CMS missionaries in north-western British India. Even if the serai system did not originate in north-western British India, it gained added importance due to geopolitical reasons. As I will argue in Chapter Five, the CMS's chain of medical missions served the double purpose of winning north-western British India for Christ and preparing the ground for the 'Empire of Christ' in Afghanistan and Central Asia. The reports and letters of missionaries refer to many patients who visited the hospitals from Afghanistan and Central Asia and, according to these reports and letters, these patients were accompanied by their family members without whom they would refuse to stay in the hospitals.

It appears that initially this idea was developed to address the needs of women who were not willing to remain in the hospitals without their relatives. Four such rooms were built in Kashmir, and each consisted of a small yard.[88] Maxwell reported that '[i]t is found to be best to give the women separate huts, as they often bring their families with them'.[89] The hospitals of the CEZMS at Quetta and Peshawar also had family wards 'enabling many women who would not leave their husbands to go into an ordinary ward to be treated'.[90] Moreover, Dr Theodore Pennell sent plans in 1904 to add 'four houses' to the Bannu hospital to accommodate patients who came from some distant place with their family members.[91] After the construction of the Peshawar hospital, the serai system or the system of 'family wards' came to be viewed as an architectural solution to the practical problem of accommodating patients' family members who had nowhere else to stay.

In the first chapter I showed that missionaries used three caravanserais as the hospital before constructing the purpose-built structures at Peshawar. At the annual meeting of the MMA in 1899, Lankester asserted that '[o]ne great advantage of our particular style of work is that we have a great many small native rooms, and we can take in the whole family at the time, giving them a separate room and telling them to make themselves happy'.[92] This arrangement was duplicated within the new hospital (Figure 3.3). The hospital consisted of a quadrangle building named the James Serai, which was composed of thirty identical rooms designed around three sides of a courtyard, with each having only one door, like a caravanserai. It is 'a feature borrowed from the old hospital in the city', stated Lankester in 1906.[93] The serai hospital was characterised not with reference to hospital planning in Britain that was incorporated into the traditional building practices of the region. Far from being a result of an interface between indigenous and imported ways of building, it arose from an indigenous type of architecture

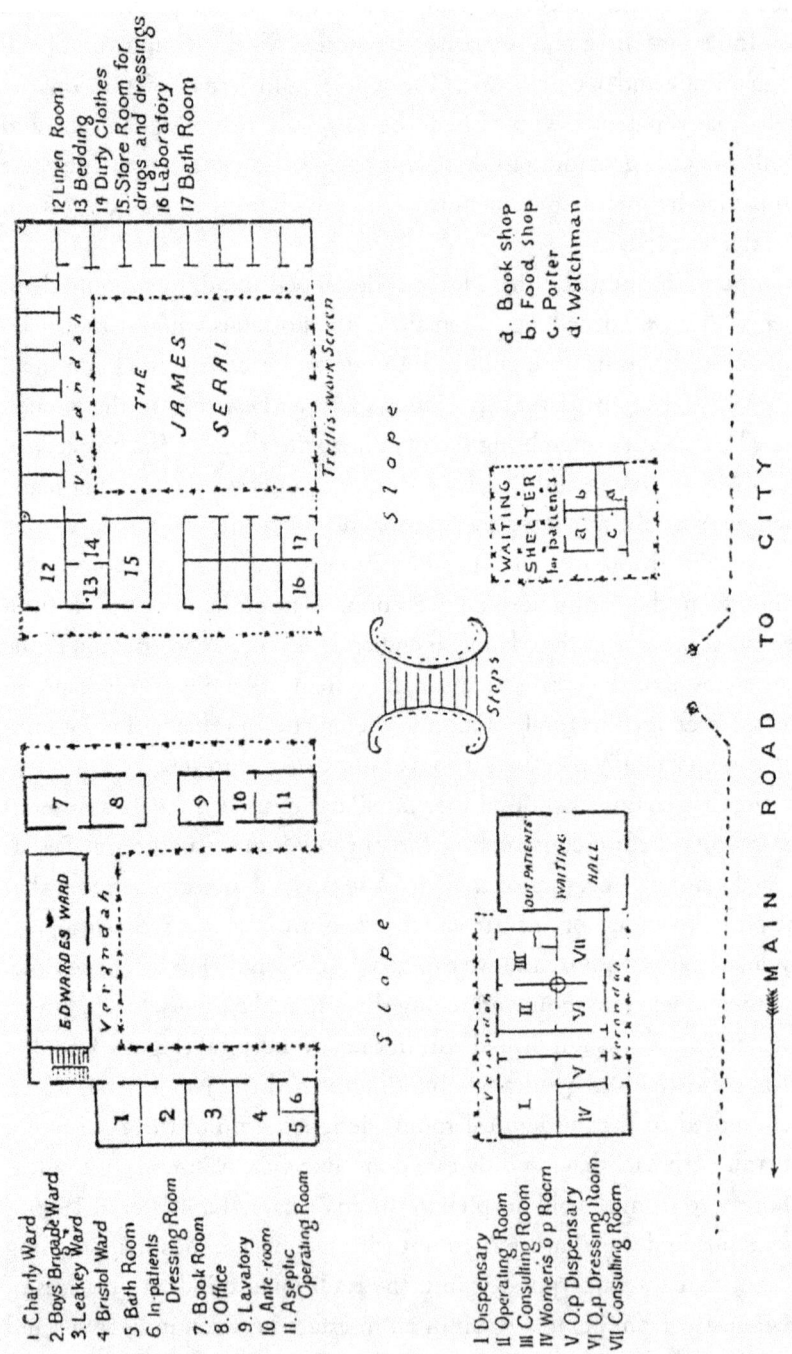

Figure 3.3 Plan of the new hospital at Peshawar.
CMS/M/EL 2/10, p. 238, Church Missionary Society Archive, Cadbury Research Library, Special Collections, University of Birmingham.

that had been associated with the region for centuries.[94] The serai hospital was not a product of an 'experiment' either, or a desire to test new ideas impossible to implement in Britain.[95] In designing the serai hospital, the missionaries disregarded their medical opinions to cultivate trust or friendship. The serai system complicates the dynamic regarding how far missionaries (consciously or otherwise) imposed dominant forms of Western culture on indigenous people.

Instead of just accepting the patient, missionaries placed one of the rooms of the serai at the disposal of the entire family. For example, when a father and mother brought a son or daughter from a village, perhaps 100 miles away, and two or three other children, missionaries took the entire family and 'put them into one of the rooms of the serai by themselves'.[96] In 1911, Dr R. J. H. Cox wrote about a woman who came to the hospital after a 'four days' journey from Bajour over the hills and far away on the north'. After explaining her case, Cox stated 'we put her up in our serai which is specially meant for trans-frontier families'.[97] A similar case was reported in 1907, when a father and a mother brought 'their little girl of six all the way from Kabul for treatment'.[98] The missionaries observed that the presence of these close associates could be irksome, but that this arrangement could 'disarm his [patients'] suspicions, whilst at the same time it brings very many more individuals under the influence of our teaching' was asserted in a pamphlet about the hospital.[99] This quote shows once more that the missionaries' prime concern was the number of patients, even if that meant they had to turn their attention from medical concerns of the time. As a 1908 report on the hospital reveals, missionaries were conscious about how the patients would perceive the hospital architecture: '[h]ow would the people regard the new hospital?' wrote Lankester. After asking this question, he assured the readers that 'the new hospital is popular' while reminding them that 'they [missionaries] were careful to not carry their foreign ideas too far' by referring to the James Serai: 'in the *Serai* portion of our hospital especially, our rough trans-frontier patients, with their families, can come and live under conditions not remotely different from those at their homes.'[100] This report indicates that the design of the James Serai involved thinking thoroughly about the requirements of certain patients and how they could preserve their way of living while in

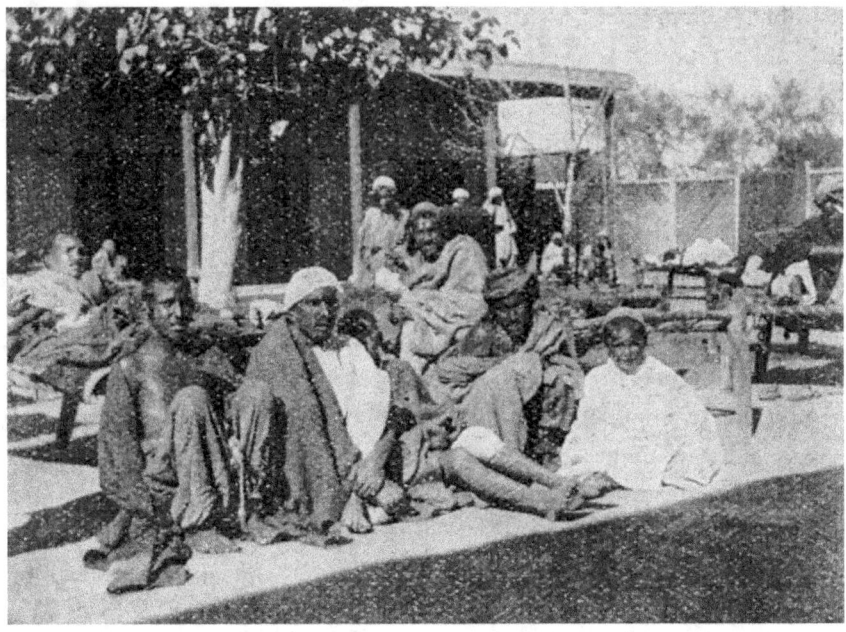

Figure 3.4 The James Serai.
CMS/M/EL 2/14, p. 173, Church Missionary Society Archive, Cadbury Research Library, Special Collections, University of Birmingham.

the hospital because there were fears that they would avoid coming to and staying in the hospital otherwise.

A photograph of the James Serai (Figure 3.4) is worthy of consideration, especially if compared with a painting of a caravanserai in Peshawar (Figure 3.5). While this painting might have been refined to illustrate the supposedly crowded and 'unsanitary' status of a caravanserai, it points to how the James Serai echoed a caravanserai not only in planning but also in the way people inhabited it. The James Serai also mimicked the adapted caravanserais in terms of construction method and materiality (as far as photographs reveal) (Figures 3.6 and 3.7), yet understanding how patients perceived the serai building requires an examination of their past experiences. As mentioned in Chapter One, the emotional charges of a caravanserai could lapse with the building being used for a hospital. Meanwhile, patients who had been to the three caravanserais were already aware of the changed circumstances and might have been able to attach certain meanings to the serai

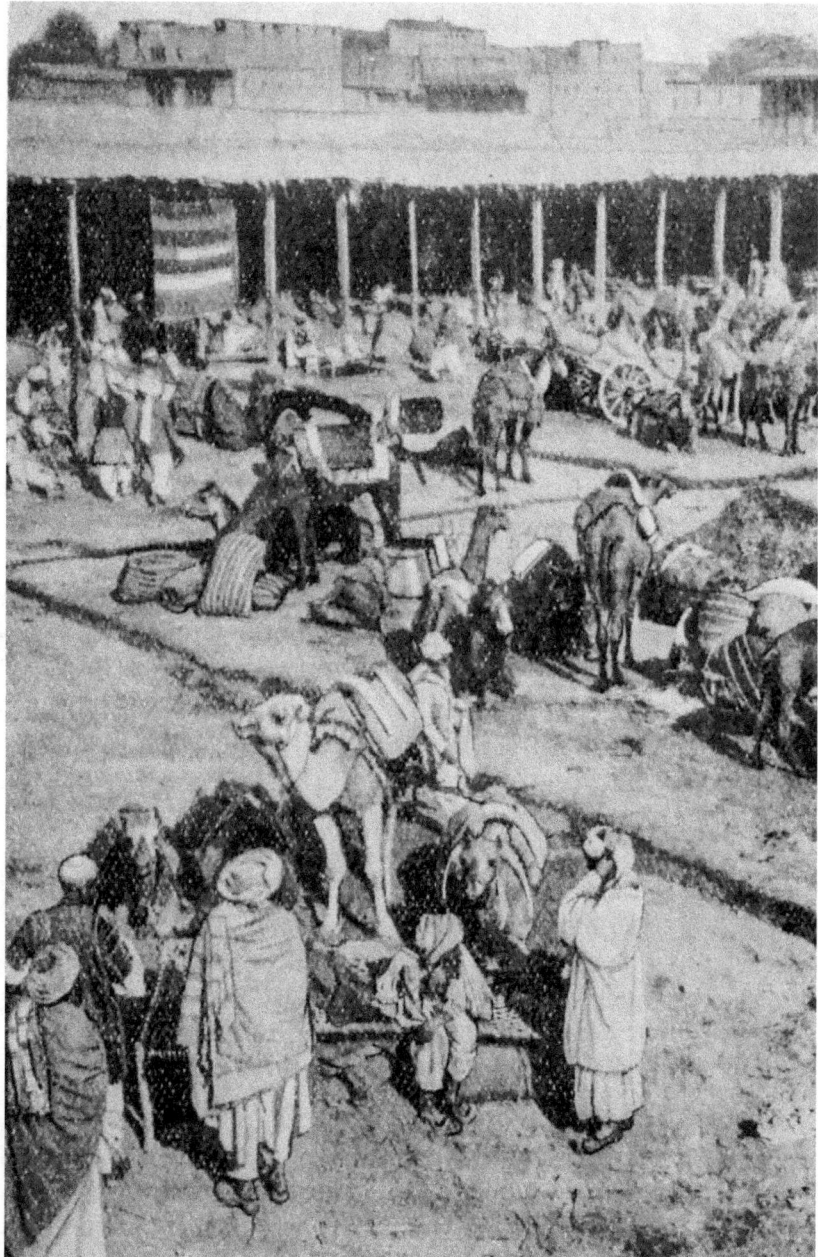

Figure 3.5 A caravanserai at Peshawar.
CMS/M/EL 2/20, p. 39, Church Missionary Society Archive, Cadbury Research Library, Special Collections, University of Birmingham.

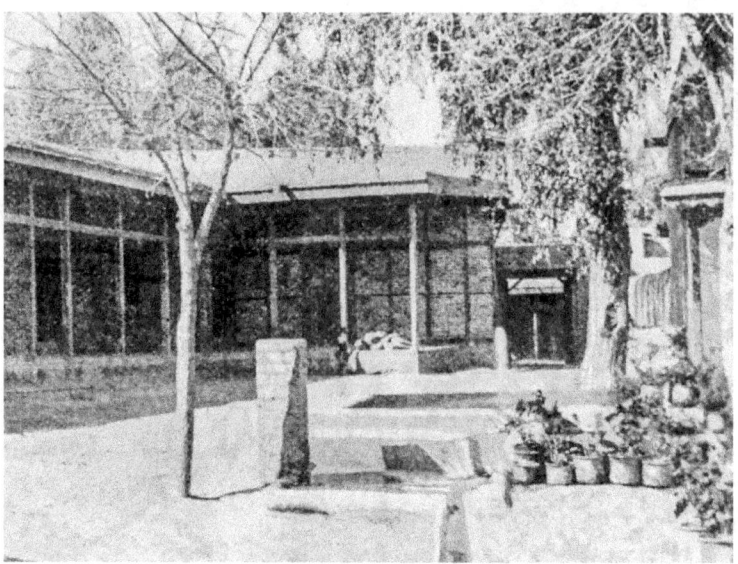

Figure 3.6 The inpatient building in adapted caravanserais.
CMS/M/EL2/2, p. 138, Church Missionary Society Archive, Cadbury Research Library, Special Collections, University of Birmingham.

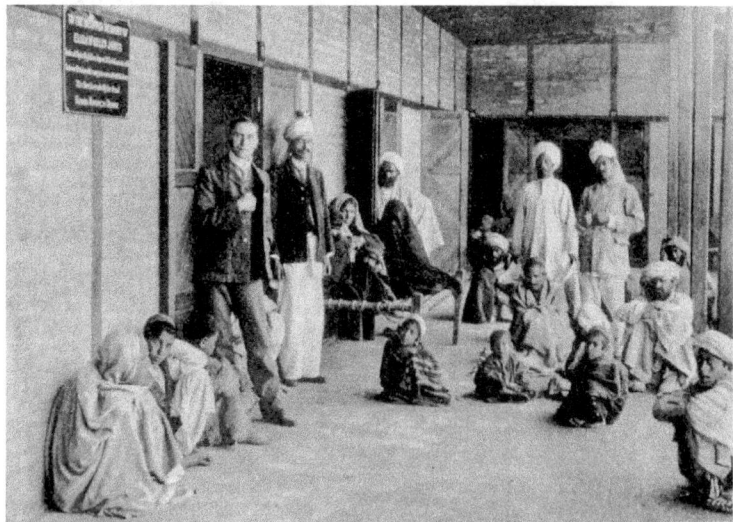

Figure 3.7 The veranda of the inpatient serai, Peshawar hospital.
CMS/M/EL 2/10, p 336, Church Missionary Society Archive, Cadbury Research Library, Special Collections, University of Birmingham.

hospital. Certainly though, the serai hospital disrupted the discursive split between 'civilised' and 'uncivilised', or 'ideal' and 'decadent' family, in missionary writing.[101] As Esme Cleall states, the family was a site for negotiating 'otherness'; that is, missionaries differentiated 'European' family from the indigenous family, considering one to be ideal and benevolent, and the other as decadent, or even non-existent, thus in need of intervention or construction. However, 'the production of a difference was always fragile, always ambivalent and always unstable' and there were multiple points of overlap and intersection.[102] Although the CMS missionaries perceive indigenous families with concern, they hoped to bring family members under the locus of their project of intervention in this way.

In his speech at the annual meeting of the MMA in 1912, Lankester pointed to the serai hospital as one of the 'needs of the N. W. Frontier',[103] indicating that by this time the design of hospitals according to the caravanserai model had become a system of hospital architecture in north-western British India (Figures 3.8, 3.9 and 3.10).[104] Besides attaching a regional weight to the serai hospital, Lankester's speech brought this type of hospital planning to the attention of other missionaries. Lankester also talked about this system in his 1905 speech at the annual meeting of the MMA.[105] Moreover, as shown earlier, missionaries, including missionaries of other denominations, sometimes toured medical missions.[106] These events and activities gave prominence to the serai hospital. Lankester claimed in his 1905 speech that the serai system had become known 'all over the country [Britain]'.[107] Whether true or not, the 'Indian block', added to the Mengo hospital in Uganda in 1915, highlights that the serai hospital at least became known in other mission fields. This block, which was built for the remaining Sikhs recruited to develop the Ugandan Railway project in the later years of the nineteenth century,[108] consisted of several small rooms, but it did not have a courtyard.

The 'Indian block' can serve as an important case study for understanding missionaries' stance on 'Indian colonisation' of East Africa.[109] An examination of the events that led to the construction of this block might also reveal important new links between British India and East Africa. However, these considerations do not explain why the missionaries copied this model instead of other types. The idea of the serai hospital was also replicated in

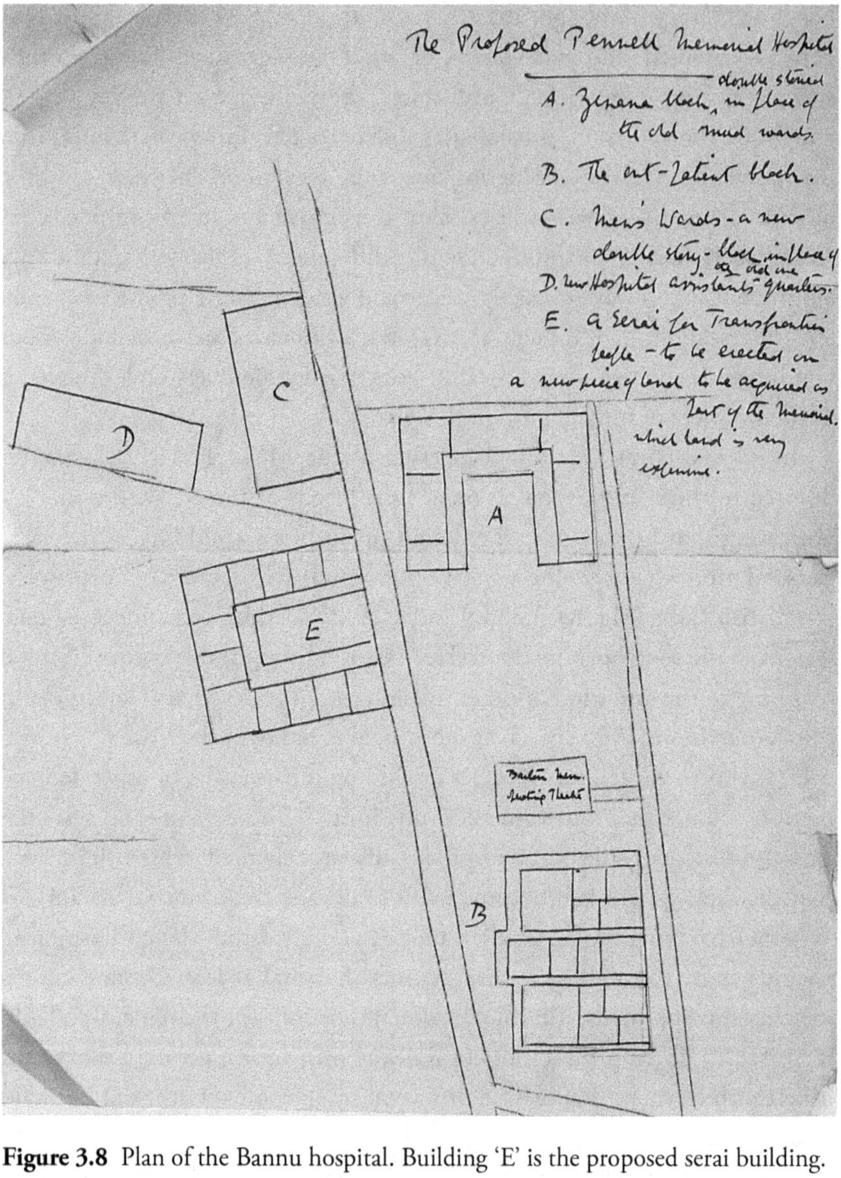

Figure 3.8 Plan of the Bannu hospital. Building 'E' is the proposed serai building. CMS/M/FL 1/I 2/8, Church Missionary Society Archive, Cadbury Research Library, Special Collections, University of Birmingham.

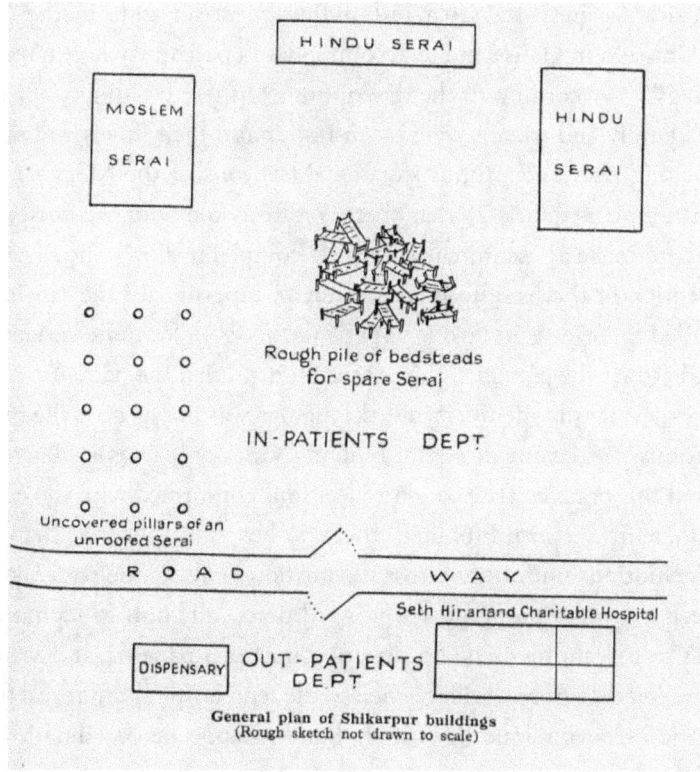

Figure 3.9 Rough plan of the Seth Hiranand inpatient serais.
CMS/M/EL 2/40 p. 77, Church Missionary Society Archive, Cadbury Research Library, Special Collections, University of Birmingham.

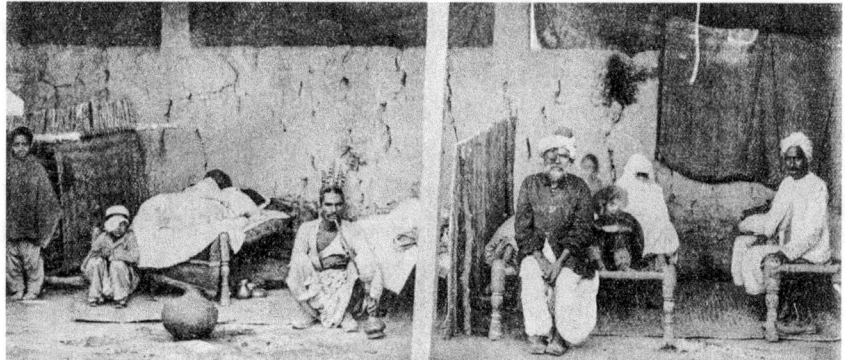

Figure 3.10 Two cubicles in the inpatient department in the Seth Hiranand hospital.
CMS/M/EL 2/14, p. 147, Church Missionary Society Archive, Cadbury Research Library, Special Collections, University of Birmingham.

West Africa, where three separate buildings were set aside in the Gierku medical mission in Hausaland to accommodate a patient's 'whole family and belongings'.[110] According to the descriptions of these buildings, not only a patient's family and friends were taken in but also their 'fowls and goats'[111] and 'cooking pots and primus stove'.[112] Ms Lyons of the Mengo medical mission complained in 1928 that 'there is scarcely room for the doctor when he comes to make an examination'.[113] Her complaint shows once again that the invention of the serai hospital was not an experiment; The missionaries disregarded their ideas in favour of patients' needs to facilitate certain practices and attract the patients. This means, in turn, that the patients' decision to bring their family members and belongings was not against the grain of expectations; the layout of a serai building was key here as it allowed and facilitated this practice. The patients' decisions conformed with the expectations inherent in a serai building. The serai hospital could not shape local people's emotions uniformly across the mission fields. Some patients might have been able to appropriate a serai ward practically but, to rephrase Sara Ahmed's words, another serai hospital or some other patients, and 'we might even have another story'.[114] Nevertheless, the serai hospital can reveal further information – beyond questions about building appearance, climatic conditions and sanitary concerns – as to why the pavilion plan was not always privileged. The serai hospital was a strategy for gaining patients' trust or affection – or for evoking the interest of the people.

Conclusion

Visiting mission hospitals involved the coming and going of local people, European residents and explorers, British administrators and patients' family and friends. According to published reports of missionaries, local people only had a chance to visit the hospitals at the opening ceremonies, which were occasions for garnering interest and bringing people into a more unified emotional community with missionaries. Other public members, such as British residents or fellow missionaries, visited the hospitals beyond opening ceremonies largely for financial gains. Their reports referred to the potential benefits of these visits for boosting patients' morale, yet they were aimed at a 'home' audience to raise money. British officials and local chiefs were among the main home visitors who contributed to the management of the hospitals by way of donation. Home visitors to mission hospitals also included audience or readers at home. Although they did not visit the hospitals physically, they could 'walk through' the hospitals by reading published reports or attending exhibitions.

Neither of these groups was regular visitors to mission hospitals; The family and friends of the patients regularly crossed the walls of the hospitals. Although historians of the mission argue that family members were permitted inside the walls of the hospitals merely due to the lack of nursing staff, three points demonstrate otherwise. Firstly, close associates included not only immediate family members and friends but also servants, children and pupils. Secondly, their number sometimes exceeded that of the patients. Thirdly, and most importantly, missionaries developed an architectural solution to accommodate patients with their family members known as the serai system. A serai hospital was designed similarly to a caravanserai for traveller patients and their family and friends. It gained currency with the construction of the Peshawar hospital and was used in other hospitals thereafter. Importantly, this system was transferred to Uganda and Nigeria.

Notes

1. Graham Mooney and Jonathan Reinarz, 'Hospital and Asylum Visiting in Historical Perspectives: Themes and Issues', in Graham Mooney and Jonathan Reinarz (eds), *Permeable Walls: Historical Perspectives on Hospital and Asylum Visiting* (Amsterdam and New York: Rodopi, 2009), 8.
2. Eleanor Abdella Doumato, 'An "Extra Legible Illustration" of the Christian Faith: Medicine, medical ethics and missionaries in the Arabian Gulf', *Islam and Christian-Muslim Relations* 13, no. 4 (2002): 385
3. Mooney and Reinarz, 'Hospital and Asylum Visiting in Historical Perspectives', 9.
4. Jonathan Reinarz, 'Receiving the Rich, Rejecting the Poor: Towards a History of Hospital Visiting in Nineteenth-century Provisional England', in *Permeable Walls* (see note 1), 31.
5. Jane L. Stevens Crawshaw has since briefly examined this topic in relation to plague hospitals in early modern Venice. See Jane L. Stevens Crawshaw, *Plague Hospitals: Public Health for the City in Early Modern Venice* (Farnham: Ashgate, 2012), 147–9; see also Jane L. Stevens Crawshaw, Irena Benyovsky Latin and Kathleen Vongsathorn (eds), *Tracing Hospital Boundaries: Integration and Segregation in Southeastern Europe and Beyond, 1050–1970* (Leiden and Boston: Brill, 2020).

6. Catharine Coleborne, *Madness in the Family: Insanity and Institutions in the Australasian Colonial World, 1860–1914* (Basingsroke: Palgrave Macmillan, 2010); James H. Mills and Sanjeev Jain, '"A Disgrace to a Civilised Community": Colonial Psychiatry and the Visit of Edward Mapother to South Asia, 1937–8', in *Permeable Walls* (see note 1), 223–42.
7. Mooney and Reinarz, 'Hospital and Asylum Visiting in Historical Perspectives', 11.
8. Michelle Renshaw, '"Family-Centred Care" in American Hospitals in Late-Qing China', in *Permeable Walls* (see note 1), 58.
9. Kevin Siena, 'Stage-Managing a Hospital in the Eighteenth Century: Visitation at the London Lock Hospital', in *Permeable Walls* (see note 1), 183–5.
10. Renshaw, '"Family-Centred Care" in American Hospitals in Late-Qing China', 58.
11. Ibid., 61.
12. Mooney and Reinarz, 'Hospital and Asylum Visiting in Historical Perspectives', 8.
13. Ibid., 9.
14. Mrs A. Lankester, 'The New Hospital at Peshawar', *Mercy and Truth* 10, no. 113 (May 1906): 145.
15. Dr Heywood, 'The New Hospital at Dera Ismail Khan', *Mercy and Truth* 7, no. 75 (March 1903): 81.
16. 'Ten thousands of people trooped through the new isolation hospitals in Oldham, Nottingham, and Edinburgh for their openings in the 1870s, 1890s and 1900s respectively, . . .', Mooney and Reinarz, 'Hospital and Visiting in Historical Perspectives', 14.
17. Mark Seymour, 'Emotional Arenas: From Provincial Circus to National Courtroom in Late Nineteenth-century Italy', *Rethinking History: The Journal of Theory and Practice* 16, no. 2 (2012): 177–97.
18. D. W. Carr, 'Progress in Persia', *Mercy and Truth* 9, no. 103 (July 1905): 209.
19. Harjot Oberoi, *The Construction of Religious Boundaries: Culture, Identity, and Diversity in the Sikh Tradition* (Chicago: The University of Chicago Press, 1994), 139–203.
20. Miss E. Sykes, 'The Hospital at Kerman', *Mercy and Truth* 8, no. 85 (January 1904): 16–18.
21. 'Items: Home and Foreign', *Mercy and Truth* 5, no. 52 (April 1901): 76.
22. Miss Finney, 'A Visit to the Hospital in Amritsar', *Mercy and Truth* 9, no. 105 (1905): 280.
23. Miss Wauton, 'A Visit to the Hospital; Amritsar', *Mercy and Truth* 7, no. 83 (November 1903): 340.
24. A. R. Cavalier, *In Northern India: A Story of Mission Work in Zenanas, Hospitals, Schools and Villages* (London: S. W. Partridge, 1899), 98.

25. Mooney and Reinarz, 'Hospital and Asylum Visiting', 14.
26. Wauton, 'A Visit to the Hospital; Amritsar', 340.
27. Finney, 'A Visit to the Hospital in Amritsar', 280–3.
28. 'Items: Home and Foreign', *Mercy and Truth* 6, no. 62 (February 1902): 36.
29. For example, see how the UMCA chapel in Chinisas village (Malawi) was altered: G. A. Bremner, 'The Architecture of the Universities' Mission to Central Africa: Developing a Vernacular Tradition in the Anglican Mission Field, 1861–1909', *Journal of the Society of Architectural Historians* 68, no. 4 (2009): 218.
30. E. Goffman, *Asylums: Essays on the Social Situation of Mental Patients and Other Inmates* (Chicago: Aldine, 1962).
31. Mooney and Reinarz, 'Hospital and Asylum Visiting', 15.
32. Ibid., 17.
33. Jennifer Scarce, 'Isabella Bird Bishop (1831–1904) and her Travels in Persia and Kurdistan in 1890', *Iranian Studies* 44, no. 2 (2011): 244.
34. 'A Traveller's Testimony', *Mercy and Truth* 1, no.6 (June 1897): 133.
35. Ibid.
36. 'Home News', *Mercy and Truth* 2, no. 18 (June 1898): 123.
37. Gili Adair, 'The "Feringhi Hakim": medical encounters and colonial ambivalence in Isabella Bird's travels in Japan and Persia', *Studies in Travel Writing* 21, no. 1 (2017): 69.
38. 'John Bishop Memorial Hospital 1902–1935', Minnie Gomery Fonds, P 170, Osler Library of the History of Medicine, McGill Library, McGill University.
39. Jeffrey Cox, *Imperial Fault Lines: Christianity and Colonial Power in India, 1818–1940* (Stanford: Stanford University Press, 2002), 32.
40. C. H. Stilmen, 8 September 1904, CMS/M/C 2/1 4, no. 83, CRL.
41. H. White, 'Five Journeys in Persia', *Mercy and Truth* 5, no. 59 (November 1901): 253; See also H. White, 28 April 1903, CMS/M/C 2/1 4, no. 75, CRL.
42. For 'emotional scripts' see Elizabeth Elbourne, 'A Complicated Pity: Emotion, Missions, and the Conversion Narrative', in Claire McLisky, Daniel Midena and Karen Vallgårda (eds), *Emotions and Christian Missions: Historical Perspective* (Basingstoke: Palgrave Macmillan, 2015), 123–50.
43. Stephen Cummins and Joel Lee, 'Missionaries: False Reverence, Irreverence and the Rethinking of Christian Mission in China and India', in Benno Gammerl, Philipp Nielsen and Margrit Pernau (eds), *Encounters with Emotions: Negotiating Cultural Differences since Early Modernity* (New York and Oxford: berghahn, 2019), 47.
44. Sykes, 'The Hospital at Kerman', 16–18.

45. Wilhelmina Eger, 'A Walk Through the Wards of the Women's Hospital, Multan', *Mercy and Truth* 13, no. 153 (September 1909): 302–5; 'A Walk Through the Wards of A Mission Hospital', *Mercy and Truth* 8, no. 88 (April 1904): 109–11.
46. Steven Maughan, '"Mighty England do good": the major English denominations and organisation for the support of foreign missions in the nineteenth century', in Robert A. Bickers and Rosemary Seton (eds), *Missionary Encounters: Sources and Issues* (Richmond: Curzon Press, 1996), 31.
47. 'Home News', *Mercy and Truth* 2, no. 18 (June 1898): 123; 'Things to be noted', *Mercy and Truth* 2, no. 21 (September 1898): 205–6.
48. Emma Sandon, 'Projecting Africa: two 1920s British travel films', in Elizabeth Hallam and Brian Street (eds), *Cultural Encounters: Representing Otherness* (London and New York: Routledge, 2013), 135.
49. 'Things to be Noted', *Mercy and Truth* 3, no. 30 (June 1899): 121.
50. 'Medical Wants Department', *The Mission Hospital* 29, no. 332 (September 1925): 252.
51. 'Things to be Noted', *Mercy and Truth* 3, no. 29 (May 1899): 98.
52. 'Rules for Medical Sub-Conferences', 4 April 1899, CMS/M/AP 2/1, CRL.
53. Reinarz, 'Receiving the Rich, Rejecting the Poor', 37–8.
54. Arthur Neve, 'A Visit to Dera Ismail Khan', *Mercy and Truth* 7, no. 70 (July 1903): 205–9; Arthur Neve, 'A Visit to Quetta', *Mercy and Truth* 7, no. 76 (April 1903): 109–11; 'Editorial Notes', *Mercy and Truth* 14, no. 161 (May 1910): 129.
55. Arthur Neve, 'Memorandum on the CMS Medical Missions of the Punjab & N.W. Frontier', CMS/M/C 2/1 4, no. 64, CRL.
56. Reinarz, 'Receiving the Rich, Rejecting the Poor', 38–40.
57. John Chircop, 'Management and Therapeutic Regimes in Two Lunatic Asylums in Corfu and Malta, 1837–1870', in Laurinda Abreu and Sally Sheard (eds), *Hospital Life: Theory and Practice from the Medieval to the Modern* (Oxford: Peter Lang, 2013), 179–208.
58. Doumato, 'An "Extra Legible Illustration" of the Christian Faith', 385.
59. John R. Stanley, 'Professionalising the Rural Medical Mission in Weixian, 1890–1925', in David Hardiman (ed.), *Healing Bodies, Saving Souls: Medical Missions in Asia and Africa* (Amsterdam, New York: Rodopi, 2006), 122.
60. David Hardiman, 'Christian Therapy: Medical Missionaries and the Adivasis of Western India, 1880–1930', in *Healing Bodies, Saving Souls* (see note 59), 147.

61. For 1894, see 'Things to be Noted', *Mercy and Truth* 5, no. 49 (January 1901): 2; for 1898, see 'Nurses Working in CMS Hospitals', *Mercy and Truth* 2, no. 24 (December 1898): 281 and 'Things to be Noted', *Mercy and Truth* 3, no. 25 (January 1899): 1.
62. For 1899 see, 'Medical Mission Auxiliary Annual Meeting, May 4th, 1899', *Mercy and Truth* 3, no. 30 (June 1899): 128; Medical Committee Minutes, vol. 1, CMS/M/C1/1 1891–1914, no. 36, CRL.
63. Charles F. Harford to the members of the Medical Committee, 7 December 1911, Medical Committee Minutes, vol. 1, CMS/M C1/1 1891–1914, no. 88, CRL.
64. 'Nurses Working in CMS Hospitals', *Mercy and Truth* 2, no. 24 (1898): 281.
65. A. R. Blackett, 'A Hospital Chaplain', *Mercy and Truth* 2, no. 20 (August 1898): 201.
66. Donald W. Carr, 'Julfa Medical Mission', *Medical Mission Quarterly*, no. XIII (January 1896): 7.
67. Carol Helmstadter and Judith Godden, *Nursing before Nightingale, 1815–1899* (London and New York: Routledge, 2011).
68. T. L. Pennell. 'The Afghan – How Can We Reach them?' *Mercy and Truth* 1, no. 1 (January 1897): 10.
69. Wauton, 'A Visit to the Hospital; Amritsar', 340.
70. Florence M. James, 'Kerman Then and Now', *The Mission Hospital* 42, no. 482 (March 1938): 62.
71. Ibid.
72. 'Punjab and Sindh Mission', *Mercy and Truth* 11, no. 130 (1907): 238.
73. Henry White, 'The Governor of Yezd and His Prisoners', *Mercy and Truth* 14, no. 164 (August 1910): 268.
74. Mooney and Reinarz, 'Hospital and Asylum Visiting in Historical Perspectives', 11.
75. Catherine Ironside, 'Open Doors in Persia', *Mercy and Truth* 20, no. 235 (August 1916): 151.
76. T. L. Pennell, 'The Afghan – How Can We Reach them?' *Mercy and Truth* 1, no. 1 (January 1897): 11.
77. Renshaw, 'Family-Centred Care', 70.
78. E. F. Pennell, 'Some patients at Bannu', *Mercy and Truth* 3, no. 30 (June 1899): 145.
79. Arthur Neve, 'A Day at Kashmir Hospital', *Mercy and Truth* 1, no. 3 (March 1897): 60.
80. Marcus Eustace, 'News from Quetta', *Mercy and Truth* 1, no. 1 (January 1897): 17.

81. Florence M. James, 'Kerman Then and Now', *The Mission Hospital* 42, no. 482 (March 1938): 62.
82. Renshaw, 'Family-Centred Care', 60.
83. Doumato, 'An "Extra Legible Illustration" of the Christian Faith', 385
84. Catherine Ironside, 'In the Women's Hospital, Ispahan', *Mercy and Truth* 19, no. 228 (December 1915): 390.
85. Cynthia Imogen Hammond, 'Reforming Architecture, Defending Empire: Florence Nightingale and the Pavilion Hospital', *Studies in Social Sciences* 38 (2005): 41.
86. Preeti Chopra, *A Joint Enterprise: Indian Elites and the Making of British Bombay* (Minneapolis and London: University of Minnesota Press, 2011), 146–7.
87. Cathy Keys, 'Designing hospitals for Australian conditions: The Australian Inland Mission's cottage hospital, Adelaide House, 1926', *The Journal of Architecture* 21, no. 1 (2016): 83.
88. T. Maxwell, 'The Opening of the Door in Kashmir, 1873–1876', *Mercy and Truth* 1, no. 9 (September 1897): 201.
89. 'The Kashmir Medical Mission', *The Church Missionary Gleaner* (1876): 26.
90. 'What Others are Doing and Saying', *Mercy and Truth* 58, no. 5 (October 1901): 223
91. Copy of letter from Dr T. L. Pennell dated 10 May 1904, group 2, no. 257, CMS/M/FL 1/I 2 4, CRL.
92. 'Medical Mission Auxiliary Annual Meeting, May 4th, 1899', *Mercy and Truth* 3, no. 30 (June 1899): 143.
93. A. Lankester, 24 August 1904, CMS/M/C 2/1 4, no. 135, CRL.
94. For a study of the interface between indigenous and imported ways of building, see Mark Crinson, *Empire Building: Orientalism and Victorian Architecture* (London and New York: Routledge, 2013).
95. This line of enquiry show how new ideas were often adopted more quickly beyond Europe due to the lack of monitoring. For one of the earliest studies in this regard, see Gwendolyn Wright, *The Politics of Design in French Colonial Urbanism* (Chicago: The University of Chicago Press, 1991).
96. A. Lankester, 'The Needs of the N. W. Frontier', *Mercy and Truth* 16, no. 189 (1912): 299.
97. R. J. H. Cox, 'More Notes from Peshawar', *Mercy and Truth* 15, no. (1911): 268–9.
98. Mrs A. Lankester, 'A letter from Peshawar', *Mercy and Truth* 11, no. 127 (July 1907): 211.

99. 'Peshawar Medical Missions', 1904, CMS/M/FL 1/I 7, CRL.
100. 'A Frontier Hospital: Peshawar Medical Mission of the Church Missionary Society', CMS/ACC 7/O 10, CRL.
101. Several historians, such as Patrishia Grimshaw and Esme Cleall, have examined the importance of 'family', broadly defined, for missionaries. See Patricia Grimshaw, 'Faith, Missionary Life, and the Family', in Philippa Levine (ed.), *Gender and Empire* (Oxford: Oxford University Press, 2007), 260–80; Esme Cleall, *Missionary Discourses of Difference: Negotiating Otherness in the British Empire, 1840–1900* (Basingstoke: Palgrave Mcmillan, 2012), 25–73.
102. Cleall, *Missionary Discourses of Difference*, 48–9.
103. A. Lankester, 'The Needs of the N. W. Frontier', *Mercy and Truth* 16, no. 189 (1912): 297.
104. The hospitals at Quetta, Bannu and Multan all had a serai building or family wards. See 'Items: Home and Foreign', *Mercy and Truth* 13, no. 146 (1909): 38; R. J. H. Cox, 2 June 1912, no. 110, CMS/M/C2 1/10 1912–1914, CRL.
105. 'The Annual Meeting', *Preaching and Healing: The Report of the CMS Medical Mission Auxiliary for 1905–1906* (1906): 23–6.
106. For example, see Cavalier, *In Northern India*.
107. 'The Annual Meeting', *Preaching and Healing* (see note no. 105): 24.
108. Darshan Singh Tatla, 'Sikh free and military migration during the colonial period', in Robin Cohen (ed.), *The Cambridge Survey of World Migration* (Cambridge: Cambridge University Press, 1995), 71.
109. Thomas R. Metcalf, *Imperial Connections: India in the Indian Ocean Arena, 1860–1920* (Berkeley: University of California Press, 2007), 165–203.
110. 'Keswick Convention Medical Mission Meeting', *Mercy and Truth* 9, no. 106 (October 1905): 296.
111. Ibid.
112. Miss S. Lyon, 'Glimpses of Work at Mengo Hospital', *The Mission Hospital* 32, no. 369 (1928): 272.
113. Ibid.
114. Sara Ahmed, *The Cultural Politics of Emotions* (Edinburgh: Edinburgh University Press, 2004), 7.

4

FEMALE MISSIONARIES AND THE ARCHITECTURE OF WOMEN'S HOSPITALS

I started the Introduction with the story of the Kashmir medical mission. To recall: it tells that Reverend Robert Clark and his wife, Elizabeth Mary Browne, visited Kashmir to find an 'opening' for evangelistic work in 1864. They were greeted with 'opposition', yet Mrs Clark opened a dispensary which 'was largely attended', and this signified the need for a medical mission. This story demonstrates the centrality of Mrs Clark to the foundation of the Kashmir hospital and the history of medical mission work more generally. In 1904, Robert Clark even acknowledged that his wife's dispensary 'was the commencement of the present Kashmir Medical Mission'.[1] However, missionary publications credited Dr William Jackson Elmslie as the founder of the Kashmir hospital. Some thirty years later, Dr Henry White of the Yazd medical mission recognised Dr George Dodson as the sole designer of the Kerman hospital, disregarding the involvement of Dr Winifred Westlake completely. While the work of female missionaries like Mrs Clark and Westlake was acknowledged in mission accounts, the history of missions was written in a way as though male missionaries were the solo actors. These cases recall Jeffrey Cox's statement that 'interpreting missionary records requires constant attention to the multiple levels of exclusion in the narratives'.[2]

This chapter builds on works of feminist scholars and historians of missionary women.[3] It highlights some of the different ways female missionaries were active agents in Persia and British India. It provides information about several female missionaries whose names and activities have remained unknown in scholarship. Moreover, it demonstrates that there was more to female missionary work than most scholarship has recognised. More specifically, it argues that women's work in mission should include their involvement in the construction of the hospitals (and mission buildings more generally). Female missionaries were not only educators, doctors, nurses, traveller writers and collectors but were also 'amateur' architects.[4] It also shows that scholarship on women and architecture in the late nineteenth and early twentieth centuries should include women who set sail for different countries across the British Empire. Their inclusion deepens our understanding of the relationship between women and the material and spatial environment. According to Lynne Walker, houses and churches were two building types that were 'thought appropriate for women to design' in the nineteenth century.[5] In contrast, I illuminate that many female missionaries designed not only houses and churches but also hospitals.[6] They contributed to the built environment by drawing plans, supervising building construction and renovating existing buildings solely and jointly with their male colleagues.

It is essential to examine the architecture of mission hospitals for women to understand how missionaries sought to change their sensory relationship with local people through architecture. As noted in the Introduction, there were differences in how building trust was understood and practised based on the missionaries' gender, national affiliation and the country they worked in. In particular, building trust concerned female missionaries in a different way and quality than male missionaries.[7] While coming into close contact with indigenous people was relevant to both male and female missionaries, it took on an extra shape for female missionaries in the form of 'familial connections' or 'sisterhood' with (potential) converts.[8] Thus, mission hospitals for women played a crucial role in changing the sensory relationship between missionaries and the local people, resulting in a new architectural solution known as the 'purdah hospital'. This type is another indication of why there were a variety of hospitals with diverse spatial and material forms and arrangements across the mission fields. It also shows the extent to which missionaries disregarded their ideas to cultivate trust. Like the serai system, the purdah hospital was a place where the boundaries between missionaries and local women were intentionally breached.

Women in Mission in the Nineteenth Century

Mrs Clark belonged to the 'helpmates' or 'helpmeet' phase of female missionary activity abroad when missionary societies accepted women mainly as wives.[9] This phase, as Emily Manktelow notes, 'was not an assumed presence in the missionary endeavour, but rather grew out of early mission experience'.[10] Eighteenth- and nineteenth-century Protestant missionary enterprise was predominantly male-orientated. While missionary organisations occasionally sent married men to the mission field, the early conceptualisation of mission masculinity had as little room for the personal as mission femininity had for the professional. There were also practical considerations; missionary wives, and missionary families, were viewed as a setback for the evangelical missionary movement because they could increase costs and distract male missionaries from their spiritual work. Some missionary societies, such as the LMS, even initially encouraged intermarriage. The CMS introduced a period of celibacy to measure 'altruism and character building'.[11] A force for change emerged from concerns over religiously mixed marriages – single missionary men marrying 'heathen' women.[12] Missionary societies reacted and changed their position. Missionary wives gradually surfaced as a source of moral support, protection and comfort for male missionaries.[13] But changing policies as regards missionary children and widows, and thus integrating missionary families into the mission field as a practical necessity, would take several decades.[14] At the time of Mrs Clark's marriage to Reverend Clark, missionary couples had become the primary mission agents within mission enterprise, but not everywhere. In some places, such as Madagascar and Uganda, the missionary family only took root in the final decades of the nineteenth century due to practical and safety reasons. It was only after the formation of the Uganda Protectorate in 1895 that the CMS permitted male missionaries to take wives with them.[15]

Mrs Clark's career is not as well known as the career of some other missionary wives, such as Ann Hamilton, the wife of the LMS missionary, Robert Hamilton of the Kuruman mission (South Africa). It is not my intention to examine her career in detail.[16] Instead, I aim to highlight the multi-layered nature of female professionalism within the mission circles in the first half of the nineteenth century by drawing on her career and a few other female medical missionaries. Although the involvement of female missionaries, such as Mrs Clark and Westlake, was not adequately acknowledged, this was not always the case. Seeing gender as central to understanding the complexities at work does not mean that it had the same influence in all mission stations. As Phillipa Levine states, '[o]ne of the lessons of feminist history has been about the dangers of too readily assuming that group identification always works: that all men, for example, opposed greater female participation in the public sphere or liked to play sports.'[17] According to Robert Clark's biography, '[t]he causes of mission . . . appealed powerfully to [Mrs Clark's (Miss Browne)] heart'. Like Hamilton, she may have viewed 'her marriage as a means to missionary activity'.[18] However, the early nineteenth-century missionary enterprise was not entirely a 'male noun'. Independent female missionary agency was possible.[19] Female-led societies, including the Ladies' Female Education Society and the Society for Promoting Female Education in China, India and the East (FES), sent many single women to the mission field in the first half of the nineteenth century, whose work as educators was even reported in several journal and books and was hence visible to the public in Britain.[20] Moreover, some missionary societies recruited single women as missionaries in the first half of the nineteenth century. For example, the CMS began to recruit single women on their own right before the establishment of the female-led societies, and there were names of single women in the CMS's *Register of Missionaries* published in the 1820s.[21]

Neither did all missionary wives played subordinate roles. The primary role of a missionary wife was breeding and housekeeping,[22] yet there were missionary wives, if only a handful, who went against this 'patriarchal structure' of missions by venturing beyond the boundaries of the domestic sphere and publicising domestic Christian culture or, like Mrs Clark, offering basic educational and medical work to local women and children.[23] Others were able to bring a sense of vocation and service to their domestic activities.[24] While these women were not paid, their actions did not go unnoticed, as evident from their memoirs. Written often by the missionary husbands, these memoirs 'celebrated missionary wives as female missionaries'.[25] They trouble the use of the salaried/unpaid ancillary work binary in describing the role of missionary wives in the middle decades of the nineteenth century.[26]

At the very least, efforts of early female missionaries demonstrated their accessibility to spaces otherwise closed to missionaries' religious influences, such as the exclusively female quarters of houses in British India and Persia. As a result, the second half of the nineteenth century brought the rhetoric of 'women's work among women'. This rhetoric remained the slogan of women's missionary endeavours until the First World War.[27] An increasing number of single women were accepted as missionaries on their own rights, initially as teachers and then as medical doctors and nurses in the last two decades of the nineteenth century. They also participated and delivered speeches at mission conferences.[28] By 1888, the number of European and North American female missionaries was 1,000. This number grew to 10,735 by 1910.[29] A trend that grew out of concerns over the morality of male missionaries and the exploitation of the fault lines of evangelical ideology by female missionaries became about the 'gendered needs of "heathen" women' and eventually the civilising role of female missionaries by the late nineteenth century.[30] Indeed, mission societies reframed their gender norms in such a way that they no longer projected marriage and vocation as two different aspects of the same evangelistic work.[31]

It would take almost thirty years from the departure of Mrs Clark to British India for the CMS to recruit a female missionary doctor. As we already know, the CMS was slow to adopt medical work. While some missionary societies, such as the LMS, sent female medical missionaries to the field in the 1880s,[32] the CMS recruited its first female medical missionary in 1895: Henrietta Cornford. Cornford took the degree of Doctor of Medicine in Brussels and attained the LRCS and LRCP (Edin.) diplomas.[33] After her, the Society recruited Miss Emmeline Stuart, a graduate of the University of Glasgow, and Mrs S. Synge, a graduate of the University of Brussels. Of forty-eight medical missionaries the CMS accepted between 1865 and 1897, only three were women. Nevertheless, the CMS's 'sister societies' sent medical doctors in the 1880s. A note in 1892 stated, 'the medical work of the Church Missionary Society is thus supplemented by that of the two sister societies [CEZMS and Indian Female Normal School Society (IFNS)], and the bond between the three is a close one.'[34]

Only Stuart's life and career have been studied among the first three female medical missionaries of the CMS. Scholarship on mission work in British India and Persia has also examined the life and career of the following female missionaries: Fidelia Fiske, the first female educator who worked in the 'Nestorian

Mission' in 1843–57[35] and was highly regarded for establishing a popular girl's school and securing many converts;[36] Dr Clara Swin, the first female medical doctor that was sent from the US to British India by the Methodist Women's Foreign Missionary Society (WFMS);[37] Fanny Butler who set sail for British India under the auspices of the CEZMS; Mary Bird, whose contribution to medical work at Isfahan granted her the status of the first female medical missionary to Persia;[38] and Alice M. Sorabji Pennell of the Punjab mission.[39] Cornford has entirely remained unknown in scholarship, perhaps because she stayed in Old Cairo for a short period of seven or eight months and left the mission in August 1896.[40] The CMS required female missionaries to wait at least one year before marrying and, like Miss K. Potter of the Uganda mission, Henrietta may have married without permission and thus been discharged from the Society.[41]

Cornford is unknown mainly because the focus of scholarship has been primarily on female medical missionaries in British India. British India was the locus of female missionary doctors, yet the first medical missionaries of the CMS were appointed to Egypt, Persia and China, respectively.[42] On 11 July 1899, the General Committee of the CMS approved a scheme whereby they took over much of the work and workers of the FES. Among the mission work and female missionaries thus transferred was the Multan Medical Mission and Dr Winifred Eger, who became the first female medical missionary of the Society in north-western British India.[43] After Eger, the CMS accepted Dr Minnie Gomery as a medical missionary in December 1900. As I will explain below, she established the Islamabad medical mission.[44] The CMS sent more female medical missionaries to Persia in the 1900s than it sent to north-western British India: after Bird and Stuart, the following female doctors arrived in quick succession: Dr Urania Latham in 1898, Dr Elsie Taylor in 1902, Dr Winfred Westlake in 1903[45] and Dr L. Molony and Dr Catherine Ironside in 1904. These five women were to be the only female doctors in the Persia Mission until 1910 when Dr Alicia P. Aldous arrived in the country.[46] In Egypt, Mrs MacInnes (who was a sister of Dr Carr of the Isfahan hospital and qualified doctor) succeeded Cornford in 1899 and worked single-handedly. No female medical doctors were sent to work in Palestine and Turkish-Arabia Missions until the mid-1900s. To put it another way, north-western British India and Persia became the focal point of the CMS female doctors' ambition in the Muslim world in the late nineteenth and early twentieth centuries.

These instances show that female missionaries participated in the mission in diverse ways. They used their home activities as examples, worked as single teachers, and joined missions as doctors and nurses. Notwithstanding the ability of women to navigate structures of patriarchy, as stated by Rhonda Anne Sample, 'women's labour in Christian missions, as in the secular British Empire and domestic society, remained undervalued in terms of both remuneration and administrative advancement, until well into the twentieth century.'[47] Mrs Clark is an exemplary instance of female exclusion from official mission histories. Mrs Clark was a hospital worker (a sister of St John at King's College Hospital) before marrying Reverend Clark in 1858. Moreover, her father was a medical doctor, Dr Robert Browne, who had worked in Calcutta for forty-five years.[48] She was also instrumental in the foundation of the CEZMS hospital in Amritsar, which was known as the St Catherine Hospital.[49] The implication is that she administered medicine or accompanied Reverend Clark not merely because of her access to the zenana but because of her medical knowledge. Yet, the CMS publications deny her any role. In 1939, the CMS medical magazine, *The Mission Hospital*, published an article entitled 'CMS Medical Missions: Our Yesterdays'. After stating that the medical work of the CMS is focused in 'seventy-seven hospitals, 200 welfare centres, and thirty-three leper colonies', the article asked, 'How did it all begin?' Although it recognised the vision and achievement of 'giant men and women', it only referred to male missionaries when explaining 'the first days'.[50] It especially mentioned Elmslie and Abdul Massih. It even referred to Massih as the first medical missionary of the Society,[51] while failing to recognise Mrs Clark's contribution altogether.

Moreover, the offer of some single women missionaries to work was rejected or resisted. For example, the foreign secretary endorsed Miss Alice Gill's capability to live and work in Duddhi only after she had worked in British India for twenty years.[52] Similarly, there were appeals for opening a medical mission in Shiraz in 1903. Reverend W. A. Rice and Carr both wrote letters stating that 'a lady medical missionary should be sent before a medical man'.[53] However, Bishop Stuart questioned this proposal.[54] Bird also faced opposition from a male colleague and was not an exception. Reverend Arthur Russell Blackett of the Kerman mission was against Bird's work in Kerman.[55] It is telling to note that guidelines for the recruitment and training of women candidates were only formally presented at the Edinburgh Missionary Conference in 1910.[56] Moreover, the CMS accepted women to its General Committee for the first time in 1917.[57] The contribution of female (medical) missionaries to building construction was another excluded area, which I shall address in the next section.

Dr Minnie Gomery and the John Bishop Memorial Hospital

Dr Minnie Gomery is among the female medical missionaries who contributed to building construction. Gomery is a lesser known female missionary of the CMS, and hence it would be helpful first briefly to examine her career. Gomery was born in Birmingham in 1875 and was the third child of Henry Gomery (formerly Gumery) and Sarah Smith. When Minnie was nine years old the family immigrated from England to Canada and, in 1892, they settled in Montréal. Minnie was accepted to study medicine at the Bishop's Medical School two years later, graduating with M.D. in 1898. She was sent to Kashmir in 1900 after theological training at The Willows, one of the CMS's private schools for women.[58] She established the John Bishop Memorial Hospital in Islamabad (Anantnag), where she worked until her retirement in 1935, after which she returned to Kashmir first as a medical missionary for another twelve years and then as a superintendent and teacher at a girl's school until 1953.[59] Overall, she worked in Kashmir for nearly fifty years. In her obituary, E. H. Bensley, the head of the Faculty of Medicine at McGill University, stated the following regarding Minnie's academic record:

> The records of Bishop's Medical School show that she was a superior student. At the close of her first academic session in 1895 she won two prizes, one in botany, the other in practical anatomy. The following year she was awarded the David Silver Medal for the highest marks in the primary examination and the Senior Dissector's Prize. She graduated in 1898, receiving the degree of M.D., C.M. from Bishop's University, and the Wood Gold Medal; this medal was the senior medical undergraduate award given annually to the graduating student who had attained the highest aggregate number of marks in all subjects.[60]

Bensley portrayed Gomery as an excellent medical student. Nevertheless, obituaries were written 'to demonstrate a "good life" and death'.[61] Moreover, referees and mission committees used criteria other than, and as well as, academic excellence to access female candidates.[62] Besides having a class-based attitude, missionary societies evaluated female candidates' commitment to chapel and community, their knowledge of church doctrine and history and their ability to communicate complex ideas and feelings to diverse audiences. The attitude of mission organisations did not change even after the demand for women with university education increased by the late nineteenth century.[63] As Elizabeth Prevost states, mission societies continued to 'place the highest value for missionary success on deeper levels of spirituality and religiosity'.[64] Some mission societies such as the LMS also continued to emphasise 'ladylike' qualities over professional qualifications.[65] Furthermore, professional and familial links, as well as informal church ties, played a crucial role in the recruitment of female candidates.[66] Women in nineteenth-century Britain supported themselves and their institutional efforts through creating informal networks.[67] These networks took on a unique more close-knit characteristic in religious societies. Referees of the candidates to the Scottish Presbyterian did not even feel the need to spell out commitment to chapel and community.[68] Such was the case with Gomery. Her father acted as the British and Foreign Bible Society's secretary from 1892–98 in Montreal and as the Canadian agent of the SPCK from 1898–1900.[69] Meanwhile what drew her to medical mission cause, like many other female missionaries, was a meeting with another missionary (a lady doctor) who was on leave from British India.[70] This meeting convinced her of the employment and career prospects that a missionary career would offer to women independent of metropolitan pressures.[71] At the time of Gomery's graduation, only a few hospitals in Canada would accept female medical graduates and her application to Western Hospital was turned down.[72] This incident made her pursue a medical missionary career.

Upon arrival in British India, Gomery worked in the Kashmir medical mission until March 1902, when she moved to and commenced the John Bishop Memorial Hospital in Islamabad (Anantnag). The hospital was located, according to Gomery, 'just outside the town, having a lovely view over the hidden valley, with grand snowy mountains in the distance'.[73] However, the hospital's origin goes back to the 1880s; it bears the names of several people and connects across nations and continents. The hospital was named after the Scottish doctor, John Bishop, who was the husband of the well-known explorer Isabella Bird. Bishop died eight years after their marriage in 1886, and Bird established the John Bishop Memorial hospital in her husband's name in Kashmir. As mentioned in the previous chapter, before travelling to Kashmir, Bird had at least engaged in medical work in Persia.[74] The hospital also bears Dr Fanny Butler of the CEZMS's name, who acted as the physician in charge of the hospital.[75] A severe flood damaged this hospital in 1891[76] and the John Bishop Memorial hospital in Islamabad took the place of this hospital. Furthermore, a Scottish nurse, Miss C. A. Newnham, accompanied Gomery. Newnham was initially sent to British India by CEZMS and worked in the Kashmir hospital for several years. In 1900, she was transferred to the CMS and accompanied Gomery to Islamabad.[77]

To return to the obituary, Bensley also explained about Gomery's time in Islamabad and her life after retirement but left out her involvement in the construction process of the John Bishop Memorial hospital. This omission mirrors missionary publications, which played down the role of female missionaries in building construction, referring to their involvement, at the very best, only in passing. According to Annmarie Adams, women's role as 'regulators' of household systems 'fitted well with Victorian theories of sexual difference, which claimed that because of the smallness of their brains, women were better at arranging or finishing work started by men rather than initiating the work themselves'.[78] Moreover, as Lynne Walker writes, designing chapels or churches 'reinforced the idea of women's supposedly superior moral and spiritual nature'.[79] These beliefs underwent a change with the acceptance of women as professional architects by the late nineteenth century. But female missionaries, many of whom were not from middle-class backgrounds, were involved in planning, repairing and supervising buildings long before this period. Their range of activities fell outside the contemporary accepted definition of women's capacity. As early as the middle decades of the nineteenth century, Bessie Price, the daughter of the LMS missionary to South Africa, Robert Moffat, lent a hand in repairing buildings when needed.[80] By the late nineteenth century female missionaries were sharing the design of the buildings with their male colleagues. Gomery did not initiate building construction, a task that was left to the

Neve brothers of the Kashmir medical mission, but she designed the buildings with their help. She and Miss Newnham also 'marked out on the site the proposed position of the buildings, according to plans'.[81] Additionally, she looked after the 'plastering, flooring, &c' upon the completion of building construction.[82] Moreover, in a 1902 report, Gomery stated that 'I carefully planned a window for one of our bedrooms'.[83]

Similarly, the houses for the Kerman hospital were repaired and altered based on plans 'drawn up by Drs Griffith and Day and Miss Bird'.[84] Again when the decision was made to build a separate hospital for women in Kerman, Dodson and Westlake drew the plan of the hospital together: 'Enclosing preliminary plan of new women's hospital drawn by himself and Dr Westlake,' wrote Dodson in a letter on 7 June 1904.[85] The female missionaries of the SPG and the ABCFM also left their mark on the architectural landscape. A few examples include Eva Swift of the ABCFM and Jenny C. Muller, Emily Lawrence and Ethel Margaret Phillips of the SPG. After her proposal to establish a training school for Indian women was rejected, Swift raised money and first started a school in a rented room and then purchased land for a purpose-built structure.[86] Muller 'carefully and skilfully planned' St Stephen's hospital in Delhi and the hospital in Karnal.[87] The 1934 report of SPG called her 'the creator St Stephen's Hospital'.[88] Phillips drew the plans of St Agatha's hospital for women in Shandong, China and superintended the construction of the buildings.[89] And Lawrence oversaw the construction of the first medical mission on Madagascar's eastern coast.[90] Their involvement in building design and construction demonstrates, what Prevost has described, the 'highly independent nature of single missionary activity'.[91] Female missionaries were able to escape metropolitan pressures and gain professional experience while stretching the 'boundaries of socially sanctioned notions of femininity', thus experiencing 'opportunities normally reserved for men'.[92]

In her examination of the design of Australian Inland Mission's cottage hospitals, Cathy Keys argues that nursing sisters' 'knowledge of social and climatic conditions' influenced their design. They did not only offer advice on building materials, number of doors and windows, and the size of verandas, but also sought to 'combine nursing, medical and social work in a single plan under one roof'.[93] In other words, they acted as reformers while innovating new architectural designs.

Purdah Hospital

The John Bishop Memorial hospital was one of the active ninety-three mission hospitals for women in British India in 1927. Under colonial health policies, the provision of medical relief to Indian women was most conspicuously inadequate. As Rosemary Fitzgerald states, 'Western responses to Indian women's health needs came largely from philanthropic organizations, and, most notably, the missionary societies'.[94] The ninety-three mission hospitals for women that were recorded in *A Survey of the Status and Conditions of Women in India* represented more than half of all women's hospitals in India.[95] This statistic demonstrates once more that mission hospitals are an essential lens through which we can explore architectural and medical histories of British imperialism.

As already mentioned, the history of the Islamabad hospital demonstrates the global interconnectedness of the Protestant missionary enterprise. By contrast, the hospital's architecture disconnects it from other hospitals of the CMS that I have examined. I explained in Chapter Two that the Neve brothers designed a pavilion plan hospital in Kashmir. The first John Bishop Memorial hospital was also a pavilion plan hospital. It consisted of 'an outpatient department, a waiting-room, consulting-room, operating room, dispensary; two pavilions, fifty feet long, to hold thirty-two patients'.[96] Indeed, if there was one place where missionaries should have built a pavilion hospital, or at least a 'miniature pavilion hospital',[97] it was in Islamabad. Yet, they opted instead for two bungalows, one containing four small wards for twelve inpatients, and the other having the operating room, the consulting and dressing rooms and dispensary for outpatients (Figure 4.1).[98] Although not in layout and appearance, being a bungalow, the hospital was a variation of the Dera Ismail Khan or the Bannu hospitals, both of which were not all that different from PWD's bungalows.[99] In other words, they can be examined side by side if the topic is the global production of the bungalow. But if the topic is hospital architecture, then the Islamabad hospital is aligned with cottage or small local hospitals. In Britain, the cottage hospital originated in the mid-nineteenth century and, in time, became the ideal type for meeting the medical and surgical needs of rural districts, small towns or specific communities.[100] Gomery and the Neve brothers might have drawn on such pattern books as *A Handy Book of Cottage Hospitals* (1870), which describes existing

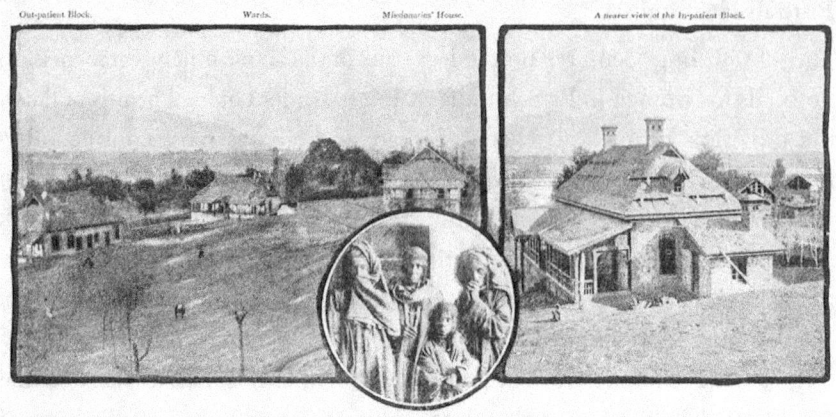

Figure 4.1 The Islamabad hospital.
CMS/M/EL 2/6, p. 362, Church Missionary Society Archive, Cadbury Research Library, Special Collections, University of Birmingham.

cottage hospitals in Britain.[101] Henry Burdett's *Cottage Hospitals – General, Fever and Convalescent* (1896) also contains many plans and illustrations.[102]

According to Gomery, Islamabad had 'no English residents' at the time of her arrival there and had 'never had a resident missionary except for a few weeks'.[103] Thus, building a hospital straight away after her arrival went against the grain of medical missionaries' standard practice. Gomery wanted to build a hospital as fast as possible and opted for a cottage hospital due to financial constraints. Gomery and the Neve brothers might have also been motivated by the fact that a cottage hospital was small in scale and could be constructed using 'domestic-scale' details, and hence could fit into its surrounding.[104] Indeed, they sourced stone from the surrounding mountains, and Neve described the hospital as 'unpretentious' in his 1904 report.[105]

The three free-standing buildings (including the missionary house) built out of rough stone with their tiled roof and chimneys might have appeared different to people as Gomery was quick to note in her report in 1902.[106] The hospital's architecture, together with its location away from the town of Islamabad, might point to the role of missionaries as guardians of social and cultural change in the imperial enterprise. They viewed the 'native city' as a source of illness and disease, and the spatial separation was supposed to bring change.[107]

But Islamabad, according to Neve, was 'a populous district, and on all sides, we see flourishing villages and scattered homesteads. Within a twenty-mile radius must be a quarter of a million people, for whom Islamabad is a commercial centre.'[108] If buildings like those of the John Bishop hospital were new in Islamabad, they were not in many other parts of the country. They could neither have 'amused' nor could they have had a 'civilising' influence on everyone.

Moreover, the hospital was not merely a cottage hospital. Arthur Neve's 1904 report indicated that the hospital had, in fact, a distinct design, where it described the hospital as a purdah hospital: 'It is a *Purdah* hospital, kept strictly for women, but the waiting-room is by the roadside, and is occasionally used for men.'[109] Purdah (it means literally 'a curtain') is the term that is commonly used for referring to the system of secluding women through clothing and architecture in the Middle East and South Asia. It is practised among both Muslims and Hindus, although each has a different understanding of the practice, meaning that they observe or keep purdah differently and in varying degrees.[110] By purdah, Neve might have merely meant that the hospital was strictly for women. Yet, the location of the inpatient block on the steep slope part of the compound behind the outpatient block ensured that it was, to some extent, invisible from the road (see Figure 4.1).

The idea of a purdah hospital was executed on a different, more tangible level, in the design of the Multan hospital, which was described as having an 'extreme purdah arrangement' (Figure 4.2).[111] Eger established the Multan hospital in 1885 under the auspices of FES. Like Elmslie and Carr, she faced 'opposition' and 'prejudice' for some time until she managed to secure a small house and opened a dispensary in 1886. This dispensary was closed in 1891 when Eger went on leave. As hinted at in Chapter One, she took a medical degree while on leave and returned to Multan in 1894. After experiencing again 'a great deal of opposition', Eger managed to secure first a small house, then a government building and eventually a ground to construct a hospital.[112] When the CMS took over the FES's work and workers in 1899, the Multan hospital was transferred to the CMS.[113] The hospital was divided between Muslims and Hindus, with each group having their own compound that consisted of wards and a courtyard (Figure 4.3). The hospital also had an inner, walled, area and an outer section. The interior space was composed of an entrance block and an inpatient block and the outpatient department,

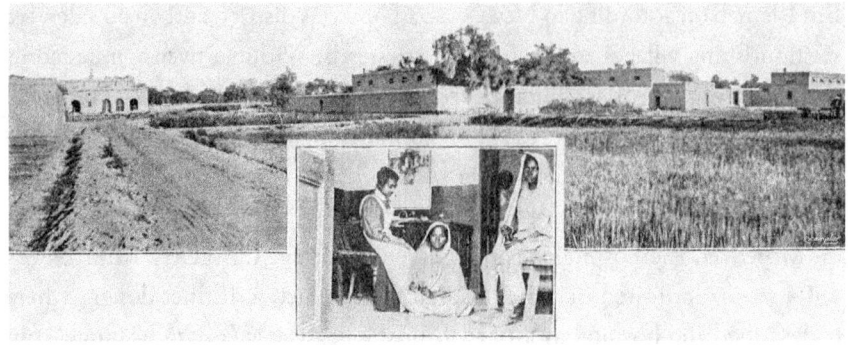

Figure 4.2 The medical mission at Multan.
CMS/M/EL 2/ 5, p. 180, Church Missionary Society Archive, Cadbury Research Library, Special Collections, University of Birmingham.

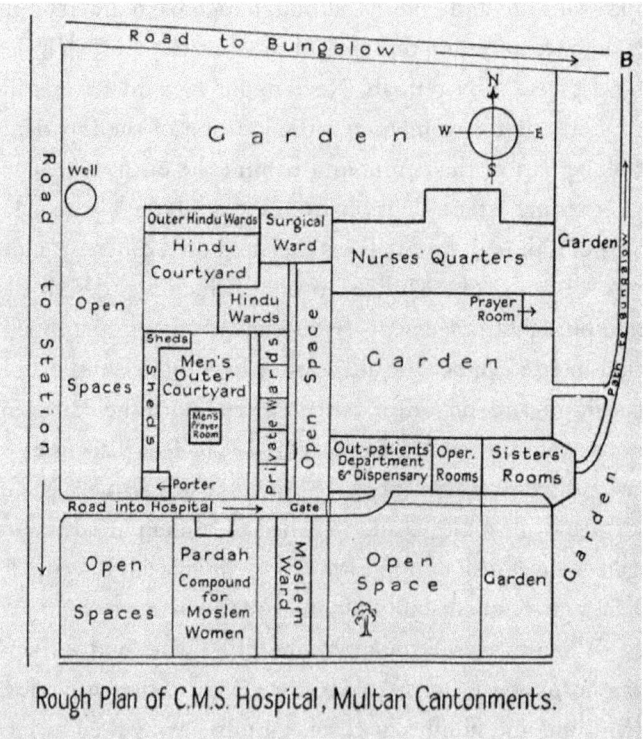

Figure 4.3 Rough plan of the Multan hospital.
CMS/M/EL 2/40, p. 104, Church Missionary Society Archive, Cadbury Research Library, Special Collections, University of Birmingham.

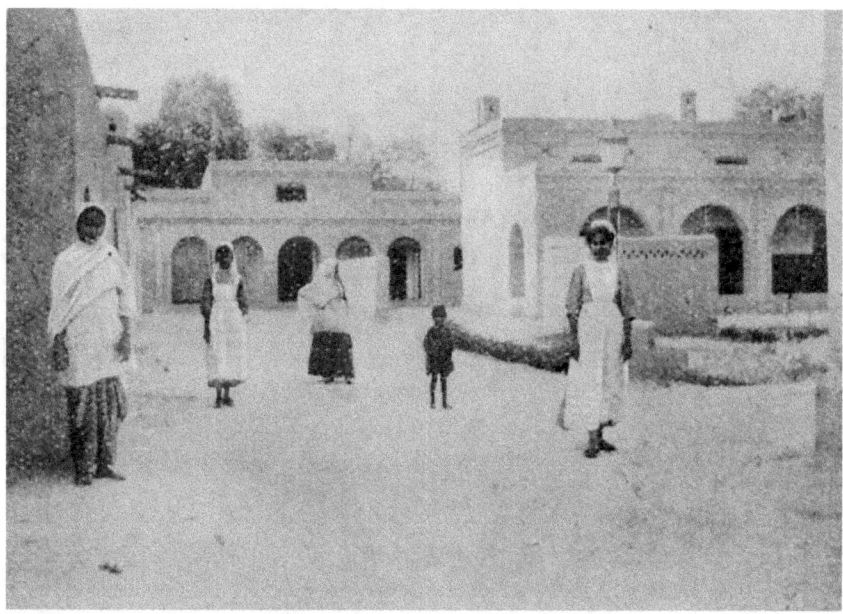

Figure 4.4 Part of inner section of the Multan hospital.
CMS/M/EL 2/19, p. 44, Church Missionary Society Archive, Cadbury Research Library, Special Collections, University of Birmingham.

with 'operating-room and special surgical and private wards, besides a large hall where the out-patients assemble for Bible teaching' (Figure 4.4).[114] The outer section consisted of rooms, or a caravanserai, for male relatives of the female patients (Figure 4.5). In other words, like houses in some parts of Persia and India, the hospital had an *andarūni* (inner quarter) and a *birūni* (outer quarter). The only difference was that the hospital's *andarūni* was not a family quarter and was reserved for women.[115]

While purdah had been practised for centuries and had even found echoes in literary and artistic traditions, it achieved a certain 'fashionableness' in the nineteenth century, at least in British India. According to Eliza Kent, this 'coincided with the interest that Europeans showed in the "exotic" custom of purdah, suggesting that such interest may have given strength or social significance to this so-called traditional custom'.[116] Kent states that missionaries in British India generally did not aim to force women to disregard purdah. Their goal was instead to transform their identification of women with home, so that they could be 'preservers of the home' based on ideals of

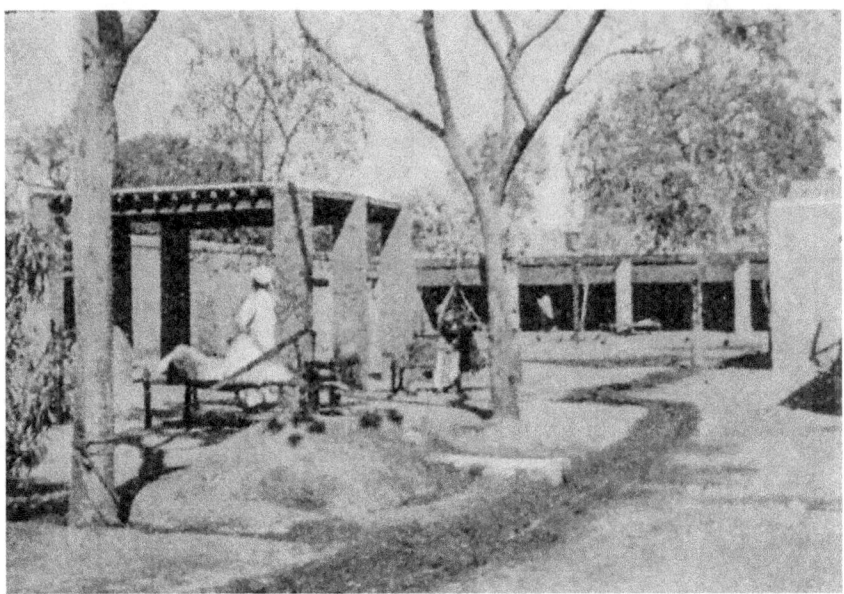

Figure 4.5 Serai outside the Multan hospital which accommodated patients' families. CMS/M/EL 2/35, p. 51, Church Missionary Society Archive, Cadbury Research Library, Special Collections, University of Birmingham.

Christian faith.[117] Kent refers to Annal Satthianadhan's child-rearing manual, *Nalla Tay* (The Good Mother). She shows how Satthianadhan established links with the existing Tamil literary genre to communicate 'Western ideals of feminine domesticity through idioms and illustrations that were meaningful to their Indian audience'.[118] The CMS missionaries might have been thinking along similar lines when designing the Multan hospital. Eger's statement in 1901 is telling:

> One very purdah Mohammedan woman whom, with great difficulty, I got into the hospital, explained on arrival, 'Oh, keep me here; I have come from their own tiny dark rooms!' ... After her recovery her husband told me he was looking for a house built after the hospital patter, as his wife had been so happy there![119]

Medical missionaries sought to teach new ideas about health and hygiene through a pre-existing architecture that was meaningful to the women.

Nevertheless, Sister A. R. Simmonds made a statement in 1937 that contradicts that of Eger: '

> This may sound strange to those who only know English hospitals, but in the East our patients like to be out on the veranda or open compound until the sun gets hot; then every one [sic] goes into the ward, and the fierce heat is shut out.[120]

Simmonds does not present wards as airy and bright and the hospital as similar to an English hospital (Figure 4.6). In fact, in layout and appearance, the buildings resembled those of the Dera Ismail Khan and Bannu hospitals which, as I showed in Chapter Two, were dark and were not cross-ventilated. Simmonds' statement is comparable to Miss Eardley's regarding the Isfahan hospital, where patients practically lived in the hospital

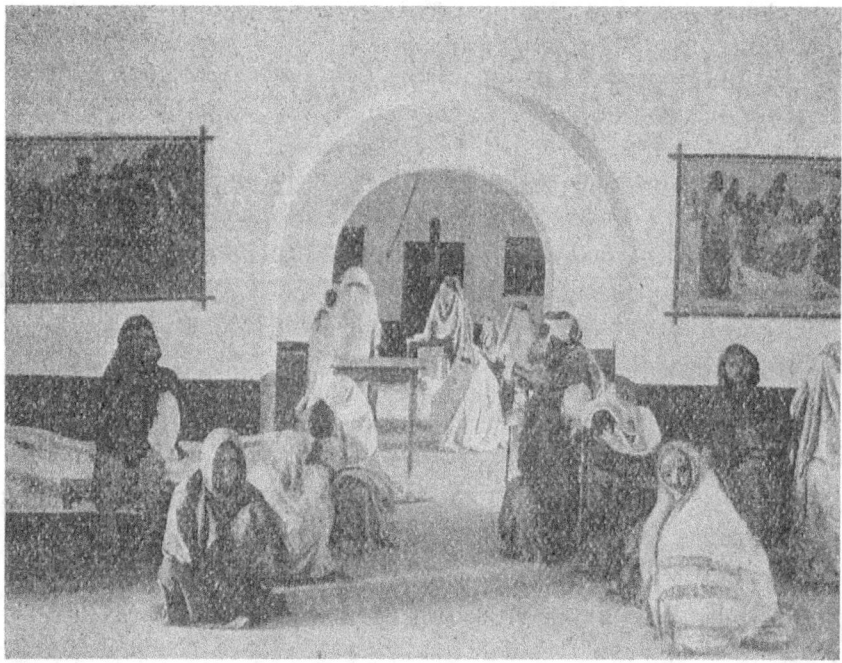

Figure 4.6 Inside of a ward in Multan hospital.
CMS/M/EL 2/14, p. 17, Church Missionary Society Archive, Cadbury Research Library, Special Collections, University of Birmingham.

compound. Like Eardley, she was not talking about open-air treatment, which again demonstrates the shifting balance between outside and inside spaces in mission hospitals and thus the extent to which they could display surveillance and order.

Analysing the Multan hospital as simply a hybrid structure overlooks how male and female missionaries experienced spaces and places differently, which could influence their architectural decisions. Female missionaries had access to women and their sex-segregated private and domestic realm. In her examination of Lady Mary Wortley Montagu's *Turkish Embassy Letters*, Ambereen Dadabhoy shows how Wortley was able to challenge the Orientalist discourse, at the same time as employing it, and thus rescue women's spaces from 'the realm of European male fantasy', investing themselves and local women with agency.[121] Considering Dadabhoy's argument, female missionaries offered a 'corrective vision' of the veil through the purdah hospital. In this way, they hoped to strengthen their identification with women. The purdah arrangement could facilitate certain practices. An outer section for male relatives welcomed many women who 'would not [have been] able to stay with us [missionaries] unless provision was made for their men', stated Eger in 1901.[122] This statement illustrates that designing a purdah hospital was linked to the missionaries' desire to attract as many people as possible. It could also assure the male relatives that their wives or daughters would be protected and separated from the eyes of male strangers. Eger's statement also recalls missionaries' views on the serai system. As explained in the previous chapter, it seems that the serai system was originally developed to address the needs of women who were not willing to stay without their male relatives. It was probably female missionaries who pushed for the invention of family wards, which means that the serai system might have been a product of women's role as well.

This idea of a separate space might have been essential to the female patients' experience. Take, for example, Eger's statement regarding 'unappreciative Hindus' in 1906:

> Picture No. 1 shows the interior of the large wards – it was built in three rooms connected by large arches in the hope that Hindu patients would occupy a

part of it, and also to make it easy to hold a service for a number of patients together. But we cannot get Hindus to see with us in this matter. They do not like our large, tiled room, but prefer small mud rooms on the outside of the purdah wall, where they can squeeze in various members of their family, and which they can on taking possession cleanse to their own satisfaction from all ceremonial defilement of the last inhabitant.[123]

While Eger's language is racially charged because of her use of the term 'unappreciative', it highlights how the material arrangement of the hospital allowed the Hindu patients to make a special provision for themselves. They were permitted to bring their utensils and cook their food in the hospital. A picture of 'friends of Hindu patients cooking in hospital' accompanied Simmonds' report, showing patients and their female family members surrounded by pots and pans (Figure 4.7). The decision of the Hindu patients was not a form of transgression; the design of the hospital encouraged this activity.[124]

Returning to Sister Simmonds' report, she also described part of the 'inner working of' the Multan hospital: 'the whole hospital is quiet, the

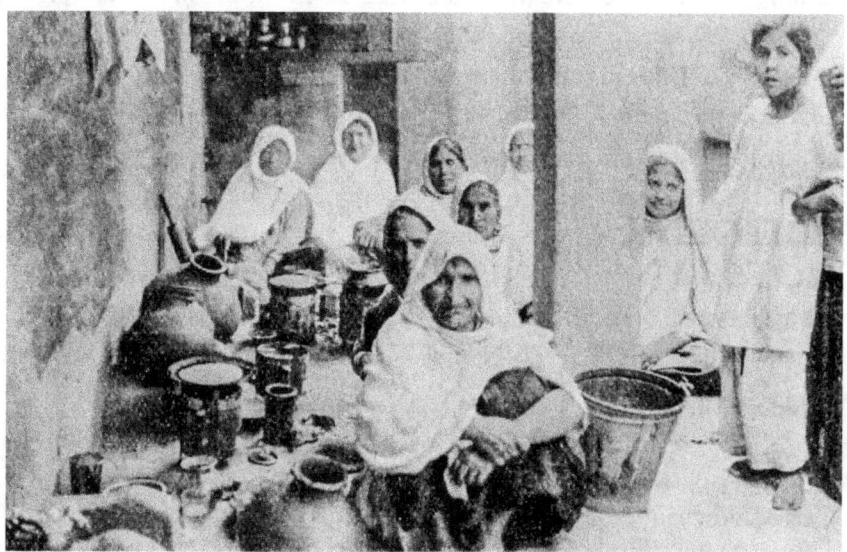

Figure 4.7 Friends of Hindu patients cooking in the hospital.
CMS/M/EL 2/41, p. 29, Church Missionary Society Archive, Cadbury Research Library, Special Collections, University of Birmingham.

porter is asked to prevent men at the gate calling to their wives inside . . . for it is so disturbing when this happens, and the wife calls back "*Andi pai*" (I am coming) and goes!'[125] This statement demonstrates that female missionaries' evaluations of the purdah system collided with that of indigenous women.[126] Meanwhile, public areas such as the hammam, where women could gather, were also subject to strict rules, social conventions and religious laws.[127] Some female patients might have understood missionaries' prescriptions according to their previous experiences.

Nevertheless, purdah was not a meaningful practice among all members of a community.[128] Some women did not favour the purdah system and would manipulate the meanings and representations associated with this system. Others, who observed purdah, could also act as religious leaders, storytellers, healers and even promote women's welfare and education.[129] As Ann Grodzins Gold states, '[w]omen may think of purdah . . . as a cover behind which they gain the freedom to follow their own lights, rather than as a form of bondage or subordination.'[130] How women observed purdah could also vary between rural and urban areas and between elite and non-elite families. In other words, there were internal differences in the emotional charges of purdah based on religion, profession and class.

Notably, the purdah hospital was a new type of hospital architecture, unknown in Britain. Hospital wards in Britain were separated based on gender but did not have a separate walled section for women. The purdah hospital was another need of north-western British India: the women's hospital opened in Bannu was also described as a purdah hospital; it was separated from the men's block by a small by-road.[131] Moreover, in 1923, a new building was added to the Peshawar hospital consisting of 'three private wards', where 'a purdah family could be housed and remain separate from the rest of the patients' (Figure 4.8).[132] The building, which resembled the outpatient and the main inpatient blocks in terms of details and ornamentations, consisted of three small walled sections built side by side. Each section had one or two rooms, a kitchen and a bathroom.

The missionaries did not disseminate the design of the Multan hospital widely and did not build a purdah hospital in other mission fields. Yet, providing privacy was as much of a concern in Persia and Palestine as in north-western British India. As Philippe Bourmand has stated regarding the

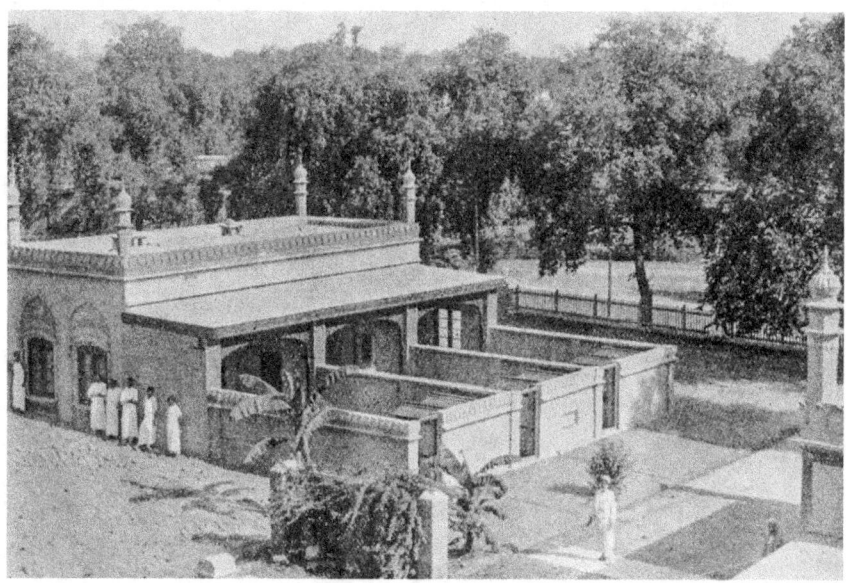

Figure 4.8 New block of wards at Peshawar.
CMS/M/EL 2/ 28, p. 3, Church Missionary Society Archive, Cadbury Research Library, Special Collections, University of Birmingham.

Nablus hospital, besides being 'finance-related' and 'hygiene-concerned', discussions regarding the design of the hospital were 'part of a moral agenda: where were the women's wards and their toilets, or the entrances of the hospital and to the consultation room, so as to create as much gender separation as possible, and prevent an occasion for scandal?'[133] The women's hospitals built in these regions might be described as purdah-like. The entrance arrangement to the Isfahan hospital demonstrates, for example, concerns with providing privacy for female patients. While access to the men's section was direct, access to the women's hospital was indirect (Figure 4.9). The men's hospital had two entrances: one for outpatients and one for inpatients. The recessed portal of the inpatient department had a central location. Once passing this main entrance gate, the first noticeable building was the inpatient block. Unlike the men's hospital, the women's hospital had only one entrance which served both inpatient and outpatient departments. It was planned at a distance from the inpatient section and was connected to it by an L-shape passageway. This arrangement was similar to

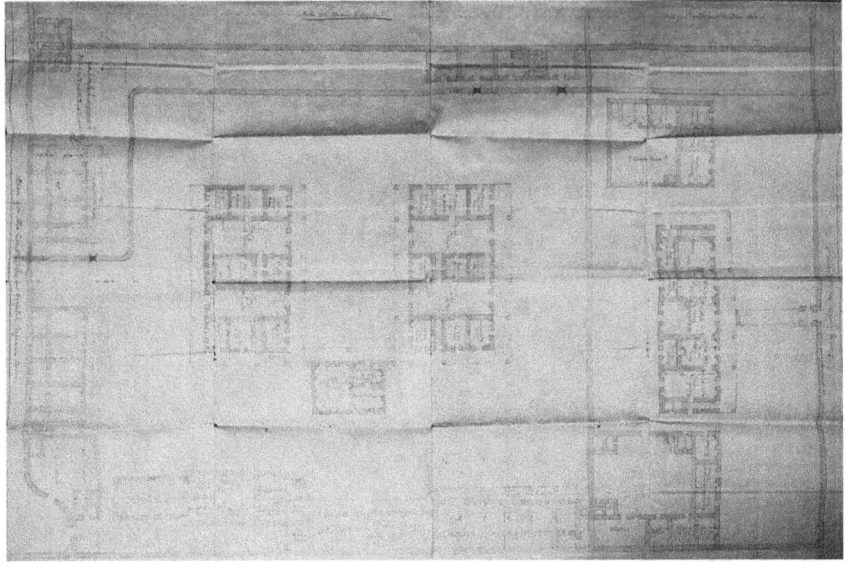

Figure 4.9 Plan of the Isfahan women's hospital. Note the L-shaped passageway from the entrance to the inpatient section.
CMS/M/FL1/PE 1-1, Church Missionary Society Archive, Cadbury Research Library, Special Collections, University of Birmingham.

courtyard houses where the entrance was set at a distance from the central yard to prevent a direct view of the interior, thereby providing privacy.[134] Access to the women's hospital in Kerman was also indirect. As explained in Chapter Two, the entrance to the inpatient sections in the Kerman hospital was at the end of a narrow blind alley that ran between the two hospitals. The patients would enter a domed area; turning to the left, they would enter a long, straight arcade that led to the men's hospital's inpatient section. Turning to the right, they had to pass a winding archway to reach the women's hospital's inpatient section. Female missionaries were familiar with these architectural features because of their access to the female quarter of the houses. Thus, it was them who most likely pushed for these architectural features or even handled their execution.

Conclusion

This chapter focused on female missionaries and their involvement in the construction process of mission hospitals. It first provided an overview of women in mission in the nineteenth and early twentieth centuries, highlighting that there existed multiple layers of exclusion and inclusion in official histories and reports of mission societies. For example, these publications failed to mention the central role of Mrs Clark in the history of medical mission work, who should be credited as the founder of the Kashmir medical mission instead of Elmslie. Especially, these publications failed to acknowledge the contribution of female medical missionaries to the built environment.

One of the female medical missionaries who was involved in building construction was Dr Minnie Gomery. Gomery, who was among the first female medical missionaries that the CMS sent to north-western British India, was the founder of the John Bishop Memorial hospital in Islamabad. This hospital took the place of the hospital that the well-known nineteenth-century explorer Isabella Bird built in the name of her husband in Kashmir. Gomery shared the design of the hospital with the Neve brothers. Although she did not supervise building construction, there were female medical missionaries who were involved in planning, repairing and superintending the construction of the buildings as early as the middle decades of the nineteenth century and it is possible to speculate about their role and contribution by analysing the hospitals' layout.

In appearance, the women's hospitals were either like models in Britain, such as the Islamabad hospital, which was modelled after cottage hospitals, or mimic the rest of the hospitals. Even a first glance at the hospitals' layout may not suggest otherwise. However, they were designed to provide women with a private and segregated space. The missionaries in north-western British India employed the term 'purdah hospital' to highlight this distinctive feature of women's hospitals and, in fact, the Multan hospital had a purdah arrangement. Consisting of an outer section for male relatives and an inner section, the plan of the Multan hospital was not that dissimilar to traditional courtyard houses. The outer section was in the form of a caravanserai, and I suggested that the idea of the serai hospital might have even been a product of women's agency. The purdah arrangement of the hospitals was essential to the experience of female patients. While the purdah system was not a meaningful practice to every woman, it could, at the very least, prevent 'occasions of scandal'.

Notes

1. Robert Clark, *The Missions of the Church Missionary Society and the Church of England Zenana Missionary Society in the Punjab and Sindh* (London: Church Missionary Society, 1904), 168.
2. Jeffrey Cox, *Imperial Fault Lines: Christianity and Colonial Power in India, 1818–1940* (Stanford: Stanford University Press, 2002), 5.
3. For example, see Dana Lee Robert, *American Women in Mission: A Social History of Their Thoughts and Practice. The Modern Mission Era, 1792–1992* (Macon, GA: Mercer University Press, 1996); Delia Davin, 'British Women Missionaries in Nineteenth-Century China', *Women's History Review* 1, no 2 (1992): 257–71; Diana Langmore, *Missionary Lives: Papua 1874–1914* (Honolulu: University of Hawaii Press, 1989); Patricia Grimshaw, *Paths of Duty: American Missionary Wives in Nineteenth-Century Hawaii* (Honolulu: University of Hawaii Press, 1989); Margaret Jolly and Martha Macintyre (eds), *Family and Gender in the Pacific Domestic Contradictions and the Colonial Impact* (Cambridge: Cambridge University Press, 1989); Ruth A. Tucker, *Guardians of the Great Commission: The Story of Women in Modern Mission* (Grand Rapids: Zondervan, 1988); Robin W. Winks, 'The Future of Imperial History', in Robin W. Winks (ed.), *The Oxford History of the British Empire*, Vol. V, Historiography (Oxford: Oxford University Press, 1999): 665; Rhonda Anne Sample, *Missionary Women: Gender, Professionalism and the Victorian Idea of Christian Mission* (Rochester: The Roydell Press, 2003); Patricia Grimshaw and Peter Sherlock, 'Women and Cultural Exchange', in Norman Etherington (ed.), *Missions and Empire* (Oxford: Oxford University Press, 2005), 173–93.
4. For female missionaries as traveller writers and collectors, see, for example, Inbal Livne, 'The Many Purposes of Missionary Work: Annie Royle Taylor as Missionary, Travel Writer, Collector and Empire Builder', in Hilde Nielssen, Inger Marie Okkenhaug and Karina Hestad Skeie (eds), *Protestant Missions and Local Encounters in the Nineteenth and Twentieth Centuries: Unto the Ends of the World* (Leiden and Boston: Brill, 2011), 43–70.
5. Lynne Walker, 'Women and Architecture', in Judy Attfield and Pat Kirkham (eds), *A View from the Interior: Feminism, Women and Design* (London: The Women's Press, 1989), 94.
6. For the contribution of female missionaries to church architecture, see Desmond Keith Martin, 'The Churches of Bishop Robert Gray & Mrs Sophia Gray', PhD diss. (University of Cape Town, 2002).

7. To read about how emotions are gendered, see Ute Frevert, *Emotions in History – Lost and Found* (Budapest: Central European University Press, 2013), 87–247.
8. Long before mission historians engage with emotion history, the 'emotive' participation of women in mission work had been highlighted. For example, Sample, *Missionary Women: Gender, Professionalism*, 3; Heleen Murre-van den Berg, 'Dear Monther of My Soul: Fidelia Fiske and the Role of Women Missionaries in Mid-Nineteenth Century Iran', *Exchange* 30, no. 1 (2001). For sisterhood, see Robert, *American Women in Mission*, 133.
9. The term 'helpmate' appeared in the publications of many missionary societies such the United Presbyterian Church of North America. See Healther J. Sharkey, *American Evangelicals in Egypt: Missionary Encounters in an Age of Empire* (Princeton and London: Princeton University Press, 2008), 83; and the LMS. See also Sample, *Missionary Women: Gender,* Professionalism, 52. Helpmeet was used in Charlotte Brontë's novel *Jane Eyre* (1847), which has been the topic of several studies.
10. Emily J. Manktelow, *Missionary Families: Race, gender and generation on the spiritual frontier* (Manchester: Manchester University Press, 2013), 24.
11. T. O. Beidelman, 'Alturism and Domesticity: Images of Missionizing Women among the Church Missionary Society in Nineteenth-Century East Africa', in Mary Taylor Huber and Nancy C. Lutkehaus (eds), *Gendered Missions: Women and Men in Missionary Discourse and Practice* (Ann Arbor: University of Michigan Press, 1999), 119.
12. Manktelow, *Missionary Families*; Patricia Grimshaw, 'Faith, Missionary Life, and the Family', in Philippa Levine (ed.), *Gender and Empire* (Oxford: Oxford University Press), 265.
13. Grimshaw, *Paths of Duty*, 6–7; see also Beidelman, 'Alturism and Domesticity', 122.
14. Manktelow, *Missionary Families*. The CMS had a more comprehensive welfare service for the family members of missionaries. See Beidelman, 'Alturism and Domesticity', 122.
15. Elizabeth E. Prevost, *The Communion of Women: Missions and Gender in Colonial Africa and the British Metropole* (Oxford: Oxford University Press, 2010), 14–15.
16. For Anna Hamilton, see Manktelow, *Missionary Families*, 56–9; Doug Stuart, 'Of Savage and Heroes: Race, Nation and Gender in the Evangelical Mission to Southern Africa in the Early Nineteenth Century' (PhD diss., University of London, 1994), 185–7.
17. Phillipa Levine, 'Introduction: Why Gender and Empire?', in *Gender and Empire* (see note 12), 2.

18. Stuart, 'Of Savages and Heroes', 185.
19. For example, Valentine Cunningham's pioneering scholarship emphasised that independent female missionary activity was an impossibility in the early nineteenth century: Valentine Cunningham, '"God and nature intended you for a missionary life": Mary Hill, Jane Eyre and other missionary women in the 1840s', in F. Bowie, D. Kirkwood and S. Ardener (eds), *Women and Missions: Past and Present: Anthropological and Historical Perspectives* (Oxford: Berg Publishers, 1993), 85–108.
20. Clare Midgley, 'Can Women be Missionaries? Envisioning Female Agency in the Early Nineteenth-Century British Empire', *Journal of British Studies* 45, no. 2 (2006): 339–40.
21. Douglas, *The Feminization of American Culture*; Jocelyn Murray, 'The Role of Women in the Church Missionary Society, 1799–1917', in Kevin Ward and Brian Stanley (eds), *The Church Mission Society and World Christianity, 1799–1999* (London and New York: Routledge, 2019), 71.
22. Jeffrey Cox, *The British Missionary Enterprise since 1700* (London and New York: Routledge, 2008), 111.
23. Rosemary Fitzgerald, 'Rescue and redemption: The rise of female medical missions in colonial India during the late nineteenth and early twentieth centuries', in Anne Marie Rafferty, Jane Robinson and Ruth Elkan (eds), *Nursing History and the Politics of Welfare* (London and New York: Routledge, 1997), 67.
24. Manktelow, *Missionary Families*, 58.
25. Midgley, 'Can Women be Missionaries?', 358.
26. As Richard Price states, there was 'always a tension between ideology and the reality'. Richard Price, *Making Empire: Colonial Encounters and the Creation of Imperial Rule in Nineteenth-Century Africa* (Cambridge: Cambridge University Press, 2008), 18.
27. Grimshaw and Sherlock, 'Women and Cultural Exchanges', 184.
28. Eliza F. Kent, *Converting Women: Gender and Protestant Christianity in Colonial South India* (Oxford: Oxford University Press, 2004), 81. For example, Miss Mary Bird of the Persia Mission delivered a speech at the annual meeting of the MMA in 1904. See 'The Annual Meeting', *Preaching and Healing: The Annual Report of the CMS Medical Mission Auxiliary for 1903–04* (1904): 27–30; and Dr Emmeline Stuart of the Persia Mission delivered a speech at the annual meeting of the MMA in 1903. See 'The Annual Meeting', *Preaching and Healing: The Annual Report of the CMS Medical Mission Auxiliary for 1902–03* (1903): 15–19.
29. Fitzgerald, 'Rescue and redemption', in *Nursing History* (see note 23), 68.

30. Elizabeth Prevost, 'Married to the Mission Field: Gender, Christianity, and Professionalization in Britain and Colonial Africa, 1865–1914', *Journal of British Studies* 47, no. 4 (2008): 797.
31. Ibid., 798.
32. Fanny Butler is considered as the first fully trained female medical missionary. She was sent by the Church of England Zenana Missionary Society to India in the 1880s. See Rosemary Seton, *Western Daughters in Eastern Lands: British Missionary Women in Asia* (Santa Barbara, Denver, Oxford: Praeger, 2013), 150.
33. 'CMS Medical Missions, July 1896', *Medical Mission Quarterly*, no. 15 (July 1896): 80.
34. 'Women's Medical Missions in India', *The Church Missionary Gleaner* (1892): 101.
35. Amanda Porterfield, *Mary Lyon and the Mount Holyoke Missionaries* (New York and Oxford: Oxford University Press, 1997), 68–86. Porterfield considers Fiske's work among Assyrian women as the overriding factor in destabilising the relationship between the Assyrian and Muslim communities. Heleen Murre-van den Berg, however, disagrees with Porterfield's argument. Murre-van den Berg makes the point that the Assyrian-Muslim relationship had been tense before the arrival of missionaries and their work contributed to further deterioration of their relationship. Murre-van den Berg, 'Dear Mother of My Soul', 34.
36. Porterfield, *Mary Lyon and the Mount Holyoke Missionaries*, 68–84.
37. Kumari Jayawardena, *The White Woman's Other Burden: Western Women and South Asia During British Rule* (New York and London: Routledge, 1995).
38. Gulnar Eleanor Francis-Dehqani, *Religious Feminism in an Age of Empire: CMS Women Missionaries in Iran, 1869–1934* (Centre for Comparative Studies of Religion and Gender, 2000).
39. C. L. Innes, *A History of Black and Asian Writing in Britain, 1700–2000* (Cambridge: Cambridge University Press, 2004), 142–66; Antoinette Burton, *At the Heart of the Empire: Indians and the Colonial Encounter in Late-Victorian Britain* (Berkeley: University of California Press, 1998).
40. According to a short note in October 1896, Cornford resigned her position because of her marriage. See 'Editorial Notes', *Medical Mission Quarterly*, no. 16 (October 1896): 83.
41. Prevost, 'Married to the Mission Field', 821.
42. H. G. Harding, *The Story of CMS Medical Missions* (London: Church Missionary Society, 1915), 14; see also 'Report for 1895–96', *Medical Mission Quarterly*, no. 15 (July 1896): 59.

43. 'Things to be Noted', *Mercy and Truth* 3, no. 32 (August 1899): 182
44. 'Things to be Noted', *Mercy and Truth* 4, no. 37 (January 1900): 4.
45. 'Things to be Noted', *Mercy and Truth* 6, no. 64 (April 1902): 97.
46. 'Persia Mission', *Mercy and Truth* 14, no. 163 (1910): 222.
47. Semple, *Missionary Women: Gender, Professionalism*.
48. Henry Martyn Clark, *Robert Clark of the Punjab: Pioneer and Missionary Statesman* (London: Andrew Melrose, 1907), 139–40.
49. 'Women's Medical Missions in India', *The Church Missionary Gleaner* (189): 100.
50. 'CMS Medical Missions. Our Yesterdays', *The Mission Hospital* 43, no. 492 (January 1939): 15; Graham Kings, 'Abdul Masih: Icon of Indian Indigeneity', *International Bulletin of Missionary Research* 23 (1999): 69.
51. Arvil A. Powell, 'Creating Christian Community in Early nineteenth-century Agra', in Richard Fox Young (ed.), *India and the Indianness of Christianity: Essays on Understanding Historical, Theological, and Bibliographical – in Honour of Robert Eric Frykenberg* (Grand Rapids: William B. Eerdmans, 2009), 100.
52. Semple, *Missionary Women: Gender, Professionalism*, 79.
53. Rev. W. A. Rice, 21 January 1903, CMS/M/C 2/1 4, no. 23, CRL; D. W. Carr, 31 January 1903, CMS/M/C 2/1 4, no. 24, CRL.
54. Bishop Stuart, 19 February 1903, CMS/M/C 2/1 4, no. 37, CRL.
55. Francis-Dehqani, *Religious Feminism in an Age of Empire*.
56. Semple, *Missionary Women: Gender, Professionalism*, 2.
57. Kenneth John Trace Farrimond, 'The Policy of the Church Missionary Society Concerning the Development of Self-Governing Indigenous Churches, 1900–1942' (PhD diss., University of Leeds, 2003), 45.
58. 'Items: Home and Foreign', *Mercy and Truth* 4, no. 39 (1900): 52. The CMS had two such establishments, The Willows and The Olives, as well as a hostel. They provided basic practical and religious training for women. Beidelman, 'Altruism and Domesticity', 134.
59. Minnie Gomery Fonds, P170, Biographical/Folder 2, Osler Library of the History of Medicine, McGill Library, McGill University.
60. Ibid.
61. Linda Wilson, 'Nonconformist Obituaries: How Stereotyped was their View of Women?', in Anne Hogan and Andrew Bradstock (eds), *Women of Faith in Victorian Culture: Reassessing the Angle in the House* (Basingstoke: Palgrave, 1998), 145.
62. Semple, *Missionary Women: Gender, Professionalism*, 17.

63. G. A. Spottiswoode (ed.), *The Official Report of the Missionary Conference of the Anglican Commission* (London, 1894), 584. Elizabet Prevost has referred to this report: Prevost, 'Married to the Mission Field', 803 and 806.
64. Prevost, 'Married to the Mission Field', 806.
65. Semple, *Missionary Women: Gender, Professionalism*, 57.
66. As Manktelow states, 'For missionaries, the best blessing on their parenting style was the continuation of the missionary endeavour into the next generation.' Manktelow, *Missionary Families*, 98.
67. Philippa Levine, *Feminist Lives in Victorian England: Private Roles and Public Commitment* (Oxford: Basil Blackwell, 1990), 62–3.
68. Semple, *Missionary Women: Gender, Professionalism*, 19–20.
69. Minnie Gomery Fonds, P 170, Biographical/Folder 2, Osler Library of the History of Medicine.
70. For example, read about Claudius Buchanan, who, after his return to England from India, became an advocate of missionary work: Stuart Piggin, *Making Evangelical Missionaries, 1789–1858: The Social Background, Motives and Training of British Protestant Missionaries to India. Evangelicals & Society from 1750*, vol. 2 (Abingdon: Sutton Courtney Press, 1984), 19.
71. Hilary Ingram, 'A Little Learning is a dangerous thing: British overseas medical missions and the politics of professionalisation', in Jonathan Reinarz and Rebecca Wynter (eds), *Complaints, Controversies and Grievances in Medicine: Historical and social science perspectives* (London and New York: Routledge, 2015), 80.
72. Minnie Gomery Fonds, Folder 2, P 170, Osler Library Archive.
73. Minnie Gomery, 'Islamabad', *Mercy and Truth* 5, no. 53 (1901): 107.
74. Gigi Adair, 'The "Feringhi Hakim": medical encounters and colonial ambivalence in Isabella Bird's travel in Japan and Persia', *Studies in Travel Writing* 21, no. 1 (2017): 63–75.
75. 'CMS Medical Missions: A Comparative Survey', *Mercy and Truth* 18, no. 215 (1914): 378.
76. 'The Mission-Field', *Church Missionary Intelligencer* (1891): 769.
77. 'Items: Home and Foreign', *Mercy and Truth* 4, no. 39 (1900): 52.
78. Annmarie Adams, *Architecture in the Family Way: Doctors, Houses, and Women, 1870–1900* (Montreal and Kingston: McGill-Queen's University Press, 1996), 152.
79. Walker, 'Women and Architecture', 94.
80. Deborah Gaitskell, 'Rethinking Gender Roles: The Field Experience of Women Missionaries in South Africa', in Andrew Porter (ed.), *The Imperial Horizons of*

British Protestant Missions 1880–1914 (Grand Rapids: William B. Eerdmans, 2003), 134–5.

81. From Dr Minnue Gomery, *Extracts from the Annual Letters of the Missionaries for the year 1901* (London: Church Missionary Society, 1902), 553
82. 'Items: Home and Foreign', *Mercy and Truth* 6, no. 61 (January 1902): 6.
83. Minnie Gomery, 'Work in the New Hospital at Islamabad', *Mercy and Truth* 6, no. 72 (1902): 362.
84. Rev. C. H. Stillman, 8 April 1903, CMS/M/C 2/ 1 4, no. 65, CRL.
85. G. E. Dodson, 7 June 1904, CMS/M/C 2/1 4, no. 56, CRL.
86. Kent, *Converting Women: Gender and Protestant Christianity*, 115–16.
87. Edited by her mother, *Letters of Marie Elizabeth Hayes, M. B. Missionary Doctor, Delhi, 1905–8* (London: Marshall Brothers, 1909), 218–19.
88. *The Eternal Purpose*, 1934, Being the Report of the Year 1934 of the Society for the propagation of the Gospel in Foreign Parts, 96. http://nla.gov.au/nla.obj-1550594854
89. Clifford H. Phillips, *The Lady Named Thunder: A Biography of Dr. Ethel Margaret Phillips (1876–1951)* (Edmonton: The University of Alberta Press, 2003), 131–44.
90. Prevost, 'Married to the Mission Field', 814.
91. Ibid.
92. Janet Lee, 'Between Subordination and She-tiger: Social Constructions of White Femininity in the Lives of Single, Protestant Missionaries in China, 1905–1930', *Women's Studies International Forum* 19, no. 6 (1996): 624.
93. Cathy Keys, 'Designing hospitals for Australian conditions: The Australian Inland Mission's cottage hospital, Adelaide House, 1926', *The Journal of Architecture* 21, no. 1 (2016): 82–3.
94. Fitzgerald, 'Rescue and redemption', 63.
95. M. Balfour and R. Young, *The Work of Medical Women in India* (London: Oxford University Press, 1930), 45–79; referred to in Fitzgerald, 'Rescue and redemption', 64.
96. Anna M. Stoddart, *The Life of Isabella Bird (Mrs Bishop)* (London: John Murray, 1906), 206.
97. Jeremy Taylor, *Hospital and Asylum Architecture in England 1840–1914: Building for Health Care* (London: Mansell, 1991), 73.
98. Minnie Gomery, 'The New John Bishop Memorial, Islamabad', *Mercy and Truth* 6, no. 65 (1902): 146.
99. Anthony D. King, *The Bungalow: The Production of a Global Culture* (New York and Oxford: Oxford University Press, 1995).

100. Taylor, *Hospital and Asylum Architecture in England*, 73. See also R. M. S. McConaghey, 'The Evolution of the Cottage Hospital', *Medical History* 11, no. 2 (1967): 128–40. DOI: https://doi.org/10.1017/S0025727300011984
101. Horace Swete, *Handy Book of Cottage Hospitals, Issue 133* (London: Hamilton, Adams, and Co., 1870).
102. Henry C. Burdett, *Cottage Hospitals: General, Fever, Convalescent: Their Progress, Management, and Work in Great Britain and Ireland and the United States of America*, 3rd ed. (London: The Scientific Press, 1896).
103. Gomery, 'Islamabad', 107.
104. Taylor, *Hospital and Asylum Architecture in England*, 73.
105. A. Neve, 'John Bishop Memorial Hospital, Islamabad', *Mercy and Truth* 8, no. 91 (1904): 199.
106. Gomery, 'The New John Bishop Memorial, Islamabad', 147.
107. Anthony D. King, *The Bungalow: The Production of a Global Culture*, 35.
108. Neve, 'John Bishop Memorial Hospital, Islamabad', 199.
109. Ibid., 200.
110. Hannah Papanek, 'Purdah: Separate Worlds and Symbolic Shelter', *Comparative Studies in Society and History* 15, no. 3 (1973): 289; Sabir Khan, 'Memory Work: The Reciprocal Framing of Self and Place in Emigre Autobiographies', in Eleni Bastea (ed.), *Memory and Architecture* (Albuquerque: University of New Mexico Press, 2004), 127.
111. Wilhelmina Eger, 'The Mission Hospital at Multan', *Mercy and Truth* 5, no. 56 (1901): 180.
112. 'CMS Medical Missions: A Comparative Survey', *Mercy and Truth* 18, no. 214 (1914): 347.
113. 'Things to be noted', *Mercy and Truth* 8, no. 32 (1899): 182.
114. Annie W. Eger, 'The Mission Hospital at Multan', *Mercy and Truth* 5, no. 56 (1901): 180.
115. Gholamhossein Memarian and Frank Brown, 'The shared Characteristics of Iranian and Arab courtyard houses', in Brian Edwards, Magda Sibley, Mohamad Hakmi and Peter Land (eds), *Courtyard Housing: Past, Present, and Future* (London and New York: Taylor & Francis, 2006), 35.
116. Kent, *Converting Women: Gender and Protestant Christianity*, 137.
117. Ibid., 128.
118. Ibid., 146.
119. Annie W. Eger, 'The Mission Hospital at Multan', *Mercy and Truth* 5, no. 56 (1901): 180.

120. Sister A. R. Simmonds, 'Pressing Forward in Multan', *The Mission Hospital* 41, no. 469 (1937): 28.
121. I am inspired here by Ambereen Dadabhoy's examination of Lady Mary Wortley Montagu's *Turkish Embassy Letters*. Montagu is known for her poems, her contribution to the fight against smallpox and, last but not least, her life in Turkey where her husband worked as the British ambassador. See Ambereen Dadabhoy, '"Going Native": Geography, Gender, and Identity in Lady Mary Wortley Montagu's *Turkish Embassy Letters*', in Mona Narain and Karen Gevirtz (eds), *Gender and Space in British Literature, 1660–1820* (London and New York: Routledge, 2016), 52.
122. Eger, 'The Mission Hospital at Multan', 180.
123. Wilhelmina Eger, 'Some of Our Multan Patients', *Mercy and Truth* 10, no. 118 (1906): 301.
124. Rob Boddice, *The History of Emotions* (Manchester: Manchester University Press), 170–1. See also Roy Kozlovsky, 'Architecture, Emotions and the History of Childhood', in Stephanie Olsen (ed.), *Childhood, Youth and Emotions in Modern History: National, Colonial and Global Perspectives* (Basingstoke: Palgrave Macmillan, 2015), 95–118.
125. Sister A. R. Simmonds, 'Pressing Forward in Multan', *The Mission Hospital* 41, no. 469 (1937): 28.
126. Sara Mills, 'Gender and Colonial Space', *Gender, Place and Culture: A Journal of Feminist Geography* 3, no. 2 (1996): 142.
127. Dadabhoy, '"Going Native": Geography, Gender, and Identity', 54.
128. To read about the highly differentiated voices and viewpoints of Muslim women on any social and political issue, see Ghazi-Walid Falah and Caroline Nagel (eds), *Geographies of Muslim Women: Gender, Religion, and Space* (New York and London: The Guilford Press, 2005).
129. Begum Wali-ud-Dowla was the president of the Hyderabadi Women's Association. Satyasikha Chakraborty, 'European Nurses and Governesses in Indian Princely Households: "Uplifting that impenetrable veil"?', *Journal of Colonialism and Colonial History* 19, no. 1 (2018). doi:10.1353/cch.2018.0001
130. Ann Grodzins Gold, 'Purdah is As Purdah's Kept: A Storyteller's Story', in Gloria Goodwin and Ann Grodzins Gold (eds), *Listen to the Heron's Words: Reimagining Gender and Kinship in North India* (Berkey, University of California Press, 1994), 164. See also Joyce Burkhalter Flueckiger, *In Amma's Healing Room: Gender and Vernacular Islam in South India* (Bloomington and Indianapolis: Indiana University Press, 2006).

131. Miss E. Giles, 'First Impressions of Bannu', *The Mission Hospital* 27, no. 396 (January 1931): 9.
132. J. H. Cox, 'Peshawar Hospital – Extension', *The Mission Hospital* 28, no. 312 (1924): 3.
133. Philippe Bourmaud, 'Public Space and Private Spheres: The Foundation of St Luke's Hospital of Nablus by the CMS (1891–1901)', in Heleen Murre-van den Berg (ed.), *New Faith in Ancient Lands: Western Missions in the Middle East in the Nineteenth and Early Twentieth Centuries* (Leiden and Boston: Brill, 2006), 140.
134. Memarian and Brown, 'The Shared Characteristic of Iranian and Arab Courtyard Houses', 26.

5

MEDICAL MISSIONS AND ANGLO-RUSSIAN RIVALRY

From the design of the Kashmir, Dera Ismail Khan and Bannu hospitals to the Peshawar, Multan, Islamabad, Isfahan, Kerman and Yazd hospitals, there were continuities, varieties, differences, as well as innovations. As I explained, these varieties and innovations mean that we need to expand our understanding of British hospital architecture in the nineteenth and early twentieth centuries. Besides, what do these variations and innovations tell us about the relationship between missionary medicine and empire? More specifically, could missionaries' agenda to gain trust overlap with the interests of 'the state'?[1] This chapter addresses this question. A statement by Lord Frederick Roberts, which was made probably sometime in the 1900s, regarding Dr Theodore Pennell would be a good starting point: 'Dr Pennell is worth a couple of regiments to the British on that frontier any day'.[2] This statement interested missionaries; they referred to it in their reports, extending it at times to include all the medical missionaries who worked in north-western British India.[3] Lord Roberts was one of the most successful British military commanders, famous for his service in both British India and South Africa. Concerning north-western British India, he is known for his standpoint and actions regarding Anglo-Russian rivalry that lasted intermittently from approximately 1807 until 1914.[4] In using the word 'regiments', Roberts associated or even equated the missionaries with his troops in the struggle against Russia. The missionaries' interest in this declaration suggests that they presented (if not partly perceived) their work as an essential component of the British Indian defence.

This chapter will shed some light on how the missionaries presented their efforts to gain trust in the context of Anglo-Russian rivalry. Eighteen years after Jeffrey Cox warned against 'the marginality of missionaries in narratives of the imperial enterprise', missionaries are now one of the main preoccupations in the 'mainstream imperial history and literature'.[5] However, the same cannot be said about the narratives of Anglo-Russian rivalry, where the missionaries are still marginalised or ignored altogether, in favour of those judged to be central to the rivalry: scholars, military officers, imperial administrators and travellers.[6] This makes defining a point of view from which to tell the story challenging, and this chapter by no means claims to provide an all-inclusive examination.

The nature of the relationship between mission and empire was equivocal. Therefore, missionaries cannot be viewed unequivocally as 'faceless imperialist agent[s]'.[7] Whether the topic is the aims and outcomes of missionaries and the colonial state, missionaries' cultural labour, or varieties of interactions that surrounded missionary labour, there were ambiguities and unintended consequences involved.[8]

Beginning in the sixteenth century, up until the early twentieth century, the relationship between home and colonial government and missionaries oscillated between cooperation, toleration and criticism.[9] However, matters were more complicated than a 'religion versus empire' formulation might suggest. Following postcolonial trends, studies have highlighted missionaries' participation in the cultural labour that underpinned colonial rules, such as the imposition of Christian order and cleanliness, and thus the spread of new ways of building and living characteristics of Western modernity – specific methods of child-rearing and monogamous marriage are but two examples.[10] The tension between Christianity and civilisation was never a resolved issue,[11] and a group of scholars have demonstrated the capability of some missionaries to assign value to indigenous cultures.[12] Scholars have also criticised the coherence of the term 'cultural imperialism'. For example, Hayden J. A. Bellenoit has demonstrated that missionaries utilised precedent traditions in othering Hinduism and India, including the approaches of Arab, Persian and Indo-Muslim scholars. As

Bellenoit states, missionaries differed from their predecessors in degree but not in essence.[13]

On a parallel but distinct track, historians have mapped, as far as possible, local people's participation and even leadership in the mission cause. Thus, they have challenged the view that missionaries universally imposed cultural changes by force and against the people's interests. Even friendship across the axis of the coloniser/colonised divide was possible. These diverse interactions could have been equally transformative for missionaries and thus unbalanced the logics of the colonial order.[14]

Lord Roberts's recognition of Pennell as worth a regiment is part of this history. Ignoring it leads to what Cox has termed 'presumption of marginality', that views missionaries as insignificant.[15] This view, as Cox states, 'has been carried over from imperial establishment to imperial history'. Roberts's opinion of Pennell was echoed in the CMS medical magazine *Mercy and Truth* and Pennell's book, biography and obituary. These publications contained 'public views' of missionaries,[16] and this chapter is concerned with the CMS missionaries' public views of Anglo-Russian rivalry. To be sure, some missionaries, such as Reverend T. Bomford, were critical of the CMS's overextended work in Punjab.[17] However, as I shall show, some missionaries talked publicly about the importance of the Punjab mission while referring to Anglo-Russian rivalry.

It was not the first time that views of this nature were being expressed or endorsed in missionaries' publications. Strong has provided an excellent account of Evangelical and non-Evangelical Anglicans, both in the metropole and colonies, of the British Empire between 1700 and 1850. He has examined the annual sermons and published extracts of the SPG and the CMS missionaries' reports of their annual meetings.[18] Although there were missionaries who were critical of the empire or whose private views may have been different, there was 'an official and conscious Anglican concern for empire'.[19] A new pattern of the close alliance between church and state was developed between 1790 and 1830. This pattern gave the Church of England an advantage to shore up imperial connections. It was partly a consequence of the American War of Independence and an antidote to French revolutionary fervour. Strong shows how Bengal, after Canada, was 'the oldest and most long-lived site of this new ecclesiastical imperialism'.[20] Many church leaders believed that Britain's conquest of India had a providential purpose; that is, India was given to Britain by God for Christianisation. They believed that the best way to achieve this was through an alliance between Church and state, arguing that official government support could create a favourable atmosphere for the growth of the Church and vice versa.[21] Though actions were slow to emerge, and the government provided little support up until the 1840s, many foundations were laid in terms of securing public and financial support.[22]

Within this providential discourse, Daniel Wilson, the bishop of Calcutta, claimed Punjab for Christ in 1836. Additionally, missionaries displayed a kind of 'geo-religious triumphalism', which viewed Punjab as an 'ecclesiastical pathway to [Afghanistan] and Central Asia'.[23] Although subject to Protestant missionary influence at various times in the nineteenth century, Afghanistan and Central Asia had remained 'closed lands'.[24] However, it would be almost twenty years before the state Churches of England or Scotland would start a regular mission in Punjab. As I explained in the Introduction, Reverend Robert Clark opened this mission in Amritsar in 1852. While providential thinking lost some of its power by the late nineteenth century, many continued to employ this language up until the 1920s.[25]

One last point needs to be unpacked; there was no one way of contemplating the providential gift of the empire. The Church leaders that Strong examines argued for a religious model of the empire and the extension of the national church. Another view linked 'English' Christianity to the spread of the 'English' race. Moreover, a group of more secular thinkers viewed religion as a unifying force in that it could assist in the dissemination of 'English' social and ethical values.[26] With the increasing emphasis on social service and medical work in the Christian missions in British India from the late nineteenth century, some missionaries reconsidered the providential purpose of the British Empire as to be the 'drawing together of the spirituality of East and West'.[27] Even though the CMS (medical) missionaries did not share this view,[28] they regarded medical work, as I have shown, as the best means of earning trust from people who would otherwise be unreceptive of or hostile to them.[29] Significantly, the importance of Pennell's work was acknowledged in this regard. In elaborating on Roberts's statement, the medical missionaries referred to their close encounters and entanglements with local communities. They claimed that their missions were worth those of a regiment to the government because they had been instrumental in obtaining people's trust and friendship.

For example, Dr Arthur Neve, the head of the Kashmir medical mission, explained how medical work changed the attitude of the Maharajah of Kashmir towards missionaries. Neve further mentioned that he was once invited, alongside Reverend Cecil Tyndale-Biscoe, to a 'great Mohammedan meeting'. Upon their arrival, Neve wrote, 'the whole mass of people stood up and received them' by playing '"God Save the King"'. He used this story to validate Roberts's statement regarding Pennell.[30]

As already stated, friendship across the axis of the coloniser/colonised divide could efface inequalities and destabilise the colonial social order. However, as Karen Vallgårda and Clare McLisky warn, it would not 'automatically and unambiguously counteract the logics of colonial rule'.[31] According to them, 'Evangelical love' had an 'ambivalent effect' and could shape power relations. As stated in the Introduction, Vallgårda highlights the importance of considering how regulating individual emotions could have been a driving force in forging a community at large. So, Neve's story of the Mohammedan meeting. In the remainder of the chapter, I will first discuss Pennell's habit of wearing local clothes and the geographical location of the hospitals. We should remember the significance of considering the buildings with objects, sound, smell, touch and (built) environment side by side. I examine Pennell's practice of adopting local clothes and the geographical location of the hospitals separately here in the interest of narrative clarity. Still, I want to show that they have to be considered when analysing buildings and discussing how they impressed people. Indeed, family wards worked together with patients' belonging, family and friends, Pennell's clothes and geographical location of the buildings to attract the patients, or rather specific patients. The chapter will then explore two ways through which securing friendship and Anglo-Russian rivalry were linked in missionaries' writings.

The Cloth

I have already mentioned that Pennell was the founder of the Bannu hospital. He added several family wards to the hospital in 1904, and after his death a purdah hospital for women was constructed. Pennell was also among missionaries who 'went native'. He received his medical training at the University College, London taking his M.B. degree in 1890 and his M.D. degree in 1891. His obituary sketched him as a distinguished medical student who won many awards, including a Bruce Medal and Morley Scholarship.[32] In 1892, he became F.R.C.S (Eng) and, in the same year, offered himself to the CMS – he was twenty-five. He was stationed first at Dera Ismail Khan before being transferred to Bannu in 1893, where he worked until his death in 1912.[33]

Lord Roberts wrote the introduction to Pennell's biography, published in 1914. After declaring that Pennell was a distinguished medical student who worked 'unceasingly for the spiritual and physical welfare' of the inhabitants of Bannu, Roberts referred to Pennell's 'striking appearance'.[34] On various occasions, Pennell adopted local dresses and costumes. One of such occasions was during the winter of 1903–4 when, instead of going to Britain on leave, he decided to tour north India as a sadhu or mendicant pilgrim. Associated with Hindu or Sikh holy men, the costume consisted of a saffron-coloured robe and turban. Based on Pennell's account of the tour, he wore this costume the entire time, but this is not certain.[35]

Around six years before Pennell's tour, Isabelle Eberhardt, born in Geneva (although with a Russian background), travelled to Bône (today Annaba, Algeria), converted to Islam and went native.[36] While Pennell might not have known Eberhardt, he probably had heard of Annie Basant, a former Church of England vicar's wife, who arrived in British India around the same time as him, in 1893, and adopted local dress.[37] Pennell had many predecessors and contemporaries among European missionaries, explorers, traders and officials. The following are a small selection of examples of Europeans who went native between the sixteenth and nineteenth centuries. Mr Day of the Dera Ghazi Khan medical mission dressed as a mullah on his tour in 1896–97.[38] Dr C. F. Harford-Battersby of Sudan and Upper Niger Mission adopted local garments in the 1890s consisting of turban, gown and loose trousers.[39] Miss Inie Newcombe of the Foo-Chow mission (East China) wore the local dress while visiting several villages for the first time in 1888.[40] General Charles Stuart, an East India Company (EIC) army officer in the early nineteenth century, also adopted local garments,[41] as well as

Lady Anne Blunt, a British woman in Arabia in the first half of the nineteenth century,[42] Arnold Zisserman, a Russian officer in the Caucasus again in the first half of the nineteenth century[43] and João Machado, a Portuguese in early sixteenth-century India.[44]

One of the main lines of enquiry refers to Europeans who went native as renegades. It argues that they caused 'fear' among colonial officials. French renegades in sixteenth-century American colonies rendered fear[45] as did British merchants in nineteenth-century North America and New Zealand, who mostly went native temporarily for economic reasons.[46] But Portuguese attitude towards renegades in the sixteenth century was a mixture of condemnation and admiration.[47] 'Nativisation' did not cause as much fear in the Eastern borderland of the Russian Empire in the seventeenth and eighteenth centuries either and, at worst, it was viewed as an example of 'cultural slippage'. According to Willard Sunderland, a shift occurred in the nineteenth century, whereby going native was increasingly considered as a mark of degeneration.[48] Still, going native was not condemned in the Russian Empire in the Caucasus in the nineteenth century. Comparing Russian military officers to their British counterparts, Mikail Mamedov argues that their rapid adoption of native clothes 'demonstrates the remarkable flexibility of Russians' imperial consciousness'.[49] Mamedov refers to Colonel Thomas Edward Lawrence, or Lawrence of Arabia, as an exception but excludes many British missionaries who went native. The point that I want to make by referring to these examples is that the things that cause emotions, such as fear, are not constant across time and space.[50] We need to refocus our attention from going native as either frightening or courageous to an emotional practice. Wearing a specific dress was a practice that could give or threaten an individual's agency and power depending on circumstances and shifting and diverse notions about 'native' clothes.[51]

The CMS may not have criticised Pennell due to the less disciplined organisational structure of the Society. Although some missionaries were against the practice of adopting the local dress,[52] 'the simple fact' was that the CMS Committee 'never dreamed of laying down the law on the subject [wearing native dress] at all', was noted in the editorial note of the *Church Missionary Gleaner* in 1890. According to this note, it was 'left to every missionary to act as circumstances seem to require'. The note even stressed that more missionaries 'than formerly are now desirous to adopt the practice habitually'.[53] The practice of adopting local dress was a personal matter. The CMS neither encouraged the missionaries to wear nor was strictly against the practice of wearing a local dress, and it was down to the missionaries to decide.

But Pennell's habit of adopting local garments was one of the reasons behind Roberts's admiration for him too. Roberts might have admired the connections that Pennell had established in north-western British India, even if they were imagined or fictional. Pennell undertook his sadhu pilgrimage partly with the aim of 'philosophizing on the role that a man's clothes play in gaining him a reception or a rejection'.[54] Besides wearing sadhu dress, he wore the costumes of an Afghan soldier, a Pathan (a Waziri), a Peshawari khan and a mullah. He wore these garments on his tours when visiting patients at their homes, at missionary conferences and in the hospital (Figure 5.1). Pennell even grew a beard and became vegetarian later in his missionary career.[55]

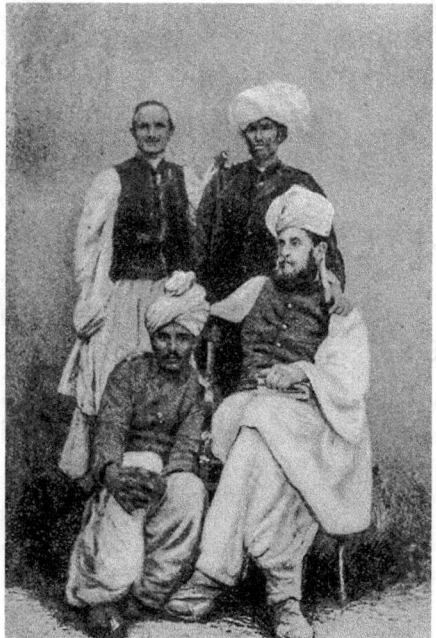

Figure 5.1 Dr Pennell siting on the right.
CMS/M/EL 2/ 1, p. 108, Church Missionary Society Archive, Cadbury Research Library, Special Collections, University of Birmingham.

He wore a native dress for diverse reasons. For example, like some of his predecessors and contemporaries, Pennell wore local dress partly out of necessity. He wore a Pathan dress while touring villages surrounding Bannu in January 1894. Writing about this tour, he stated, 'I found it not particularly uncomfortable, and got along very well. Indeed, as several streams had to be crossed, it was just as well to have no socks on.'[56] He asserted again in his 1895 annual letter that he had found wearing 'native' dress 'a very comfortable travelling costume'.[57] Pennell regarded wearing local clothes as more functional, especially en route from one village to another.

Moreover, Pennell's purpose was 'to realize more vividly what treatment is often meted out to our native brethren and how they feel under it [their dress]'.[58] In other words, as Cox notes, Pennell aimed to demonstrate 'genuine sympathy' to non-western people.[59] According to Cox, this method was suggested by Reverend Golak Nath, an Indian Presbyterian minister, at the Lahore Missionary Conference in 1863. Nath believed the missionaries should attempt to demonstrate sympathy by 'going native' not just in their clothing but also in their way of life if they aim to develop a self-supporting, self-governing and self-extending Indian Church.[60] Whether or not Pennell was influenced by Nath – given that the ideals of the native agency were abandoned in 1901 – demonstrating sympathy was one of his aims. For instance, when adopting sadhu dress, he contemplated how, as a 'Christian Sadhu', he would be perceived by British officers or other missionaries. He recalled how he had to wait for 'as long as two hours' to be received when calling on an officer or another missionary if he was not recognised as a European.[61] On another occasion, when on a train, he was rejected from staying in the European compartment.[62] Pennell thought that these ways of acting caused Indians 'pain' and aimed to acknowledge and understand this pain. As his wife, Alice Pennell, put it: 'he [Pennell] felt that for his part it gave him a just appreciation of the feelings of the people among whom he worked if he resembled them in outward appearance.'[63] It is difficult to comment on the extent to which Pennell managed to understand the feelings of the local population. The missionaries' body was always 'more or less foreign', states Eric Reinders concerning missionaries in China. According to Reinders, no matter how hard missionaries tried to go native they would be reminded of their 'foreignness' on various occasions.⁶⁴ When on the train during his pilgrimage, Pennell did not hesitate to remind an 'English soldier' that he belonged to the European 'category'. This quote also points to what a group of scholars have emphasised regarding the nature of emotions such as pity, sympathy or compassion, that they maintain inequality.⁶⁵ Pennell's experience of sympathy did not involve 'self-sacrifice' in the interest of the collective.⁶⁶

Pennell's main reason was to gain people's friendship or affection. Pennell thought about how local people felt 'restraint' or 'nervous' when visiting the missionaries and believed that these feelings could be removed if he wore local clothes. One of the activities in which he hoped to participate was the 'exchange of paggris', a 'custom on the border when friend meets friend'.⁶⁷ According to his biography, by adopting the people's dress, 'Dr Pennell could share this custom in a way that would otherwise have been possible. For this reason, he also early grew a beard, as amongst the Muhammadans of the north the beard is a sign of manhood.'⁶⁸ Even the reason Pennell became vegetarian was 'to induce the Hindus to eat with him'.⁶⁹ In other words, wearing a local dress was an emotional set-up for changing the sensory relationship between Pennell and local people. For instance, he perceived the exchange of paggris as a sign of 'affection' and by wearing local garments aimed to gain 'a speedy entry into the affections of the people'.⁷⁰ As he put it in his 1895 annual letter, wearing 'native' dress acted as 'a great disarmer of prejudice, and a giver of greater facility in going about among the people'.⁷¹ There were moments when he considered his convenience and thought about understanding people's feelings, but these reasons do not explain the prime reasoning behind his choice of clothing. By adopting local dress, Pennell took extra measures to obtain the trust of the local population.

A photograph of Pennell standing next to a patient in a ward in the Bannu hospital dressed partially in a local garment is suggestive; it recalls statements regarding the un-English nature of mission hospitals (Figure 5.2). Along with other practices – such as allowing patients to stay in the hospital with their family and friends, bring their utensils and move freely in and out of the wards – a doctor dressed in local-style clothing made the hospitals appear quite different from an English hospital. Visualising Pennell visiting a family

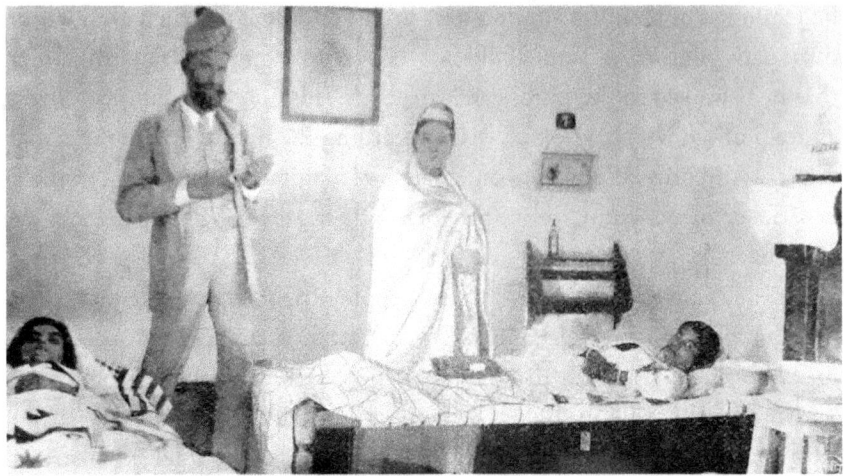

Figure 5.2 Dr Pennell in a ward in the Bannu hospital.
CMS/M/EL 2/11, p. 111, Church Missionary Society Archive, Cadbury Research Library, Special Collections, University of Birmingham.

ward in local dress provides a particularly powerful image; one cannot help thinking about a painting of a Muhammadan doctor visiting a patient at their home (Figure 5.3). Pennell, of course, would not read the Quran to the patient, but his clothes would bring the design of the family ward all together. Some patients might not have been in favour of Pennell's practice of adopting local dress. Nevertheless, a doctor dressed in a local cloth was certainly the ultimate part of the missionaries' plan to make the hospital appear familiar. Indeed, Pennell's practice of wearing local dress was part of the missionaries' overall desire to attract the patients.[72]

A 'Chain' of Missions

We also need to zoom out and consider the geographical location of the hospitals. Until now we have considered the missionaries' practice of obtaining trust at the micro level by discussing how they thought about the design of the buildings and their clothing while disregarding their own ideals. We should also look at their efforts to attract the patients at the macro level by contemplating the geographical location of the medical missions. It is only by zooming out that we can start asking questions about who missionaries aimed

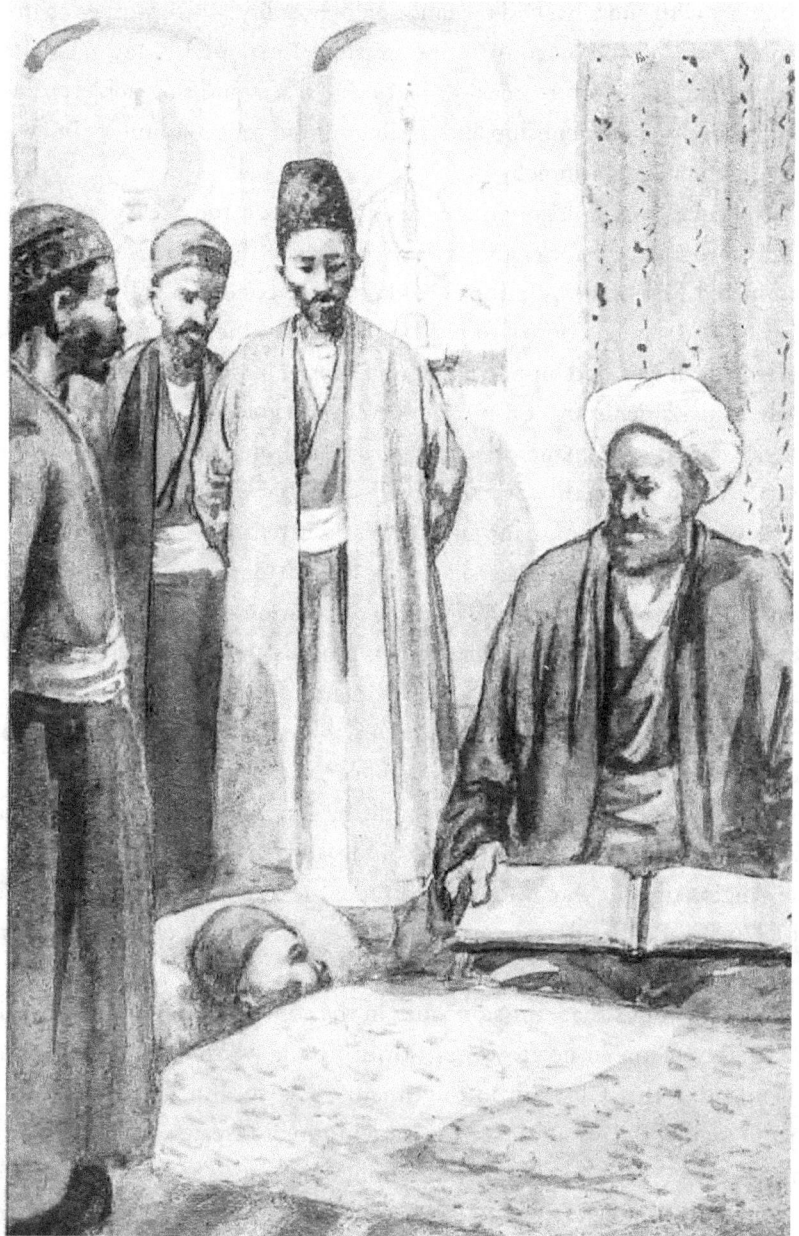

Figure 5.3 Reading the Quran to the sick.
Mrs Napier Malcolm, *Children of Persia* [Edinburgh and London: Oliphant, Anderson & Ferrier, 1911] p. 58. Author's own collection.

to contact with and why. Did the emotion of hostility, which worked to bring medical work to life by constituting mission work in crisis and missionary work in 'danger' become 'stuck' to particular spaces and thus subjects? How could gaining their friendship alter feelings of the very community in favour of the colonial establishment?[73]

Cox states that 'missionaries entered Punjab on the heels of a series of brutal military invasions, and British rule over the province was always dominated first of all by military and strategic concerns'.[74] By the 1820s, the EIC had gained control of the Indian subcontinent as far as the Indus River. The lower and upper areas of Indus, Sindh and Punjab, respectively, and Baluchistan beyond them were independent tribal regions. As Russia started to expand its territories and influences towards Central Asia in the wake of the Crimean War – making overtures with Shahs of Persia and Amirs of Afghanistan, travelling extensively and opening consulates in various cities in Persia[75] – the British started to search for solutions for what became known, after the occupation of Merv by Russians in 1884, as 'the Central Asian Question'. Opinions about a perceived Russian threat were different between the departments of the government in Britain, and between the Foreign Office and the Cabinet in London and the British Government in India (later Indian Office), resulting in a wide variety of solutions. These included a list of military campaigns: the Anglo-Afghan War of 1839–42; the annexation of Sindh and Punjab in 1843 and 1849; the Anglo-Afghan War of 1878–80; and the occupation of Baluchistan in 1876. Thus, Britain brought its north-western frontier closer to Afghanistan and Persia.[76]

Cox does not situate mission work in the context of British military and strategic concerns in north-western British India, yet he provides a pointer when stating that Clark 'from the time of his arrival in Amritsar in 1852, spent much of the rest of the century attempting to create a frontier chain of missions, as if mission stations were military outposts'.[77] The missionaries, indeed, sometimes referred to medical missions on north-western British India as a chain.[78] This discussion regarding a chain of medical missions was even extended to Persia. We can discern this from Dr S. W. Sutton's account of the visit from Reverend Henry Carless of the Persia mission in Quetta in 1895. In a report about this meeting, published in 1896, Sutton pointed out that they discussed the development of a chain of hospitals from Quetta to Isfahan:

> One of the subjects over which we talked together was the extension of our work. Why should we not hope that the Persia Mission might extend eastward and Quetta mission westwards in such a way that the two might co-operate in forming a chain of stations from Julfa and Ispahan [sic] on the west to Quetta on the east? [. . .] Might not the intermediate links of such a chain be forget [sic] in Yazd, Kirman [sic], Nasirabad, and Nushki?[79]

Sutton and Carless's proposal demonstrates that creating a chain of medical missions was a planned scheme. While no medical mission was established in Nushki or Nasirabad, the Yazd and Kerman medical missions were founded in 1899 and 1901, four and six years after this meeting.

Nevertheless, Cox goes on to explain Clark's creation of a chain of missions merely in the context of geo-religion triumphalism, or a desire to convert Asia through 'penetrating' Punjab. There are at least two clues that suggest an alternative vision. One is a statement made by Clark concerning Quetta in 1889; he stated, '[Quetta] is regarded as one of the most valuable defences of our Indian Empire'.[80] Secondly, Pennell referred to the geographical location of Bannu in a 1905 report, stating that 'politically [Bannu] is an advanced post guarding the confines of our Indian empire, situated, as it is, at the entrance of one of those great passes by which it is possible for an invader from the west to enter Indian Bannu'.[81] Quetta lies at the Bolan Pass, and the pass that Pennell was talking about is the Tochi Pass. Pennell may have meant Russia by employing the term 'invader'. The security of these passes became a subject of British foreign policy.[82] The most prominent fortified post that Britain established in the mountains of the Afghan frontier was at Quetta. However, the term invader needs to be deconstructed. It is less likely that Pennell meant an invasion of some sort by Russia to British India. Although opinions about a perceived Russian threat differed, there was common thinking that the Russian's expeditions towards the Indian frontier were mainly to inflame internal unrest, and no invasion was ever planned.[83]

These were not all; Clark had stated in an 1887 report of the Quetta medical mission that '[i]f danger threatens us, let us establish a mission and maintain it strongly. It may be our best defence against Russian aggression.'[84] Similarly, missionaries in Kashmir made the following remark in an appeal in 1895:

> Owing to the advance of the Russians, the dominions of the Maharajah of Kashmir, particularly on the north-western frontier, have been brought into special prominence of late years ... Here we are on the high road to Thibet, Yarkand, Kashghur, Khotan, Kaffiristan, and other places. This surely marks out Kashmir as quite one of the most secure points of action, from a missionary as well as from a political point of view. Such high-roads are surely 'high-roads for the Gospel of Christ' too.[85]

These quotes represent missionaries' desire to portray the medical missions as akin to an armed force. Remarks such as these indicate that north-western British India was presented as a land worthy of missionary attention because of its strategic position. The tone of these statements is in harmony with those made earlier in the century. For example, when talking about the importance of extending British religious influence among inhabitants of southern Africa in 1858, the Bishop of Oxford, Samuel Wilberforce, stated, 'it is the half-way house to India, and that the maintaining it in our strength is essential to our maintaining, unshaken, the Indian Empire which God has given to us.'[86] The presence of missionaries in north-western British India was necessary for the sake of healing bodies and saving souls as well as imperial security.

Yet not all reports, nor Clark himself, always made mention of Russians in this way. There were multiple competing understandings of the Russian presence in Central Asia. One view argued that if the British Empire was ephemeral and the Christian church was to be long lasting, then it mattered little which Christian kingdom would exercise authority.[87] Moreover, it appears that some missionaries differentiated Russia's contribution to the spread of Christianity from their claims over British India. 'We might have our own difficulties with Russia, and quarrel with that power on our account; but if the Czar were to level every mosque in Central Asia or in Mecca itself to the ground, we should not lift a little finger to avert the destruction of them,' was noted in an article *On Religious Neutrality* in 1876.[88] Notwithstanding these competing views, the chain of medical missions that the missionaries intentionally created in north-western British India was an emotional practice in and of itself. We should remember from Chapter One the vastness of the area under the influence of a medical mission and thus consider all the villages they could visit or open a dispensary in.[89] They could target specific locations and meet specific groups of people. They did not shy away from highlighting these points publicly in their speeches or writing.

A New Archive of Knowledge

If Clark argued for establishing missions, Neve proposed how missionaries could be helpful. Neve studied the physical geography of Kashmir and the regions beyond, for which he received the Back Grant from the Royal Geographical Society (RGS) in 1911.[90] In an article published in 1895, he depicted the missionaries' study of the region as crucial due to the Russian threat, believing that Salisbury's advice to politicians to study large-scale maps during a Russian scare was equally applicable to missionaries since 'mission politicians' could provide valuable 'geographical knowledge and forethought'.[91] While Neve did not provide more information, he certainly did not mean that there were secret attempts at surveying the region and that missionaries could contribute to these attempts. The assumption that there was ever an official secret expedition to collect political information derives from the 1901 novel *Kim*, and it is false. Pundits, men with a knowledge of scientific instruments, surveyed countries between British and Russian territories in the 1860s. But these men had no military and political training and could never have assessed such matters.[92] Nonetheless, there was a close relationship between imperialism and precision maps and route books. By the 1880s, such standardised intelligence forms had become sites where planning for military campaigns in little-known places was situated. There existed many maps in the secret archive of the Intelligence Branch at Simla as well as route books.[93] Neve most likely meant these and similar maps produced by colonial administrators.

Georgina Endfield remarks that 'pioneering missionaries were regularly charged with identifying the most appropriate routes to their designed field and the most suitable locations, and physically constructing mission stations'.[94] Although not all missionaries travelled and wrote about the region to the same extent as Neve, they investigated natural resources of the regions during these 'travelling experiments'.[95] A case in point is Dr Marcus Eustace's three-month itineration from 'Quetta to Persian border' in winter 1897.[96] Eustace went on this trip following the discussion between Sutton and Carless regarding the extension of medical mission work from Quetta to Persia. Sutton called the trip 'Spying the Land', believing that it would help them to identify the best location to establish a medical mission.[97] Eustace commented on the climate and water scarcity in a report about this trip. During this trip, he also took some photographs.[98] Furthermore, according to Dr Andrew Jukes, the location of the Dera Ghazi Khan hospital 'was left open' for two years. During this time, the missionaries spent the cold seasons itinerating and the hot seasons in the hills, at Fort Munro, 'studying the language and the people' to identify the best place to plant a mission.[99] Further to this was Clark's tour of Western Himalaya in 1854. In his travel journal, he commented on the geographical position and climate, animal life and vegetable production, among other things.[100] Clark's travel route was documented on a map (Figure 5.4).[101]

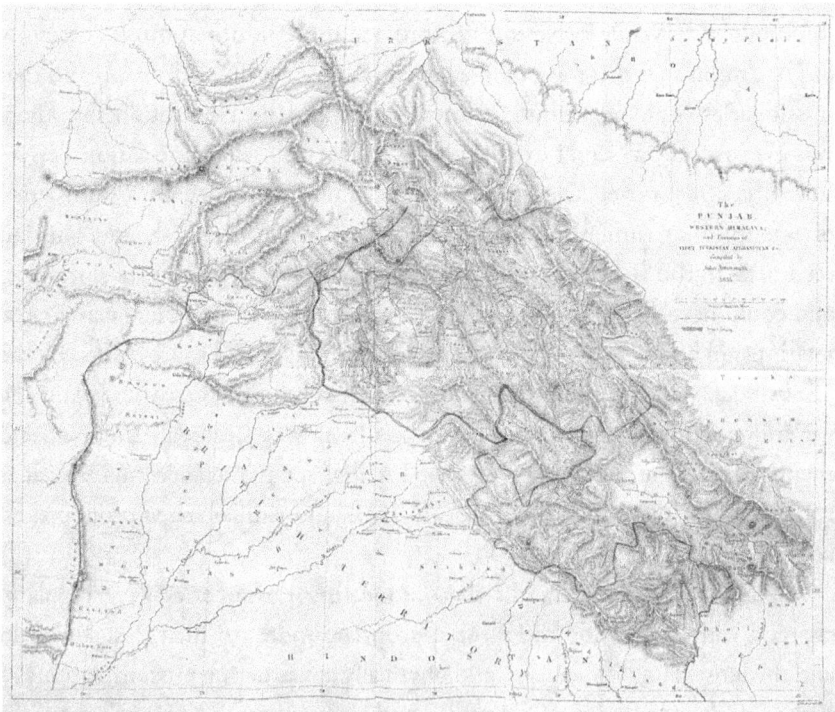

Figure 5.4 The Punjab, Western Himalaya, &c., distinguishing the routes of the Rev. Clark and Lieut Colonel Martin and of the Rev. Dr Prochnow. From the CMS Intelligencer, 1855.

The comparison that Neve drew between missionaries and politicians is particularly tantalising. As stated above, historians of British imperialism have examined the close links between imperialism and the production of knowledge about human and natural resources. James Havia has further demonstrated that not only knowledge produced by colonial administrators was essential, but also the knowledge that was collected by army intelligence.[102] There has also been some critical study of the knowledge gathered by missionaries.[103] A notable missionary is David Livingstone, who is credited for opening the interior of Africa.[104] Moreover, reports and environmental observations of missionaries such as John Croumbie and Robert Moffat influenced state conservation practices.[105] Some missionaries contributed to the processing and distribution of botanical information.[106] According to Endfield, 'the mission represented a node in the global network through which a wide variety of geographical information was circulated'.[107]

The extent to which missionaries' knowledge could underpin military planning, even if 'naively' requires a separate study.[108] Whereas the missionaries were not trained to document routes or survey the regions, as David N. Livingstone asserts, writing their knowledge out of scientific history based on 'the sense that the only science that counts is professional science', is to 'fall foul of historical particularity'.[109] There existed, in particular, a connection between missionaries and maps, with the most notable examples being the Jesuits' involvement in the mapping of China in the sixteenth century or the earth-measuring purposes in the Levant in the seventeenth century.[110] Female missionaries' texts and activities are as important in this discussion as male missionaries. As Maria-Dolors Garcia-Ramon notes, women's narratives could have sometimes been 'sites of resistance to colonialism as well as sites of complicity'.[111] Similarly, male missionaries' writing could have been about imperial expansion as well as proving 'individual manhood', or 'a particular type of colonial manhood'.[112] Anna Young Thompson was among female missionaries who was known for her knowledge of family connections in Egypt,[113] and Annie Royle Taylor of the China Inland Mission (CIM) for single-handedly 'pioneering' in Tibet, collecting and, subsequently disseminating, details 'unknown to most travellers in the Himalayas' at the time.[114] According to Inbal Livne, Taylor was a 'scholar' who provided one of the 'earliest ethnographic records of the Tibetan people for wider public consumption', and in so doing 'add[ed] to the imperial knowledge producing mechanisms of the British Empire'.[115]

As far as Neve's assertion is concerned, missionaries could generate a new archive of knowledge because they were in contact with a more significant number of people on a more intimate footing. Therefore, they could help in updating maps or route books, which was immensely significant.[116] Publications of some missionaries were presented as superior to those of travellers. An article in 1881 referred to the Reverend George Maxwell Gordon's journal of travel in Baluchistan and Afghanistan, stating that 'as an account of the country and people, these notes will be read, we believe, with very great interest, especially coming from so acute an observer and so devoted a missionary as Mr. Gordon was'.[117] This perspective was repeated regarding Neve's publications: '[h]e [Neve] had a wider knowledge of the mountain regions of Kashmir than any other single traveller,' stated Tom Longstaff in Neve's obituary.[118] Likewise, Roberts claimed that Pennell's book was superior to those of politicians and geographers because of his 'long and intimate intercourse' with people.[119]

The missionaries stayed longer in Punjab and were most likely to learn the language – Pennell did not leave India for fifteen years and learned Urdu, Pashto and Persian. This meant that they worked closer to local communities than other colonial agents. Their knowledge could act as useful sources of practical information and add to the existing understandings of north-western British India. Geoff Watson presents a similar debate concerning the writings of the missionaries of the LMS in Central Asia in the 1830s. Watson writes that compared to travellers, hunters and geographers, 'the writings of missionaries could claim to have been based upon lengthy residence and extensive day-to-day contact with the peoples of Central Asia. This, combined with their status within the community as spiritual leaders, lent their writings a particular authority.'[120] Likewise, Andrew Porter remarks, 'Residence, prolonged observation, knowledge of vernaculars, and close contacts gave missionary observations depths unmatched by early armchair ethnologists and most travellers.'[121]

Efforts of the British to avert a Russian threat were not limited to armed interventions. They also tried to develop Persia and Afghanistan as buffer states. Another scheme was centred on British supremacy in the Persian Gulf.[122] In north-western British India, this involved 'continual negotiations' with the Pashtun (Pathan) and Baloch tribal groups.[123] British officials made considerable efforts to form and maintain contact with these tribal groups, which proved to be a challenging enterprise, more so concerning the Pashtun.[124] To this must be added that the British policy in the region was not defined merely by concerns over the pre-emption of a Russian advance towards India.[125] The Pashtun and Baloch tribes presented problems of their own. Due to their eagerness to defend their independence and culture, they were considered by some as one of the 'internal enemies' of British India, whose disaffection could cause widespread riots and disturbance.[126] The importance of missionaries' effort to form emotional ties can be explored further in relation to these tribal groups.*

The Pashtun and Baloch Tribal Groups

The missionaries who worked in north-western British India highlighted their influence on Pashtun and Baloch. A Comment by Dr Arthur Neve even implies that one of the missionaries' purposes was to reach various tribal groups. Neve stated, 'there are missions, well placed [. . .], at Quetta, Bannu, and Peshawar, especially working among Afghans and Baluchis. In Persia, Missions should be placed at Kirman[sic], Yezd[sic] and Meshad[sic], with a view to eastward expansion among Persian-speaking tribes.'[127] Similarly, Fort Munro was chosen as an outpatient station because it was a 'common ground, and the representatives of all the tribes, within or beyond what was till recently the Frontier, meet to settle inter-tribal disputes in common council, or Jigrah'.[128]

The Pashtun inhabit some 400 miles (640 km), stretching from the Hindu Kush in the north to the Sulaiman range in the south and as far as the Gumal River. The missionaries regularly provided statistics concerning the number of patients from this tribal group in their reports and speeches. One of the most detailed figures was provided by Pennell himself in his 1898 report. He wrote:

> of the 438 in-patients during the year, there have been: 171 Bannuzais; 76 Waziris; 40 Khattacks; 33 Marwats; 39 Hindkis; 16 Khstols (Nyazis

---

* I use the word tribe as it was used in the missionaries' records.

and Punjabis); and of the reminder, nine Ghilzais, eight Mahsouds, eight Bangash, six Dawaris from Tochi Valley, five Jats, four Cabulis, four Zadrans, three Purbiahs, two Afridis, and one each of the Awan, Orakzai, Zaimukht, and Ningrahar tribes.[129]

This record is very detailed. The Pashtun and Baloch were divided into different tribal confederations, and Pennell specified the number of patients from each confederation.[130] He laid out a similarly detailed statistic again in 1901.[131] Pennell portrayed Pashtun and Baloch as the largest group of patients. The missionaries sometimes indicated that most of the patients were from these groups. For instance, in the 1906 annual meeting of the MMA, Arthur Lankester stated that '[t]he larger proportion of patients treated at the hospital are not inhabitants of Peshawar, but Pathans, Afridis, &c'.[132] In the same way, Dr John Summerhayes wrote in 1898 that they mainly tried to get 'jats and some plain Baluchis' at the Dera Ghazi Khan hospital.[133] Likewise, the 1911 annual report stated that '[t]he majority of patients are Pathan' in the Dera Ismail Khan hospital.[134] Although the missionaries wrote that the hospitals had patients from different parts of India, Persia and Turkistan, they mainly highlighted the number of Pashtun and Baloch. They also sometime itinerated for the sole purpose of visiting these tribes. Pennell itinerated among the hills between Bannu and Kohat because this region was inhabited by the Khattack tribe.[135] Therefore, the missionaries exposed these tribal groups as the main target of their hospitals.

Underlining their connection and ties with tribal groups was one of the ways in which the missionaries presented their work as beneficial to India's defence. It is helpful to cite a painting of Pennell in this regard, which signifies how the missionaries hoped to portray their contact with tribes as useful to India's defence (Figure 5.5). At first glance, it is difficult to distinguish Pennell in the painting. Compositionally, he is set in the middle of the picture, surrounded by tribesmen, whose stares accentuate Pennell's centrality. This composition creates an image that suggests the attachment of tribesmen to Pennell. While they were not fighting, except for two, all had their guns ready, implying they were prepared to fight for Pennell.

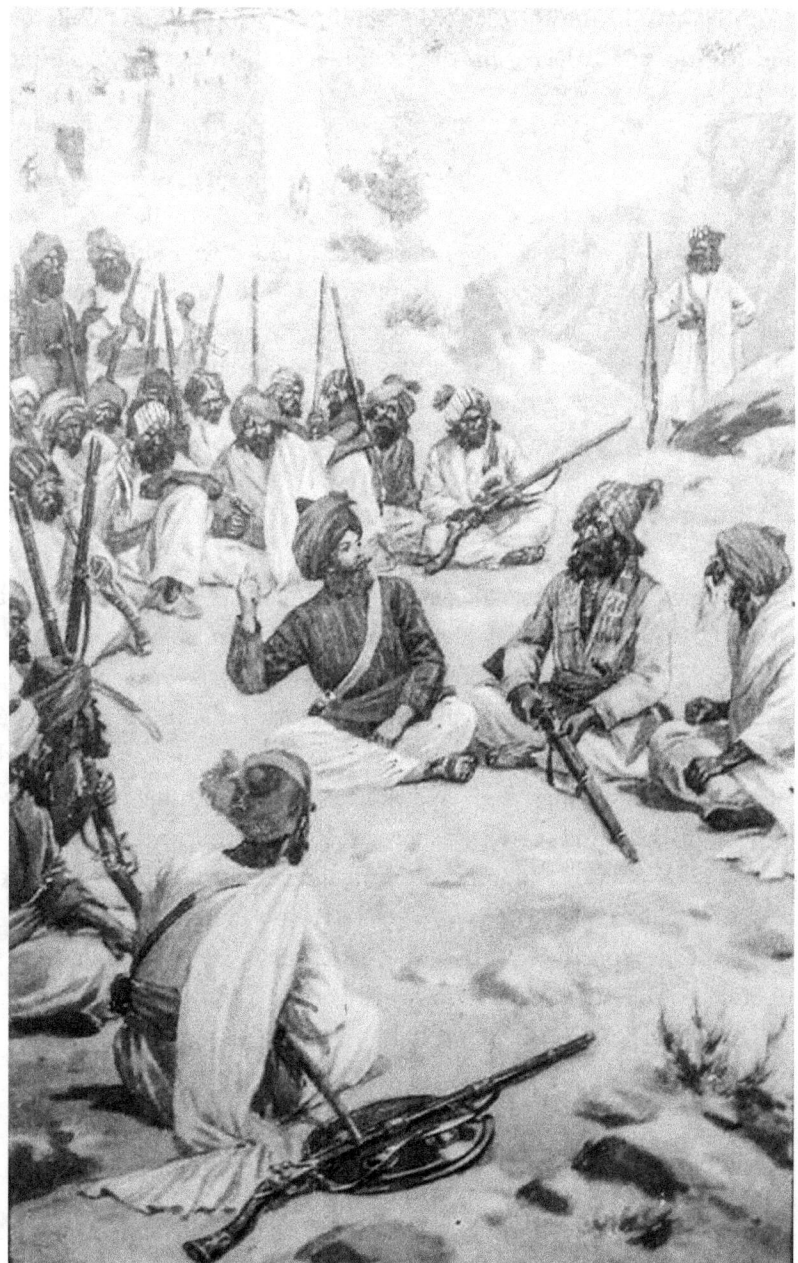

Figure 5.5 Pennell of the Indian Frontier.
Alice Pennell, *A Hero of the Afghan Frontier: Dr Pennell's Life for Boys* (1900). All reasonable steps have been taken to determine the copyright holder.

This is what the missionaries proposed in their writings and publications about Pashtun and Baloch. One of the earliest of these comments was made by Clark in 1887:

> I need hardly here refer to the peculiar circumstances of our Quetta Mission. . . . We are here standing on the ground which had been traversed by the many invaders who have poured their hordes down from the central steppes of Asia, through the mountain passes of the Bolan, or the Khurum, or the Khyber, on their way to found empires in India. We see around us the very tribes which during the last termination of whose rule we ourselves have witnessed – have established no less than eight distinct dynasties on the throne of India. All these dynasties have come from these frontiers, or beyond them; from races of whom it is said that 'whoever rules them holds the crown of India in his hand, or at any rate within his grasp'.[136]

Drilling down into Clark's statement in more detail is illuminating. At the heart of Clark's statement lies his reference to the history of north-western British India concerning invasion and empire. By the late nineteenth century, it was widely accepted that north-western British India had a background in acting as a gateway to the subcontinent – this was a reason why north-western British India was considered strategic. Through using the word 'we' and the phrase 'around us', Clark showcased the missionaries' knowledge of the region. In addition, he implied that 'ruling' tribal groups was a reason why the missionaries were in north-western British India.

Some of the reports were more explicit. A note in 1903 stated that due to their influence on tribes, medical missions were politically important and had even been backed up by British officials:

> Our Medical Mission stations, situated at the entrances to the passes into Afghanistan and Beluchistan [sic], are influencing to a remarkable degree these turbulent peoples. Willing testimony is borne by the frontier military and civil officers to the helpful work, even in the political sense, which is being accomplished by our Medical Missionaries.[137]

Similarly, Pennell referred to a statement made by a 'political officer' in the hospital log-book in his annual report in 1906:

A political officer after visiting the hospital wrote: 'I had heard a great deal about the Bannu Medical Mission Hospital before Dr. Pennell took me over it and was much interested in seeing what is now (to leave other aspects of the work out of the question) and important political factor on the Bannu frontier. I never fail to advise Tochi Waziris to go to Dr. Pennell at Bannu, and in future I shall advise them more strongly than before. This splendid work will long be remembered by all tribes and classes.'[138]

We can find another clear-cut comment in Pennell's 1908 published report, where he recalled the 1897 tribal uprising against the British. He stated that while 'all down the frontier, from Swat through Tirah down to Waziristan, every tribe was up in arms against the British Government', there was one exception. The Zaimukht tribe (one of the Pashtun sub-tribes) did not even fire a single shot 'upon any of the British' because they were the only tribe 'down all the frontier where the chief was reading the Bible and where he had had the opportunity of having a medical missionary in his own country'.[139] Likewise, a note in 1900 referred to the opening of a dispensary at Lundi Kotal on the frontier and explained how it could render excellent service politically, because medical missionaries were 'far more likely to appease turbulent tribes than to arouse their opposition'.[140] Last but not least is a story recalled in Pennell's obituary. According to this story, Neve was bicycling out from Bannu one night when he came across men with guns a little beyond the frontier. After mentioning that he was coming from 'Dr. Pennell's Hospital', those men invited him to stay with them, stating that '[w]e will make all your food; we will make you comfortable; of course, he [Pennell] is our friend'.[141] It is worth noting again that whether missionaries managed to secure people's – in this case tribes' – friendship is debatable. Regardless, these claims are crucial; they did not necessarily talk about the spread of Christianity or the dissemination of the 'English' race or ethical values. They indicated rather that they were winning the tribes for the empire of Britain by securing their friendship.

Conclusion

This chapter sheds some light on how the (medial) missionaries of the CMS in north-western British India presented their work in the context of Anglo-Russian rivalry in the late nineteenth and early twentieth centuries. The assumption that the missionaries presented their work as a defence against Russia stems from a remark made by Lord Roberts in the 1900s, who claimed that Dr Theodore Leighton Pennell was worth a 'regiment' to the British government on the frontier. This remark interested missionaries, which suggests that they presented their work as beneficial to India's defence.

This was not the first time that the missionaries publicly talked about the political significance of their work. Going back to the early nineteenth century, a new pattern of close alliance between the Church and the state started to develop, when many church leaders talked about the providential gift of the empire. They declared that India was given to Britain by God for Christianisation, an idea that for them was as much a cultural and religious as a political vision. However, the CMS medical missionaries considered the providential gift of the empire in an entirely new way. Instead of being concerned with Christianisation per se or the spread of the English race or ethical values, they highlighted their effort and success in cultivating friendship with local populations. They claimed that their missions were worth a regiment because they had been instrumental in obtaining people's trust and justified this view on at least two grounds.

The CMS created a chain of hospitals in north-western British India. Some missionaries asserted that this was due to fears of a Russian threat. Dr Arthur Neve specifically talked about their role in contributing knowledge about the region, comparing missionaries' study of the area to politicians'. Even though the extent to which the missionaries managed to secure people's friendship is debatable, they stayed in the regions longer and worked closer with the local population than other colonial agents. Thus, their observation and publications could enjoy a certain authority.

One of the main themes in the missionaries' report was Pashtun and Baloch tribal groups. Britain undertook a list of political campaigns to avert a Russian threat, one of which centred on establishing contacts with Pashtun and Baloch, who inhabited north-western British India. To highlight their political importance, the missionaries depicted Pashtun and Baluch tribal groups as the main target of the hospitals in north-western British India. Some of the missionaries went even further, claiming that they were winning tribes for the empire of Britain by obtaining their friendship.

Notes

1. G. A. Bremner, 'The Expansion of England? Rethinking Scotland's place in the architectural history of the wider British world', *Journal of Art Historiography* 18 (2018), https://arthistoriography.files.wordpress.com/2018/05/bremner.pdf
2. Arthur Neve, 'Medical Work on the Indian Frontier', *Mercy and Truth* 15, no. 177 (1911): 309. See also Miss E. E. S. Hill, 'First Impressions of an Indian Frontier Hospital', *The Mission Hospital* 30, no. 345 (1926): 268; *Medical Missions* (London: Church Missionary Society, 1928), 25.
3. Arthur Neve, 'A Word from the N. W. Frontier of India', *Mercy and Truth* 19, no. 224 (2015): 277; 'Obituary: Theodore Leighton Pennell', *The British Medical Journal* 1 (1912): 761
4. Jennifer Siegel, *Endgame: Britain, Russia and the Final Struggle for Central Asia* (London: I. B. Tauris, 2002); M. A. Yapp, 'The Legend of the Great Game', *Proceedings of the British Academy* 111 (2001): 179–98.
5. Jeffrey Cox, *Imperial Fault Lines: Christianity and Colonial Power in India, 1818–1940* (Stanford: Stanford University Press, 2002), 8.
6. James, Hevia, *The Imperial Security State: British Colonial Knowledge and Empire-Building in Asia* (Cambridge: Cambridge University Press, 2012); B. D. Hopkins, *The Making of Modern Afghanistan* (Basingstoke: Palgrave Macmillan, 2008); Elena Andreeva, *Russia and Iran in the Great Game: Travelogues and Orientalism* (London: Routledge, 2007); Siegel, *Endgame: Britain, Russia*.
7. Dana L. Robert, 'Introduction', in Dana L. Robert (ed.), *Converting Colonialism: Visions and Realities in Mission History, 1706–1914* (Grand Rapids: William B. Eerdmans, 2008), 3.
8. For example, see Patricia Grimshaw and Andrew May, 'Reappraisals of Mission History: An Introduction', in Patricia Grimshaw and Andrew May (eds), *Missionaries, Indigenous Peoples and Cultural Exchange* (Eastbourne: Sussex Academic Press, 2010), 1–9; Jeffrey Cox, *The British Missionary Enterprise since 1700* (London: Routledge, 2008); John Stuart, 'Mission and Empire', *Social Sciences and Missions* 21, no. 1 (2008): 1–5.
9. Cox, *The British Missionary*; Andrew Porter, *Religion versus Empire? British Protestant Missionaries and Overseas Expansion, 1700–1914* (Manchester: Manchester University Press, 2004).
10. John L. Comaroff and Jean Comaroff, *Of Revelation and Revolution: The Dialectics of Modernity on a South African Frontier*, 2 vols (Chicago: The University of Chicago Press, 1997); Zoë Crossland, 'Signs of Mission: Material Semeiosis

and Nineteenth-Century Tswana Architecture', *Signs and Society* 1, no. 1 (2013): 79–113.
11. Cox, *The British Missionary*, 13.
12. Emily Turner, 'The Church Missionary Society and Architecture in the Mission Field: Evangelical Anglican Perspectives on Church Building Abroad, c. 1850–1900', *Architectural History* 58 (2015): 197–228. doi:10.1017/S0066622X0000263X; G. A. Bremner, 'The Architecture of Universities' Mission to Central Africa: Developing a Vernacular Tradition in the Anglican Field, 1861–1909', *Journal of the Society of Architectural Historians* 68, no. 4 (2009): 514–39; Peter Williams, 'Healing and Evangelism: The Place of Medicine in later Victorian Protestant Missionary Thinking', *Studies in Church History* 19 (1982): 271–85; Cox, *Imperial Fault Lines*, 39–40; Sara H. Sohmer, 'Christianity without Civilization: Anglican Sources for an Alternative Nineteenth-Century Mission Methodology', *Journal of Religious History* 18, no. 2 (1994): 174–97.
13. Hayden J. A. Bellenoit, *Missionary Education and Empire in Late Colonial India, 1860–1920* (London: Routledge, 2015).
14. For example, see Tony Ballantyne, *Entanglements of Empire: Missionaries, Māori, and the Question of the Body* (Durham, NC: Duke University Press, 2014); Elizabeth Elbourne, 'Word Made Flesh: Christianity, Modernity and Cultural Colonialism in the Work of Jean and John Comaroff', *The American Historical Review* 108, no. 2 (2003): 435–59; Steven Feierman, 'A Century of Ironies in East Africa', in Phillip D. Curtin, Steven Feierman, Leonard Thompson and Jan Vansina (eds), *African Cities from Earliest Times to Independence* (New York, 1995); Elizabeth Prevost, 'Married to the Mission Field: Gender, Christianity, and Professionalization in Britain and Colonial Africa, 1865–1914', *Journal of British Studies* 47, no. 4 (2008): 808.
15. Cox, *Imperial Fault Lines*, 6.
16. Rowan Strong, *Anglicanism and the British Empire c. 1700–1850* (Oxford: Oxford University Press, 2007).
17. Christopher Harding, *Religious Transformation in South Asia: The Meanings of Conversion in Colonial Punjab* (Oxford: Oxford University Press, 2008), 76.
18. While the CMS was a voluntary society, its members were of a church established by law in both England and India and its founders were linked to men of significant governmental and imperial experience. While diverse in their approach, the SPG and the CMS were devoted to co-operation and their work complemented each other in many ways; they both contributed to the creation of Anglican mission culture. See Howard Le Couteur, 'Anglican High Churchmen and the Expansion of Empire', *Journal of Religious History* 32, no. 2 (2008):

193–215; Elizabeth Elbourne, 'The Foundation of the Church Missionary Society: the Anglican Missionary Impulse', in John Walsh, Colin Haydon, and Stephen Taylor (eds), *The Church of England c. 1689–c. 1833: From Toleration to Tractarianism* (Cambridge: Cambridge University Press, 1993), 247–64.
19. Strong, *Anglicanism*, 6.
20. Ibid., 120.
21. Strong, *Anglicanism*, 118–97. See also Julie Evans et al., *Equal Subjects, Unequal Rights: Indigenous Peoples in British Settler Societies, 1830–1910* (Manchester: Manchester University Press, 2003).
22. Hilary M. Carey, *God's Empire: Religion and Colonialism in the British World, c. 1801–1908* (Cambridge: Cambridge University Press, 2011), 45–54.
23. Cox, *Imperial Fault Lines*, 26.
24. Charles R. Bawden, *Shamans, Lamas, and Evangelicals: The English Missionaries in Siberia* (London: Routledge and Kegan Paul, 1985).
25. Stewart J. Brown, 'Providential Empire? The Established Church of England and the Nineteenth-Century British Empire in India', *Studies in Church History* 54 (2018): 255–9.
26. Carey, *God's Empire*, 28–33.
27. Brown, 'Providential Empire? The Established Church', 253–4.
28. Eugene Stock, the historian of the CMS, disregards this view in his supplement of the history of the society, calling it an 'imperfect' recognition of the objects of mission. See Eugene Stock, *The History of the Church Missionary Society: Supplementary Volume* (London: Church Missionary Society, 1916), 137.
29. Williams, 'Healing and Evangelism'; the term hostile was used by missionaries which itself requires historical analysis. See, for example, Erik Freas, *Muslim-Christian Relations in Late Ottoman Palestine: Where Nationalism and Religion Intersects* (Basingstoke: Palgrave Macmillan, 2016).
30. Arthur Neve, 'A Word from the N. W. Frontier of India', *Mercy and Truth* 19, no. 224 (1915): 278.
31. Karen Vallgårda, 'Tying Children to God with Love: Danish Mission, Childhood, and Emotions in Colonial South India', *Journal of Religious History* 39, no. 4 (2015): 595–613; C. McLisky, 'Professions of Christian Love: Letters of Courtship between Missionaries-to-be Daniel Matthew and Janet Johnston', in Amanda Barry, Joanna Cruickshank, Andrew Brown-May and Patricia Grimshaw (eds), *Evangelicals of Empire? Missionaries in Colonial History* (Melbourne: University of Melbourne eScholarship Research Centre, 2008), 173–85.
32. 'Theodore Leighton Pennell, M.D., B.Sc. (Lond), F.R.C.S (Eng.): A Memorial Sketch', *Mercy and Truth* 16, no. 185 (May 1912): 140.

33. Ibid.
34. Alice M. Pennell, *Pennell of the Afghan Frontier* (New York: E. P. Dutton and Company, 1914), viii.
35. T. L. Pennell, *Among the Wild Tribes of the Afghan Frontier*, 6th ed. (London: Seeley, Service & Co. Limited, 1922), 241–56.
36. Rebecca Weaver-Hightower, *Empire Islands: Castaways, Cannibals, and Fantasies of Conquest* (Minneapolis and London: University of Minnesota Press, 2007), 133.
37. Brown, 'Providential Empire?', 255–9.
38. J. O. Summerhayes, 'Among the Biloches', *Mercy and Truth* 1, no. 7 (July 1897): 159.
39. 'The Soudan and Upper Niger Mission', *The Church Missionary Intelligencer and Record* 15 (October 1890): 694.
40. 'A Year of Labour in our Foreign Mission Field', *India's Women and China's Daughters* IX, no. 54 (November–December 1889): 332.
41. Jörg Fisch, 'A Solitary Vindicator of the Hindus: The Life and Writings of General Stuart (1757/58–1828)', *The Journal of the Royal Asiatic Society of Great Britain and Ireland*, no. 1 (1985): 35–57.
42. Lisa McCracken Lacy, *Lady Anne Blunt in the Middle East: Travel, Politics, and the Idea of Empire* (London and New York: I. B. Tauris, 2018).
43. Mikail Mamedov, '"Going Native" in the Caucasus: Problems of Russian identity, 1801–64', *The Russian Review* 67, no. 2 (2008): 275–95.
44. Sanjay Subrahmanyam, *The Portuguese Empire in Asia, 1500–1700: A Political and Economic History* (Chichester: Wiley & Sons, 2012).
45. Frank Lestringant, 'Going native in America (French-style)', *Renaissance Studies* 6, nos 3 and 4 (1992): 325–35.
46. Daniel Thorp, 'Going native in New Zealand and America: Comparing Pakeha Maori and white Indians', *The Journal of Imperial and Commonwealth History* 31, no. 3 (2003): 1–23.
47. Subrahmanyam, *The Portuguese Empire in Asia*.
48. Willard Sunderland, 'Russians into Iakuts? "Going Native" and Problems of Russian National Identity in the Siberian North, 1870s–1914', *Slavic Review* 55, no. 4 (1996): 806–25.
49. Mamedov, '"Going Native" in the Caucasus', 280.
50. I specifically engage with Rob Boddice's work here. See Rob Boddice, *The Science of Sympathy: Morality, Evolution, and Victorian Civilization* (Urbana and Chicago: University of Illinois Press, 2016), 3–6.

51. Anu Korhonen, 'Beauty, Masculinity and Love between Men: Configuring Emotions with Michael Drayton's *Peirs Gaveston*', in Jonas Liliequist (ed.), *A History of Emotions, 1200–1800* (Oxford and New York: Routledge, 2012), 136–51.
52. See 'CMS Medical Missions', *Medical Mission Quarterly*, no. IV (October 1893): 3.
53. 'Editorial Notes', *The Church Missionary Gleaner* XVII, no. 196 (April 1890): 51.
54. Pennell, *Among the Wild Tribes*, 253.
55. Pennell, *Pennell of the Afghan*, 17.
56. *Extracts from the Annual Letters of the missionaries for the year* 1895 (1896), 220.
57. Pennell, *Pennell of the Afghan*, 46.
58. Pennell, *Among the Wild Tribes*, 253.
59. Jeffrey Cox, *The British Missionary Enterprise since 1700* (London and New York: Routledge, 2008), 205.
60. Jeffrey Cox, 'Going Native: Missionaries in India', in William Roger Louis (ed.), *More Adventures with Britannia: Personalities, Politics and Culture in Britain* (London and New York: I. B. Tauris, 2003), 309.
61. Pennell, *Among the Wild Tribes*, 255.
62. Ibid., 254.
63. Pennell, *Pennell of the Afghan*, 87.
64. Eric Reinders, *Borrowed Gods and Foreign Bodies: Christian Missionaries Imagine Chinese Religion* (Berkeley, Los Angles and London: University of California Press, 2004), 176.
65. Lauren Berlant, 'Introduction: Compassion (and Withholding)', in Lauren Berlant (ed.), *Compassion: The Culture and Politics of an Emotion* (New York and London: Routledge, 2004), 1–13.
66. Neillie Hoad, 'Cosmetic Surgeons of the Social: drawing, Freud, and Wells and the Limits of Sympathy on The Island of Dr. Moreau', in *Compassion* (see note 65), 191.
67. Pennell, *Pennell of the Afghan*, 87.
68. Ibid.
69. Ibid., 17.
70. Ibid., 87.
71. *Extracts from the Annual Letters*, 220.
72. I am grateful to an anonymous reviewer of my book for requesting me to develop the part on Pennell's dress further by adding this paragraph.
73. Sara Ahmed, 'Affective Economics', *Social Text* 22, no. 2 (2004): 117–39.
74. Cox, *Imperial Fault Lines*, 23.

75. M. A. Yapp, 'British Perception of the Russian Threat to India', *Modern Asian Studies* 21, no. 4 (1987): 647–65, doi:10.1017/S0026749X00009264.
76. Robert Johnson, '"Russians at the Gates of India"? Planning the Defence of India, 1885–1900', *Journal of Military History* 67, no. 3 (2003): 702–3.
77. Cox, *Imperial Fault Lines*, 26.
78. 'Medical Missions', *Mercy and Truth* 1, no. 11 (November 1897): 249; H. White, 'The Crescent and the Cross', *Mercy and Truth* 13, no. 153 (1909): 305–12.
79. S. W. Sutton, 'Jotting from Quetta', *Mercy and Truth* 1, no. 6 (1897): 126–9.
80. 'The New Mission at Quetta', *The Church Missionary Gleaner* 16, no. 190 (1889): 152–4.
81. T. L. Pennell, 'A Special Plea, for a Special Need, at Bannu', *Mercy and Truth* 9, no. 99 (1905): 72.
82. Hamin Goren, *Dead Sea Level: Science, Exploration and Imperial Interest in the Near East* (London: I. B. Tauris, 2011), 10.
83. Yapp, 'The Legend of the Great Game', 179–98.
84. R. Clark, 'The New Mission at Quetta', *The Church Missionary Intelligencer and Record* 12 (1877): 166.
85. 'An Appeal to the Church Missionary Society. Issued by the Missionaries in Kashmir', *The Church Missionary Intelligencer* xx new series (1895): 351–2.
86. Quoted in G. A. Bremner, *Imperial Gothic: Religious Architecture and High Anglican Culture in the British Empire* (New Haven: Yale University Press, 2013), 9.
87. Cox, *Imperial Fault Lines*, 23–51.
88. 'On Religious Neutrality', *The Church Missionary Intelligencer and Record* 1, new series (1876): 194.
89. Dr S. Gaster emphasised this point in his annual letter in November 1903. *Extracts from the Annual Letters of Missionaries for the year 1903* (London: Church Missionary Society, 1904), 499. CRL.
90. In 1896, he went on a two-month tour in the country of Baltis, which was, according to him, 'but little known to Europeans, and even Punjab Missionaries might be forgiven for asking where Baltistan is.' See A. Neve, 'Kashmir Medical Mission: A Tour in Baltistan', *Medical Mission Quarterly*, no. XV (1896): 73.
91. Arthur Neve, 'The Unevangelized Countries of Asia', *The Church Missionary Intelligencer* 20 (1895): 247.
92. Gerald Morgan, 'Myth and Reality in the Great Game', *Asian Affairs* 4, no. 1 (1973): 57.
93. Hevia, *The Imperial Security State*, 2–5.

94. Georgina Endfield, 'The Mission', in John Agnew and David N. Livingston (eds), *The Sage Handbook of Geographical Knowledge* (London: Sage Publications, 2011), 205.
95. F. Driver, *Geography Militant: Cultures of Exploration and Empire* (Oxford: Blackwell Publishers, 2001).
96. 'Things to be Noted', *Mercy and Truth* 1, no. 3 (1897): 51.
97. Sutton, 'Jotting from Quetta', 128.
98. Ibid.
99. A. Jukes, 'With Dr. Jukes Since 1879', *Mercy and Truth* 3, no. 25 (1899): 7.
100. 'Kashmir', *The Church Missionary Intelligence* 6 (1855): 68–72.
101. The competition with other missionary societies might have been another reason that might have made missionaries search for a best place. See Rhonda Anne Sample, *Missionary Women: Gender, Professionalism and the Victorian Idea of Christian Mission* (Rochester: The Roydell Press, 2003).
102. Hevia, *The Imperial Security*.
103. Andrew F. Walls, 'The Nineteenth-Century Missionary as Scholar', in Andrew F. Walls (ed.), *The Missionary Movement in Christian History: Studies in the Transmission of Faith* (New York: Orbis Books, 1996), 139–46; David N. Livingston, 'Scientific Inquiry and the Missionary Enterprise', in Ruth Finnegan (ed.), *Participating in the Knowledge Society: Researchers Beyond the University Walls* (Basingstoke: Palgrave Macmillan, 2005), 50–64.
104. F. Driver, *Geography Militant: Cultures of Exploration and Empire* (Oxford: Blackwell Publishers, 2001).
105. Richard Grove, 'Early Themes in African Conservation: The Cape in the Nineteenth Century', in David Anderson and Richard Grove (eds), *Conservation in Africa: People, Policies and Practice* (Cambridge: Cambridge University Press, 1897), 21–39.
106. Michael T. Bravo, 'Mission Gardens: Natural History and Global Expansion, 1720–1820', in Londa Schiebinger and Claudia Swan (eds), *Colonial Botany: Science, Commerce, and Politics in the Early Modern World* (Philadelphia: University of Pennsylvania Press, 2005), 49–65.
107. Endfield, 'The Mission', 206.
108. Robert, 'Introduction', 5.
109. Livingston, 'Scientific Inquiry', 50.
110. Ibid., 53–4.
111. Maria-Dolors Garcia-Ramon, 'Gender and the Colonial encounter in the Arab world: examining women's experiences and narratives', *Environment and Planning D: Society and Space* 21 (2003), 653.

112. Susan L. Blake, 'A Woman's trek: What difference does gender make?', *Women's Studies International Forum* 13, no. 4 (1990), 347–55; See also Sara Mills, *Gender and Colonial Space* (Manchester: Manchester University Press, 2013), 55–6.
113. Healther J. Sharkey, *American Evangelicals in Egypt: Missionary Encounters in an Age of Empire* (Princeton and London: Princeton University Press, 2008), 88.
114. Inbal Livne, 'The Many Purposes of Missionary Work: Annie Royle Taylor as Missionary, Travel writer, Collector and Empire Builder', in Hilde Nielssen, Inger Marie Okkenhaug and Karina Hestad Skeie (eds), *Protestant Missions and Local Encounters in the Nineteenth and Twentieth Centuries: Unto the Ends of the World* (Leiden and Boston: Brill, 2011), 51.
115. Ibid., 53 and 48.
116. Hevia, *The Imperial Security*, 78.
117. 'Mr. Gordon's March to Kandahar', *The Church Missionary Society Intelligence and Record* 6 (1881): 11–27.
118. Tom Longstaff, 'Obituary: Arthur Neve', *The Geographical Journal* 54, no. 6 (1919): 397.
119. T. L. Pennell, *Among the Wild Tribes of the Afghan Frontier, A Record of Sixteen Years' Close Intercourse with the Natives of the Indian Marchers*, 2nd ed. (London: Seeley, 1909), vi.
120. Geoff Watson, 'The Ultimate Evangelical Away Game: British Missionary Endeavour in Central Asia c. 1830–1930', in Ken Parry (ed.), *Art, Architecture and Religion Along the Silk Roads* (Turnhout: Brepols Publishers, 2009), 127.
121. Andrew Porter, 'Religion, Missionary Enthusiasm, and Empire', in Andrew Porter (ed.), *The Oxford History of the British Empire: Volume III: The Nineteenth Century* (Oxford: Oxford University Press, 1999), 241.
122. Yapp, 'British Perception', 650–6.
123. Hugh Beattie, 'Negotiations with the Tribes of Waziristan 1849–1914 – The British Experience', *The Journal of Imperial and Commonwealth History* 39, no. 4 (2011): 571–87.
124. Paul Titus, 'Honor the Baloch, Buy the Pushtun: Strategies, Social Organization and History in Western Pakistan', *Modern Asian Studies* 32, no. 3 (1998): 659–62.
125. B. D. Hopkins, *The Making of Modern Afghanistan* (Basingstoke: Palgrave Macmillan, 2008), 34–61
126. Yapp, 'British Perception', 649.
127. Arthur Neve, 'The Unevangelized Countries of Asia', *The Church Missionary Intelligencer* 20 (1895): 250.

128. A. Jukes, 'With Dr. Jukes Since 1897', *Mercy and Truth* 3, no. 25 (January 1899): 7.
129. T. L. Pennell, 'Among Trans-Border Tribesmen', *Mercy and Truth* 2, no. 22 (1898): 238.
130. Beattie, 'Negotiations with the Tribes of Waziristan', 572.
131. T. L. Pennell, 'Bannu Medical Mission in 1900', *Mercy and Truth* 5, no. 53 (1901): 110.
132. 'The Annual Meeting', *Mercy and Truth* 10, no. 114 (1906): 162.
133. John O. Summerhayes, 'Work at Dera Ghazi Khan and Fort Munro', *Mercy and Truth* 2, no. 17 (May 1898): 109.
134. 'Punjab and Sindh Mission', *Mercy and Truth* 15, no. 175 (1911): 228.
135. *Extracts from the Annual Letters of the Missionaries*, 497.
136. R. Clark, 'The New Mission at Quetta', *The Church Missionary Intelligencer and Record* 12 (1877): 165.
137. 'Things to be Noted', *Mercy and Truth* 12, no. 136 (1903): 97–8.
138. 'Items: Home and Abroad', *Mercy and Truth* 10, no. 118 (1906): 295.
139. T. L. Pennell, 'The Conflict of the Crescent and the Cross', *Mercy and Truth* 12, no. 140 (1908): 239–40.
140. 'Things to be Noted', *Mercy and Truth* 4, no. 42 (June 1900): 122.
141. 'Obituary: Theodore Leighton Pennell', 761; 'Theodore Leighton Pennell, M.D., B.Sc. (Lond.), F.R.C.S. (Eng.): A Memorial Sketch', 141.

CONCLUSION
AFFECTING BODIES, SAVING SOULS

The period between 1865 and 1914 witnessed concurrently the transformation of medicine and hospital architecture in Europe and North America and the rise of Protestant medical mission work overseas. Influential in the emergence of the latter was also a shared conviction among many Protestant missionary societies that administrating medicine was the best method for gaining people's trust, affection and friendship. This shared conviction emerged from a century of mission work marked by failure and frustration. Although the medical missionaries were not alone in talking about gaining local people's trust and affection, they certainly undertook work on a scale and in places that not only colonial officials but also missionaries themselves could have only dreamed of. By the second decade of the twentieth century, medical missions could be found in large numbers in Asia and Africa. Among the British missionary societies, the CMS took the lead in this regard in Persia and north-western British India, establishing a total of twelve medical missions by 1914.

Through focusing on the issue of gaining trust, affection or friendship, this study has made a case for examining medical mission work under the motto of affecting bodies, saving souls rather than healing bodies, saving souls. In making this interpretive shift, this study has drawn on methodological approaches offered by the field of the history of emotions. In so doing, it has demanded refocusing the attention from medical missions as either sentimental or coercive towards medical missions as emotional set-ups that served to change the sensory relationship between missionaries and local people. Viewing medical missions in this way has also demanded considering the missionaries, local people, the (built) environment, smell, sound and touch side by side. These points were explored by focusing on five key themes: dispensary and itineration works, the architecture of mission hospitals, hospital visiting and family wards, women's work and women's hospitals and the interaction between mission and empire.

I have highlighted that the story of a mission hospital began with itineration tours, dispensaries and local converted buildings that were established before constructing a permanent and purpose-built structure. These small-scale practices occupied a far more important place in missionaries' agenda than has hitherto been acknowledged. Many factors contributed to the development or otherwise of medical missions. Yet, undertaking itineration and opening dispensaries helped missionaries not only choose a place for a permanent hospital but also establish contact with a larger number of people. Medical missionaries sometimes visited as many as six or seven villages during a short itineration tour of one week. Moreover, they visited villages that were on a caravan route and opened and treated patients in diverse places, including mosques. Taken together, these factors make the view that itineration and dispensaries were emotional set-ups all the more apparent. They should be read less as temporary or auxiliary services than as requisites for the development of medical mission work. Without itineration tours and dispensaries, it would take longer to build a hospital and the number of mission hospitals would have been fewer.

Moreover, the underlying aim of establishing contact with as many people as possible meant that hospitals did not shape mission fields in an identifiable way. The hospitals were built when most new and rebuilt hospitals in Britain adhered to the principles of the pavilion plan. Variations of the pavilion hospital were also built in the mission fields, as evident from the cases of the Kashmir hospital and the hospital for Jews in Jerusalem. However, the medical missionaries also drew on other available models, such as standard plans developed by the Public Work Department of British India (PWD) and cottage hospitals. Moreover, as an examination of the CMS hospitals shows, they developed novel hospital designs, namely the serai hospital and the purdah hospital. Put another way, the missionaries did not use or develop a standard design but instead made and remade existing models while inventing new forms.

The serai hospital, a variation of which could also be found in Uganda and Nigeria, was designed similarly to a caravanserai, consisting of identical rooms arranged around three sides of a courtyard. The missionaries would place one of the rooms of the serai at the disposal of an entire family, who could also bring their bedding and utensils. Family members were a noteworthy feature of mission hospitals. Their importance influenced architectural decisions in diverse ways. For example, wards in mission hospitals had more than one point of entry and exit, facilitating the direct interaction between patients and their family members. Notably, the development of the serai system owed much to the role of female medical missionaries, who were involved in building design as consultants, reformers and innovators. It was also most likely due to their involvement in that the idea of the purdah hospital was born. Among all the women's hospitals examined in this study, the Multan hospital took on a purdah arrangement, consisting of two sections: an outer area for male relatives and an inner compartment with wards, operating theatre and an outpatient department for female patients. This type was not a hybrid approach developed to teach female patients new ideas about health and hygiene through a pre-existing architecture that was meaningful to them. Instead, it was meant to facilitate certain practices such as cooking in the hospital, interacting with male relatives, and moving freely in and out of the wards. The missionaries hoped to bring in a larger number of women through facilitating these practices.

These dissimilarities do not mean that mission hospitals should be examined separately from hospitals built in Britain. An updated account of British hospital architecture in the late nineteenth and early twentieth centuries should analyse how the pavilion plan was adapted to climatic conditions and show that securing cross-ventilation was not a concern everywhere while mapping diverse practices and innovations. The serai and purdah hospitals were less widespread than the pavilion plan (or subsequent approaches such as hospital-as-office-tower), but they are worthy of inclusion in histories of hospital architecture. They raise broader questions regarding the legitimacy of certain types of internationalism over others; for instance, short-lived over longer term and far-reaching internationalisms.[1] Examining the diverse ways in which internationalism in hospital architecture may or may not have been practised is essential for a better understanding of 'how we got here'.[2]

Likewise, an updated account of the interaction between Protestant missions and imperial expansion should discuss how missionaries viewed the extension of the national church as beneficial not only culturally and religiously but also emotionally. The CMS medical missionaries did not impose Christian forms of cleanliness and hygiene. Still, they claimed that their work was politically significant because it had been instrumental in obtaining local people's trust and friendship. They contemplate the issue of obtaining trust not only at the micro level but also at the macro level by establishing the hospitals at strategic locations and creating a chain of medical missions stretching from Isfahan in Persia to Kashmir in north-western British India. They claimed that they could generate a new archival of knowledge about these regions, while declaring that they were winning local people for the colonial establishment by changing their feelings.

I have tried to show that local people did not passively feel certain emotions throughout this study. There were internal variations in how missionaries, their work and their buildings were perceived by local people based on gender, age, occupation, past experiences and so on. I have also emphasised that the relationship between architecture and emotions is fluid rather than unchanging and static. For example, missionaries innovated the idea of the serai system to increase the number of patients. Given the familiar architecture of a serai hospital, patients may have found it attractive. Meanwhile, the hospital might have altered the emotional content of a caravanserai, causing uncertainty and unanticipated reactions.

This was not all; the serai hospital might have caused a different feeling as caravanserais lost currency by the mid-twentieth century and, as part of this conclusion, I make some speculations regarding the 'affective lives' of mission hospitals.[3] I do so through an especial reference to the Kerman and Yazd hospitals, both of which are listed as a national heritage by the Ministry of Cultural Heritage, Handicraft and Tourism of Iran. More precisely, I highlight the promise of emotions history to understand colonial buildings' diverse and sometimes contradictory affective lives.

In 1954, the CMS missionaries in Kerman decided to sell the hospital. This decision was faced with an opposition: Abolghāsim Rāsikh, a former assistant director of the hospital, wrote a letter to the Ministry of Health, arguing that the missionaries should not be allowed to sell the hospital because it belongs to the people of Kerman. To support his argument, Rāsikh emphasised that the people of Kerman offered the hospital's land for free, funded the construction of the buildings and paid for the installation of electricity and the purchase of an X-ray machine.[4] This episode alone may not reveal much about how the people of Kerman felt about the medical mission and missionaries, but if we consider it alongside another episode, it may point to the attachment of the people of Kerman to the hospital. When Dodson died of typhoid fever in Kerman in 1937 the local community closed the bazaar and mourned him. Given that daily bazaar life in Persia would only be suspended to mourn the death of very special individuals, more notably during Muharram, this event – which was recorded in a local newspaper – may suggest that the people of Kerman had a feeling of great respect for Dodson.[5] Moreover, as mentioned above, the Kerman and Yazd hospitals are listed as a national heritage. I explained in Chapter Two that the CMS built a hospital for men in Yazd and used a caravanserai as the women's hospital. Significantly, this caravanserai, rather than the purpose-built hospital (which was destroyed in a flood[6]), has been registered as a national heritage as the CMS hospital. Do these mean that these hospitals, as Rāsikh suggested, belong to the people of Kerman and Yazd?

In mapping how the inhabitants of Ruashi neighbourhood, built by the Office des Cites Africaines in the mining city of Lubumbashi, 'responded to a physical environment shaped according to western dwelling patterns', Sofie Boonen and Johan Lagae have made a case for the concept of an 'actively lived-in architecture'. In so doing, they have opened up alternative ways of thinking about the future of the city as an 'African, rather than a mere colonial built, legacy'.[7] Moreover, Mrinalini Rajagopalan has introduced the concept of affective lives to account for the 'parallel world of meanings' around, in the case of her study, the 'monument' in India. These concepts are helpful as they demand going beyond a mere focus on officials to examine the role of inhabitants and local communities. But I would like to suggest that they can be strengthened through an engagement with emotions history. Boonan and Johan's observation regards 'actively lived-in architecture' as timeless. It also does not consider internal variations based on gender, occupation, age and so on. If this concept demands going beyond the traditional focus on 'the origin of the design' to consider 'the moment when life takes over',[8] then assigning these buildings a fixed, transhistorical status as 'African' disregards the dynamic of their history. To put it another way, drawing on this concept to refer to the Kerman and Yazd hospitals as 'Persian' means disregarding the dynamic of what being Persian means, reducing it into an 'empirically verifiable and ontological consistent' place.[9] Rajagopalan's concept emphasises that histories of buildings are always 'contingent and never stable, polyphonous rather than monologic, and temporally dynamic rather than static'.[10] Yet, it too considers the 'local community' as homogeneous. It also does not consider the diverse emotional component of resistance over time.

A parallel cannot be made between Rāsikh's statement and the present status of the Kerman hospital as a national heritage. There were undoubtedly people who were not in favour of the hospitals. For example, Parvīs Shahrīārī, who was born into a Zoroastrian family in Kerman in 1926 and was a member of the Tūdeh party of Iran, referred to the Kerman hospital in his diary. Remembering the hospital as the 'Dodson hospital', he believed that it was just for rich people and did not think that the doctors were competent.[11] Moreover, both the Kerman and Yazd hospitals most likely owe their current status not so much to missionaries' efforts or Rāsikh's opinions than to two prominent publications. One is Abdolhoseyn Sanatīzādih Kermanī's autobiography, who was a well-known writer and dedicated a chapter to Dodson, celebrating his 'selflessness' and love for the people of Kerman.[12] And the other is the three-volume *Yādigārhāyi Yazd*, the first local history of the city by Iraj Afshār, which was published between 1968 and 1975. It referred briefly to the CMS hospital by introducing the caravanserai as the hospital.[13] Since the publication of Afshār's books, all studies have cited him regarding the CMS hospital. These examples back up Rajagopalan's argument regarding the power of actors who operate in the realm of unofficial to appropriate the 'monument'. But these two hospitals are currently entirely unknown and, as mentioned at the start of this book, I judged the Kerman hospital based on my own experience of studying architecture in Kerman. In short, these hospitals are not British (as their users have appropriated them), but neither are they wholly other than British.

This book focused on trust, friendship and affection and analysed Protestant medical mission work in the late nineteenth and early twentieth centuries. The missionaries assigned specific meanings to these terms and employed them to justify their activities, choices and behaviours. But the book's central argument has been more than just about these terms. It has shown that focusing on lack of resources, local people's opposition, absence of professional architects, climatic conditions, or these supposedly hard and rational things, makes us lose sight of some historical realities. We can offer more nuanced discussions of why male and female missionaries did what they did by turning to emotions. The history of emotions also prevents us from generalising about the relationship between architecture and emotions and instead consider how it changes over time and is different from one person to another. Like other studies on the history of emotions, this book's central goal has been to show that excluding emotions from our historical analysis leaves us impoverished.

Notes

1. Ana Antic, Johanna Conterio and Dora Vargha, 'Conclusion: Beyond Liberal Internationalism', *Contemporary European History* 25, no. 2 (1016): 359–71.
2. Annmarie Adams, 'Canadian hospital architecture: how we got here', *Canadian Medical Association Journal* 155, no. 5 (2016): 370–1.
3. Mrinalini Rajagopalan, *Building Histories: The Archival and Affective Lives of Five Monuments in Modern Delhi* (Chicago: The University Press of Chicago 2016).
4. Abolgāsim Rāsikh, 15, 03, 1331, 99/293/9729, National Library and Archive of Iran.
5. Abdolhoseyn Sanati Zade, *Ruzegari ke gozasht* [The Gone Years] (Tehran: Ebn-e Sina, 1346/1967), 200.
6. Charles Melville, 'Hazards and Disasters in Iran: A Preliminary Survey to 1950', *Iran* 22 (1984): 147. See also Harold G. Anderson, *Flying Visit: A Tour of the CMS Front in Africa and the Near East* (London: Church Missionary Society, 1946), 110.
7. Sofie Boonen and Johan Lagae, 'Ruashi, a Pessac in Congo? On the Design, Inhabitation, and Transformation of a 1950s Neighborhood in Lubumbashi,

Democratic Republic of Congo', in Martina Baker-Ciganikova, Kirsten Rüther, Daniela Waldburger and Carl-Philipp Bodestein (eds), *The Politics of Housing in (post)colonial Africa: Accommodating Workers and Urban Residents* (Berlin: De Gruyter, 2020), 74–5.
8. Ibid., 94.
9. Mana Kia, *Persianate Selves: Memories of Place and Origin before Nationalism* (Stanford: Stanford University Press, 2020).
10. Rajagopalan, *Building Histories*, 6.
11. Parviz Shahriyari, 'Parastu', *Chista*, np. 231 (1385/2006): 130.
12. Sanati Zade, *Ruzegari ke gozasht*, 198.
13. Iraj Afshar, *Yādegārhāye Yazd*, vol. 2 (Tehran: Anjoman-e Asar-e Farhangi, 1374/1995), 803.

BIBLIOGRAPHY

Primary Sources

Anderson, Harold G. (1946), *Flying Visit: A Tour of the CMS Front in Africa and the Near East*, London: Church Missionary Society.

Burdett, Henry C. (1896), *Cottage Hospitals: General, Fever, Convalescent: Their Progress, Management, and Work in Great Britain and Ireland and the United States of America*, 3rd ed., London: The Scientific Press.

Burdett, Henry C. (1891), *Hospitals and Asylums of the World: their Origin, History, Construction, Management, and Legislation*, vol. IV, Hospital Construction, with Plans and Bibliography, London: J. & A. Churchill.

Cavalier, A. R. (1899), *In Northern India: A Story of Mission Work in Zenanas, Hospitals, Schools and Villages*, London: S. W. Partridge.

Chandler, John S. (1912), *Seventy-five Years in the Madura Mission: A history of the Mission in South India*, Madras, American Madura Mission.

Church Missionary Intelligencer (1849–1906) (held at Crowther Library, Church Mission Society, Oxford), available online through subscription from http://www.churchmissionarysociety.amdigital.co.uk.

CMS/M/EL 2 – Monthly journals comprising *Mercy and Truth*, vols 1–21, 1897–1921; *The Mission Hospital*, vols 22–39, 1922–39 (held at Cadbury Research Library, University of Birmingham).

CMS/M/EL 1 – Quarterly journals comprising *Medical Mission Quarterly*, issue nos 1–16, 1892–3 and 1895–6 (held at Cadbury Research Library, University of Birmingham).

CMS printed papers, CMS/ACC7 O10 (held at Cadbury Research Library, Special Collection, University of Birmingham).

Dennis, James S. (1899), *Christian Missions and Social Progress*, vol. 2, New York, Chicago and Toronto: Fleming H. Revell Company.

Edited by her mother (1909), *Letters of Marie Elizabeth Hayes, M. B. Missionary Doctor, Delhi, 1905–8*, London: Marshall Brothers.

Galton, Sir Douglas (1893), *Healthy Hospitals: Observations on Some Points Connected with Hospital Construction*, Oxford: Clarendon Press.

Group 2 medical precis book 18 March 1898–6 January 1905, CMS/M/C 2/1/4 (held at Cadbury Research Library, Special Collection, University of Birmingham).

Hayes, Annabella (1909), *At Work: Letters of Marie Elizabeth Hayes, M.B. missionary doctor, Delhi, 1905–8*, London: Marshall Brothers.

Latham, Urania (1911), *Children of Persia*, Edinburgh and London: Oliphant, Anderson and Ferrier.

Minnie Gomery Fonds, p. 170, Osler Library of the History of Medicine, McGill Library, McGill University.

Moore, Herbert (1905), *Here and There with the SPG in India*, London: Society Office.

Mouat, Frederic J. and H. Saxon Snell (1883), *Hospital Construction and Management*, London: J. & A. Churchill.

Neve, Ernest F. (1928), *A Crusader in Kashmir: Being the Life of Dr Arthur Neve, with an Account of the Medical Missionary Work of Two Brothers & Its Later Developments Down to the Present Day*, London: Seeley.

Oppert, F. (1883), *Hospitals, Infirmaries, and Dispensaries: Their Construction, Interior, and Management*, London: J. & A. Churchill.

Pennell, Alice M. (1914), *Pennell of the Afghan Frontier*, New York: E. P. Dutton and Company.

Pennell, T. L. (1909), *Among the Wild Tribes of the Afghan Frontier, A Record of Sixteen Years' Close Intercourse with the Natives of the Indian Marchers*, 2nd ed., London: Seeley.

Rāsikh, Abolgāsim. 15, 03, 1331, 99/293/9729, National Library and Archive of Iran.

Report of the Margarat Williamson Hospital, Shanghai, China (1922), Women's Co-operating Foreign Mission Boards, Islandora Repository, Women in medicine and history of homeopathy, Drexel University, http://hdl.handle.net/1860/lca:2091

Sanati Zade, Abdolhoseyn [1346] (1967), *Ruzegāri ke gozasht* [The Gone Years], Tehran: Ebn-e Sina.

Speer, Robert E. (1911), *'The Hakim Sahib' The Foreign Doctor: A Biography of Joseph Plumb Cochran, M.D. of Persia*, New York: Fleming H. Revell Company.

Swete, Horace (1870), *Handy Book of Cottage Hospitals – Issue 133*, London: Hamilton, Adams, and Co., Raternster Row.

Tyler, Rev. W. S. (1859), *Memoir of Rev. Henry Lobdell, M.D., late Missionary of the American Board at Mosul*, Cornhill: The American Track Society.

The World Call to the Church: The Call from the Moslem World, London: The Press and Publication Board of the Church Assembly, 1926.

Wylie, A. (1897), *Memorials of Protestant Missionaries to the Chinese: Giving a List of their publications and obituary notice of the deceased*, Shanghai: American Presbyterian Mission Press.

Secondary Sources

Adair, Gili (2017), '"The 'Feringhi Hakim'": medical encounters and colonial ambivalence in Isabella Bird's travels in Japan and Persia', *Studies in Travel Writing* 21, no. 1: 63–75.

Adams, Annmarie (2016), 'Canadian hospital architecture: how we got here', *Canadian Medical Association Journal* 155, no. 5: 370–1.

Adams, Annmarie (2008), *Medicine by Design: The Architect and the Modern Hospital, 1893–1943*, Minneapolis and London: University of Minnesota Press.

Adams, Annmarie (1996), *Architecture in the Family Way: Doctors, Houses, and Women, 1870–1900*, Montreal and Kingston: McGill-Queen's University Press.

Adams, Annmarie (1995), 'The Eichler Home: Intention and Experience in Postwar Suburbia', in Elizabeth Collins Cromley and Carter L. Hudgins (eds), *Gender, Class, and Shelter: Perspectives in Vernacular Architecture*, V, Knoxville: The University of Tennessee Press, pp. 164–78

Afshar, Iraj, Narges Pedram and Asghar Mahdavi (2006), *Kerman dar asnad-e aminozarb: salhaye 1280–1351 ghamari* [Kerman according to Amin Alzarb's documents between 1289 and 1351 AH]. Tehran: Soraya.

Ahmed, Sarah (2004), *The Cultural Politics of Emotion*, Edinburgh: Edinburgh University Press.

Alavi, Seema (2008), *Islam and Healing: Loss and Recovery of an Indo-Muslim Medical Tradition, 1600–1900*, Basingstoke: Palgrave Macmillan.

Amutabi, Maurice (2012), 'Buildings as Symbols and Metaphors of Colonial Hegemony: Interrogating Colonial Buildings and Architecture in Kenya's Urban

Spaces', in Fassil Demissie (ed.), *Colonial Architecture and Urbanism in Africa: Intertwined and Contested Histories*, Farnham: Ashgate, pp. 325–46.

Anderson, Benedict (2006), *Imagined Communities: Reflections on the Origin and Spread of Nationalism*, London and New York: Verso.

Antic, Ana, Johanna Conterio and Dora Vargha (2016), 'Conclusion: Beyond Liberal Internationalism', *Contemporary European History* 25, no. 2, pp. 359–71.

Badr, Habi (2006), 'American Protestant Missionary Beginnings in Beirut and Istanbul: Policy, Politics, Practices and Response', in Heleen Murre-van den Berg (ed.), *New Faith in Ancient Lands: Western Missions in the Middle East in the Nineteenth and Twentieth Centuries*, Leiden and Boston: Brill, pp. 211–19.

Baker, Patricia (2012), 'Medieval Islamic Hospitals: Structural Design and Social Perceptions', in Patricia A. Baker, Han Nijdam and Karine van t Land (eds), *Medicine and Space: Body, Surroundings and Borders in Antiquity and the Middle Ages*, Leiden and Boston: Brill, pp. 245–72.

Ballantyne, Tony (2016), 'Moving Texts and "Humane Sentiment": Materiality, Mobility and the Emotions of Imperial Humanitarianism', *Journal of Colonialism and Colonial History* 17, no. 1, doi: 10.1353/cch.2016.0000

Bawden, Charles R. (1985), *Shamans, Lamas, and Evangelicals: The English Missionaries in Siberia*, London: Routledge and Kegan Paul.

Beattie, Hugh (2011), 'Negotiations with the Tribes of Waziristan 1849–1914 – The British Experience', *The Journal of Imperial and Commonwealth History* 39, no. 4: 571–87.

Becker, Adam H. (2015), *Revival and Awakening: American Evangelical Missionaries in Iran and the Origin of Assyrian Nationalism*, Chicago and London: The University of Chicago Press.

Beidelman, T. O. (1999), 'Alturism and Domesticity: Images of Missionizing Women among the Church Missionary Society in Nineteenth-Century East Africa', in Mary Taylor Huber and Nancy C. Lutkehaus (eds), *Gendered Missions: Women and Men in Missionary Discourse and Practice*, Ann Arbor: University of Michigan Press, pp. 113–44.

Bellenoit, Hayden J. A. (2015), *Missionary Education and Empire in Late Colonial India, 1860–1920*, London: Routledge.

Ben Prestel, Joseph (2017), *Emotional Cities: Debates on Urban Change in Berlin and Cairo, 1860–1910*, Oxford: Oxford University Press.

Boddice, Rob (2019), *A History of Feelings*, London: Reaktion Books.

Boddice, Rob (2018), *The History of Emotions*, Manchester: Manchester University Press.

Boddice, Rob (2016), *The Science of Sympathy: Morality, Evolution, and Victorian Civilization*, Urbana and Chicago: University of Illinois Press.

Boddice, Rob and Mark Smith (2020), *Emotion, Sense, Experience*, Cambridge: Cambridge University Press.

Boonen, Sofie and Johan Lagae (2020), 'Ruashi, a Pessac in Congo? On the Design, Inhabitation, and Transformation of a 1950s Neighborhood in Lubumbashi, Democratic Republic of Congo', in Martina Baker-Ciganikova, Kirsten Rüther, Daniela Waldburger and Carl-Philipp Bodestein (eds), *The Politics of Housing in (post)colonial Africa: Accommodating Workers and Urban Residents*, Berlin: De Gruyter, pp. 66–97.

Boulos, Samir (2016), *European Evangelicals in Egypt (1900–1956): Cultural Entanglements and Missionary Spaces*, Leiden and Boston: Brill.

Bourmaud, Philippe (2006), 'Public Space and Private Spheres: The Foundation of St Luke's Hospital of Namblus by the CMS (1891–1901)', in Heleen Murre-van den Berg (ed.), *New Faith in Ancient Lands: Western Missions in the Middle East in the Nineteenth and Twentieth Centuries*, Leiden and Boston: Brill, pp. 133–50.

Bravo, Michael T. (2005), 'Mission Gardens: Natural History and Global Expansion, 1720–1820', in Londa Schiebinger and Claudia Swan (eds), *Colonial Botany: Science, Commerce, and Politics in the Early Modern World*, Philadelphia: University of Pennsylvania Press, pp. 49–65.

Bremner, G. A. (ed.) (2020), *Architecture and Urbanism in the British Empire*, Oxford: Oxford University Press.

Bremner, G. A. (2018), 'The expansion of England? Rethinking Scotland's place in the architectural history of the wider British world', *Journal of Art Historiography*, no. 18, DOI: https://arthistoriography.files.wordpress.com/2018/05/bremner.pdf

Bremner, G. A. (2016), 'Nerthex reclaimed: reinventing disciplinary space in the Anglican mission field, 1847–1903', *Journal of Historical Geography* 51, 1–17.

Bremner, G. A. (2013), *Imperial Gothic: Religious Architecture and High Anglican Culture in the British Empire, c. 1840–70*, New Haven and London: Yale University Press.

Bremner, G. A. (2012), 'The Corporatisation of Global Anglicanism', *ABE Journal* [online], 2, DOI: https://doi.org/10.4000/abe.357

Bremner, G. A. (2009), 'The Architecture of the Universities' Mission to Central Africa: Developing a Vernacular Tradition in the Anglican Mission Field, 1861–1909', *Journal of the Society of Architectural Historians* 68, no. 4: 514–39.

Brown, Stewart J. (2018), 'Providential Empire? The Established Church of England and the Nineteenth-Century British Empire in India', *Studies in Church History* 54: 255–9.

Burkhalter Flueckiger, Joyce (2006), *In Amma's Healing Room: Gender and Vernacular Islam in South India*, Bloomington and Indianapolis: Indiana University Press.

Burton, Antoinette (1998), *At the Heart of the Empire: Indians and the Colonial Encounter in Late-Victorian Britain*, Berkeley: University of California Press.

Carey, Hilary M. (2011), *God's Empire: Religion and Colonialism in the British World, c. 1801–1908*, Cambridge: Cambridge University Press.

Chakraborty, Satyasikha (2018), 'European Nurses and Governesses in Indian Princely Households: "Uplifting that impenetrable veil"?', *Journal of Colonialism and Colonial History* 19, no. 1, Doi: 10.1353/cch.2018.0001

Chang, Jiat-Hwee (2010), 'Tropicalising Technologies of Environment and Government: The Singapore General Hospital and the Circulation of Pavilion Plan Hospital in the British Empire, 1860–1930', in Michael Guggenheim and Ola Söderström (eds), *Reshaping Cities: How Global Mobility Transforms Architecture and Urban Form*, London and New York: Routledge, pp. 123–42.

Chircop, John (2013), 'Management and Therapeutic Regimes in Two Lunatic Asylums in Corfu and Malta, 1837–1870', in Laurinda Abreu and Sally Sheard (eds), *Hospital Life: Theory and Practice from the Medieval to the Modern*, Oxford: Peter Lang, pp. 179–208.

Chopra, Preeti (2011), *A Joint Enterprise: Indian Elites and the Making of British Bombay*, Minneapolis and London: University of Minnesota Press, pp. 58–70.

Cleall, Esme (2012), *Missionary Discourses of Difference: Negotiating Otherness in the British Empire, 1840–1900*, Basingstoke: Palgrave Macmillan.

Colebourne, Catharine (2010), *Madness in the Family: Insanity and Institutions in the Australasian Colonial World, 1860–1914*, Basingstoke: Palgrave Macmillan.

Cope, Zachary (1969), 'The Influence of the Free Dispensaries upon Medical Education in Britain', *Medical History* 13, no. 1 (January 1969): 29–36.

Cox, Jeffrey (2008), *The British Missionary Enterprise since 1700*, New York and London: Routledge.

Cox, Jeffrey (2003), 'Going Native: Missionaries in India', in William Roger Louis (ed.), *More Adventures with Britannia: Personalities, Politics and Culture in Britain*, London and New York: I. B. Tauris, pp. 299–312.

Cox, Jeffrey (2002), *Imperial Fault Lines: Christianity and Colonial Power in India, 1818–1940*, Stanford: Stanford University Press.

Crinson, Mark (2013a), 'The Powers that be: Architectural potency and spatialized power', *ABE Journal* [online] 4.
Crinson, Mark (2013b), *Empire Building: Orientalism and Victorian Architecture*, London and New York: Routledge.
Crinson, Mark (2003), *Modern Architecture and the End of Empire*. Aldershot: Ashgate.
Crossland, Zoë (2013), 'Signs of Mission: Material Semeiosis and Nineteenth-Century Tswana Architecture', *Signs and Society* 1, no. 1: 79–113.
Croxson, Bronwyn (2001), 'The Foundation and Evolution of the Middlesex Hospital's Lying-In Service, 1745–86', *Social History of Medicine* 14, no. 1: 27–57.
Csengei, Ildiko (2012), *Sympathy, Sensibility and the Literature of Feeling in the Eighteenth Century*, Basingstoke: Palgrave Macmillan.
Cummins, Stephen and Joel Lee (2019), 'Missionaries: False Reverence, Irreverence and the Rethinking of Christian Mission in China and India', in Benno Gammerl, Philipp Nielsen, and Margrit Pernau (eds), *Encounters with Emotions: Negotiating Cultural Differences since Early Modernity*, New York and Oxford: Berghahn, pp. 37–60.
Cunningham, Valentine (1993), '"God and nature intended you for a missionary life": Mary Hill, Jane Eyre and other missionary women in the 1840s', in F. Bowie, D. Kirkwood and S. Ardener (eds), *Women and Missions: Past and Present: Anthropological and Historical Perspectives*, Oxford: Berg, pp. 85–108.
Dadabhoy, Ambereen (2016), '"Going Native": Geography, Gender, and Identity in Lady Mary Wortley Montagu's *Turkish Embassy Letters*', in Mona Narain and Karen Gevirtz (eds), *Gender and Space in British Literature, 1660–1820*, London and New York: Routledge, pp. 49–66.
Davin, Delia (1992), 'British Women Missionaries in the Nineteenth-Century China', *Women's History Review* 1, no 2: 257–71.
Davison, Kate, et al. (2018), 'Emotions as a Kind of Practice: Six Case Studies Utilizing Monique Scheer's Practice-Based Approach to Emotions in History', *Cultural History* 7, no. 2: 226–38.
Demissie, Fassil (2012), 'Colonial Architecture and Urbanism in Africa: An Introduction', in Fassil Demissie (ed.), *Colonial Architecture and Urbanism in Africa: Intertwined and Contested Histories*, Oxford and New York: Routledge, pp. 1–10.
Dixon, Thomas (2003), *From Passions to Emotions: The Creation of a Secular Psychological Category*, Cambridge: Cambridge University Press.
Driver, F. (2001), *Geography Militant: Cultures of Exploration and Empire*. Oxford: Blackwell Publishers.

Douglas, Anna (1977), *The Feminization of American Culture*, New York: Knopf.

Doumato, Eleanor Abdella (2002), 'An "Extra Legible Illustration" of the Christian Faith: medicine, medical ethics and missionaries in the Arabian Gulf', *Islam and Christian-Muslim Relations* 13, no. 4: 377–90.

Durra, Manikarnika (2021), 'The Sailors' Home and moral regulation of white European seamen in nineteenth-century India', *Cultural and Social History* 18, no. 2: 201–20.

Edwards, Brian, Magda Sibley, Mohamad Hakmi and Peter Land (eds) (2006), *Courtyard Housing: Past, Present, and Future*, London and New York: Taylor & Francis.

Elbourne, Elizabeth (2010), 'Mother's Milk: Gender, Power, and Anxiety on a South African Mission Station, 1839–1940', in Patricia Grimshaw and Andrew May (eds), *Missionaries, Indigenous Peoples and Cultural Exchange*, Brighton, Portland and Toronto: Sussex Academic Press, pp. 10–23.

Elbourne, Elizabeth (2003), 'Word Made Flesh: Christianity, Modernity and Cultural Colonialism in the Work of Jean and John Comaroff', *The American Historical Review* 108, no. 2: 435–59.

Elbourne, Elizabeth (1993), 'The Foundation of the Church Missionary Society: the Anglican Missionary Impulse', in John Walsh, Colin Haydon, and Stephen Taylor (eds), *The Church of England c. 1689–c. 1833: From Toleration to Tractarianism*, Cambridge: Cambridge University Press, pp. 247–64.

El Chami, Yasmina (2021), 'An American "Garden" in an Oriental "Desert": The Modernity of Timber at the Syrian Protestant College of Beirut', *Architectural Theory Review*: 10.1080/13264826.2021.1958354

Elgood, Cyril (1951), *A Medical History of Persia and the Eastern Caliphate from the Earliest times until the year A. D. 1932*, Cambridge: Cambridge University Press.

Endfield, Georgina (2011), 'The Mission', in John Agnew and David N. Livingston (eds), *The Sage Handbook of Geographical Knowledge*, London: Sage Publications, pp. 202–16.

English, Paul Ward (1968), 'The Origin and Spread of Qanats in the Old World', *Proceedings of the American Philosophical Society* 112, no. 3: 170–81.

Falah, Ghazi-Walid and Caroline Nagel (eds) (2005), *Geographies of Muslim Women: Gender, Religion, and Space*, New York and London: The Guilford Press.

Farrimond, Kenneth John Trace (2003), 'The Policy of the Church Missionary Society Concerning the Development of Self-Governing Indigenous Churches, 1900–1942', PhD diss. University of Leeds.

Ferry, Yaron and Efraim Lev (2003), 'The Medical Activities of the London Jews Society in Nineteenth-Century Palestine', *Medical History* 47, no. 1: 67–88.

Fisch, Jörg (1985), 'A Solitary Vindicator of the Hindus: The Life and Writings of General Stuart (1757/58–1828)', *The Journal of the Royal Asiatic Society of Great Britain and Ireland*, no. 1: 35–57.

Fitzgerald, Rosemary (2001), '"Clinical Christianity": The Emergence of Medical Mission Work as a Missionary Strategy in Colonial India, 1800–1914', in Biswamoy Pati and Mark Harrison (eds), *Health, Medicine, and Empire: Perspectives on Colonial India*, New Delhi: Orient Longman, pp. 88–136.

Fitzgerald, Rosemary (1997), 'Rescue and redemption: The rise of female medical missions in colonial India during the late nineteenth and early twentieth centuries', in Anne Marie Rafferty, Jane Robinson and Ruth Elkan (eds), *Nursing History and the Politics of Welfare*, London and New York: Routledge, pp. 63–78.

Forty, Adrian (2005), 'The Modern Hospital in England and France: the social and medical uses of architecture', in Anthony D. King (ed.), *Buildings and Society: Essays on the Social Development of the Built Environment*, London, Boston, Melbourne, and Hanley, pp. 61–93.

Francis-Dehqani, Gulnar Eleanor (2000), *Religious Feminism in an Age of Empire: CMS Women Missionaries in Iran, 1869–1934*, Bristol: Centre for Comparative Studies of Religion and Gender.

Freas, Erik (2016), *Muslim-Christian Relations in Late Ottoman Palestine: Where Nationalism and Religion Intersects*, Basingstoke: Palgrave Macmillan.

Frevert, Ute (2011), *Emotions in History – Lost and Found*, Budapest: Central European University Press.

Gaitskell, Deborah (2003), 'Rethinking Gender Roles: The Field Experience of Women Missionaries in South Africa', in Andrew Porter (ed.), *The Imperial Horizons of British Protestant Missions 1880–1914*, Grand Rapids: William B. Eerdmans, pp. 131–57.

Gammerl, Benno (2012), 'Emotional Style – concepts and challenges', *Rethinking History* 16, no. 2: 169–70.

Gammerl, Benno, Philipp Nielsen and Margrit Pernau (2019), 'Encountering Feelings – Feeling Encounters', in Benno Gammerl, Philipp Nielsen, and Margrit Pernau (eds), *Encounters with Emotions: Negotiating Cultural Differences since Early Modernity*, New York and Oxford: Berghahn, pp. 2–22.

Gammerl, Benno, Jan Simon Hutta and Monique Scheer (2017), 'Feeling differently: Approaches and their politics', *Emotion, Space and Society* 25, 87–94.

Gaube, Heinz (2008), 'Iranian Cities', in Salma K. Jayyusi, Renata Holod, Attilio Petruccioli and Andre Raymond (eds), *The City in the Islamic World*, vol. 1, Leiden and Boston: Brill, pp. 159–60.

Gill, Sean (1998), 'Heroines of Missionary Adventure: The Portrayal of Victorian Women Missionaries in Popular Fiction and Biography', in Anne Hogan and Andrew Bradstock (eds), *Women of Faith in Victorian Culture*, Basingstoke: Macmillan Press, pp. 172–85.

Goddard, Hugh (2000), *A History of Christian–Muslim Relations*, Edinburgh: Edinburgh University Press.

Goffman, Erving (1962), *Asylums: Essays on the Social Situation of Mental Patients and Other Inmates*, Chicago: Aldine.

Gold, Ann Grodzins (1994), 'Purdah is As Purdah's Kept: A Storyteller's Story', in Gloria Goodwin and Ann Grodzins Gold (eds), *Listen to the Heron's Words: Reimagining Gender and Kinship in North India*, Berkeley, University of California Press, pp. 164–81.

Grigor, Talinn (2021), *The Persian Revival: The Imperial of the Copy in Iranian and Parsi Architecture*, Pennsylvania: Pennsylvania State University.

Grimshaw, Patricia (1989), *Paths of Duty: American Missionary Wives in Nineteenth-Century Hawaii*, Honolulu: University of Hawaii Press.

Grimshaw, Patricia and Andrew May (2010), 'Reappraisals of Mission History: An Introduction', in Patricia Grimshaw and Andrew May (eds), *Missionaries, Indigenous Peoples and Cultural Exchange*, Eastbourne: Sussex Academic Press, pp. 1–9.

Grimshaw, Patricia and Peter Sherlock (2005), 'Women and Cultural Exchange', in Norman Etherington (ed.), *Missions and Empire*, Oxford: Oxford University Press, pp. 173–93.

Großmann, Till and Phillip Nielsen (eds) (2019), *Architecture, Democracy, and Emotions: The Politics of Feeling since 1945*, New York and London: Routledge.

Grove, Richard (1987), 'Early Themes in African Conservation: the Cape in the Nineteenth Century', in David Anderson and Richard Grove (eds), *Conservation in Africa: People, Policies and Practice*, Cambridge: Cambridge University Press, pp. 21–39.

Hammond, Cynthia Imogen (2005), 'Reforming Architecture, Defending Empire: Florence Nightingale and the Pavilion Hospital', *Studies in Social Sciences* 38: 1–24.

Hardiman, David (2017), *Missionaries and their Medicine: A Christian modernity for tribal India*, Manchester: Manchester University Press.

Hardiman, David (2009), 'The Mission Hospital, 1880–1960', in Mark Harrison, Margaret Jones and Helen Sweet (eds), *From Western Medicine to Global Medicine: the hospital beyond the West*, Hyderabad: Orient BlackSwan, pp. 198–220.

Hardiman, David (ed.) (2006), *Healing Bodies, Saving Souls: Medical Missions in Asia and Africa*, Amsterdam: Rodopi.

Harding, Christopher (2008), *Religious Transformation in South Asia: The Meanings of Conversion in Colonial Punjab*, Oxford: Oxford University Press.

Harrison, Mark (1994), *Public Health in British India: Anglo-Indian Preventive Medicine, 1859–1914*, Cambridge: Cambridge University Press.

Hattrick, Jane (2014), 'Seduced by the Archive: A Personal and Working Relationship with the Archive and Collection of the London Couturier, Norman Hartnell', in Anna Moran and Sorcha O'Brien (eds), *Love Objects: Emotion, Design and Material Culture*, London: Bloomsbury Academic, pp. 75–86.

Hevia, James (2012), *The Imperial Security State: British Colonial Knowledge and Empire-Building in Asia*, Cambridge: Cambridge University Press.

Hitzer, Bettina and Monique Scheer (2014), 'Unholy Feelings: Questioning Evangelical Emotions in Wilhelmine Germany', *German History* 32, no. 3: 371–92.

Hoad, Neillie (2004), 'Cosmetic Surgeons of the Social: drawing, Freud, and Wells and the Limits of Sympathy on The Island of Dr. Moreau', in Lauren Berlant (ed.), *Compassion: The Culture and Politics of an Emotion*, New York and London: Rutledge, pp. 187–218.

Hopkins, Benjamin D. (2008), *The Making of Modern Afghanistan*, Basingstoke: Palgrave Macmillan.

Hunt, Nancy Rose (1999), *A Colonial Lexicon of Birth Ritual, and Mobility in the Congo*, Durham, NC and London: Duke University Press.

Ingram, Hilary (2015), 'A Little Learning *is* a dangerous thing: British overseas medical missions and the politics of professionalism, *c.* 1880–1910', in Jonathan Reinarz and Rebecca Wynter (eds), *Complaints, Controversies and Grievances in Medicine: Historical and Social Science Perspectives*, London and New York: Routledge, pp. 75–90.

Innes, C. L. (2004), *A History of Black and Asian Writing in Britain, 1700–2000*, Cambridge: Cambridge University Press.

Jayawardena, Kumari (1995), *The White Woman's Other Burden: Western Women and South Asia During British Rule*, New York and London: Routledge.

Jennings, Michael (2008), '"Healing of Bodies, Salvation of Souls": Missionary Medicine in Colonial Tanganyika, 1870s–1939', *Journal of Religion in Africa* 38: 27–56.

Jennings, Michael (2006), 'A Matter of Vital Importance: The Place of the Medical Mission in Maternal and Child Healthcare in Tanganyika, 1919–39', in David

Hardiman (ed.), *Healing Bodies, Saving Souls: Medical Missions in Asia and Africa*, Amsterdam: Rodopi, pp. 227–50.

Johnson, Robert (2003), '"Russians at the Gates of India"? Planning the Defence of India, 1885–1900', *Journal of Military History* 67, no. 3: 697–743.

Jolly, Margaret and Martha Macintyre (eds) (1989), *Family and Gender in the Pacific Domestic Contradictions and the Colonial Impact*, Cambridge: Cambridge University Press.

Jonson, Ryan (2010), 'Colonial Mission and Imperial Tropical Medicine: Livingston College, London, 1893–1914', *Social History of Medicine* 23, no. 3: 549–66.

Kalusa, Walima T. (2014), 'Missionaries, African Patients, and Negotiating Missionary Medicine at Kalene Hospital, Zambia, 1906–1935', *Journal of Southern African Studies* 40, no. 2: 283–94.

Kent, Eliza F. (2004), *Converting Women: Gender and Protestant Christianity in Colonial South India*, Oxford: Oxford University Press.

Khan, Razek (2015), 'The Social Production of Space and Emotions in South Asia', *Journal of Economic and Social History of the Orient* 58, no. 5: 611–33.

Khan, Sabir (2004), 'Memory Work: The Reciprocal Framing of Self and Place in Émigré Autobiographies', in Eleni Bastéa (ed.), *Memory and Architecture*, Albuquerque: University of New Mexico Press, pp. 117–40.

Kheirabadi, Masoud (2000), *Iranian Cities: Formation and Development*, Syracuse: Syracuse University Press.

Kia, Mana (2020), *Persianate Selves: Memories of Place and Origin before Nationalism*, Stanford: Stanford University Press.

Kieser, Hans-Lukas (2002), 'Mission as Factor of Change in Turkey (nineteenth to first half of twentieth century)', *Islam and Christian–Muslim Relations* 13, no. 4: 391–410.

King, Anthony D. (2007), *Colonial Urban Development: Culture, Social Power and Environment*, London, Hanley and Boston: Routledge & Kegan Paul.

King, Anthony D. (1995), *The Bungalow: The Production of a Global Culture*, 2nd ed., New York and Oxford: Oxford University Press.

Kirmani, Nida (2015), 'Fear and the City: Negotiating Everyday Life as a Young Baloch Man in Karachi', in Razak Khan (ed.), 'Space and Emotions in South Asian History', special issue, *Journal of the Economic and Social History* 58, no. 5: 732–55.

Kisacky, Jeanne (2017), *Rise of the Modern Hospital: An Architectural History of Health and Healing, 1870–1940*, Pittsburgh: University of Pittsburgh Press.

Kisacky, Jeanne (2013), 'Germs are in the details: Aseptic Design and General Constructors at the Lying-In Hospital of the City of New York, 1897–1901', *Construction History* 28, no. 1: 83–106.

Kolapo, Femi J. (2019), *Christian Missionary Engagement in Central Nigeria, 1875–1891: The Church Missionary Society's All-African Mission on the Upper Niger*, Basingstoke: Palgrave Macmillan.

Korhonen, Anu (2012), 'Beauty, Masculinity and Love between Men: Configuring Emotions with Michael Drayton's *Peirs Gaveston*', in Jonas Liliequist (ed.), *A History of Emotions, 1200–1800*, Oxford and New York: Routledge, pp. 136–51.

Kozlovsky, Roy (2015), 'Architecture, Emotions and the History of Childhood', in Stephanie Olsen (ed.), *Childhood, Youth and Emotions in Modern History: National, Colonial and Global Perspectives*, Basingstoke: Palgrave Macmillan, pp. 95–118.

Laing, Catriona (2017), 'Anglican Mission amongst Muslims, 1900–1940', in William L. Sachs (ed.), *Global Anglicanism c. 1910–2000*, vol. V of *The Oxford History of Anglicanism*, Oxford: Oxford University Press, pp. 367–91.

Langmore, Diana (1989), *Missionary Lives: Papua 1874–1914*, Honolulu: University of Hawaii Press.

Lazich, Michael C. (2006), 'Seeking Souls through the Eyes of the Blind: The Birth of the Medical Missionary Society in Nineteenth-Century China', in David Hardiman (ed.), *Healing Bodies, Saving Souls: Medical Missions in Asia and Africa*, Amsterdam: Rodopi, pp. 59–86.

Le Couteur, Howard (2008), 'Anglican High Churchmen and the Expansion of Empire', *Journal of Religious History* 32, no. 2: 193–215.

Lee, Janet (1996), 'Between Subordination and She-tiger: Social Constructions of White Femininity in the Lives of Single, Protestant Missionaries in China, 1905–1930', *Women's Studies International Forum* 19, no. 6: 621–32.

Lestringant, Frank (1992), 'Going native in America (French-style)', *Renaissance Studies* 6, nos 3 and 4: 325–35.

Levine, Philippa (ed.) (2007), *Gender and Empire*, Oxford: Oxford University Press.

Levine, Philippa (1990), *Feminist Lives in Victorian England: Private Roles and Public Commitment*, Oxford: Basil Blackwell.

Livingston, David N. (2005), 'Scientific Inquiry and the Missionary Enterprise', in Ruth Finnegan (ed.), *Participating in the Knowledge Society: Researchers Beyond the University Walls*, Basingstoke: Palgrave Macmillan, pp. 50–64.

Livne, Inbal (2011), 'The Many Purposes of Missionary Work: Annie Royle Taylor as Missionary, Travel Writer, Collector and Empire Builder', in Hilde Nielssen,

Inger Marie Okkenhaug and Karina Hestad Skeie (eds), *Protestant Missions and Local Encounters in the Nineteenth and Twentieth Centuries: Unto the Ends of the World*, Leiden and Boston: Brill, pp. 43–70.
Lydon, Jane (2020), *Imperial Emotions: The Politics of Empathy across the British Empire*, Cambridge: Cambridge University Press.
McCracken Lacy, Lisa (2018), *Lady Anne Blunt in the Middle East: Travel, Politics, and the Idea of Empire*, London and New York: I. B. Tauris.
McConaghey, R. M. S. (1967), 'The Evolution of the Cottage Hospital', *Medical History* 11, no. 2: 128–40. DOI: https://doi.org/10.1017/S0025727300011984
McLisky, Claire (2008), 'Professions of Christian Love: Letters of Courtship between Missionaries-to-be Daniel Matthews and Janet Johnston', in Amanda Barry, Joanna Cruickshank, Andrew Brown-May and Patricia Grimshaw (eds), *Evangelists of Empire? Missionaries in Colonial History*, Melbourne: University of Melbourne eScholarship Research Centre, pp. 173–86.
McLisky, Claire, Daniel Midena and Karen Vallgårda (eds) (2015), *Emotions and Christian Missions: Historical Perspectives*, Basingstoke: Palgrave Macmillan.
Mahdavi, Shireen (2012), 'Everyday Life in Late Qajar Iran', *Iranian Studies* 45, no. 3: 355–70.
Mamedov, Mikail (2008), '"Going Native" in the Caucasus: Problems of Russian identity, 1801–64', *The Russian Review* 67, no. 2: 275–95.
Manktelow, Emily J. (2013), *Missionary Families: Race, Gender and Generation on the Spiritual Frontier*, Manchester: Manchester University Press.
Marland, Hilary (2004), 'The Changing role of the hospital, 1800–1900', in Deborah Brunton (ed.), *Medicine Transformed: Health, Disease, and Society in Europe, 1800–1930*, Manchester: Manchester University Press, pp. 31–60.
Matthee, Rudi (2005), *The Pursuit of Pleasure: Drugs and Stimulants in Iranian History, 1500–1900*, Princeton and Oxford: Princeton University Press.
Maughan, Steven (1996), '"Mighty England do good": the major English denominations and organisation for the support of foreign missions in the nineteenth century', in Robert A. Bickers and Rosemary Seton (eds), *Missionary Encounters: Sources and Issues*, Richmond: Curzon Press, pp. 11–37.
Memarian, Gholamhossein and Frank Brown (2006), 'The Shared Characteristics of Iranian and Arab Courtyard Houses', in Brian Edwards, et al. (eds), *Courtyard Housing: Past, Present and Future*, Abingdon: Taylor & Francis, pp. 21–30.
Mills, Sara (2013), *Gender and Colonial Space*, Manchester: Manchester University Press.
Mooney, Graham and Jonathan Reinarz (eds) (2009), *Permeable Walls: Historical Perspectives on Hospital and Asylum Visiting*, Amsterdam and New York: Rodopi.

Murray, Jocelyn (2019), 'The Role of Women in the Church Missionary Society, 1799–1917', in Kevin Ward and Brian Stanley (eds), *The Church Mission Society and World Christianity, 1799–1999*, London and New York: Routledge, pp. 66–90.

Murre-van den Berg, Heleen (2006), 'Introduction', in Heleen Murre-van den Berg (ed.), *New Faith in Ancient Lands: Western Missions in the Middle East in the Nineteenth and Twentieth Centuries*, Leiden and Boston: Brill, pp. 1–18.

Murre-van den Berg, Heleen (2005), 'The Middle East: Western missions and the Eastern churches, Islam and Judaism', in Sheridan Gilley and Brian Stanley (eds), *World Christianities c. 1815–c.1914*, vol. 8 of *The Cambridge History of Christianity*, Cambridge: Cambridge University Press, pp. 458–72.

Murre-van den Berg, Heleen (2004), 'Asahel Grant's The Nestorians or the Lost Tribes (1841)', in Piscataway, *The Nestorians or The Lost Tribe*, iv-vi. New Jersey: Gorgias Press. https://doi.org/10.31826/9781463209582-001

Murre-van den Berg, Heleen (2001), '"Dear Mother of my Soul": Fidelia Fiske and the Role of Women Missionaries in Mid-nineteenth Century Iran', *Exchange* 30, no. 1: 33–48.

Murre-Van den Berg, Heleen (1999), *From a Spoken to a Written Language: The Introduction and Development of Literary Urmia Aramaic in the Nineteenth Century*, Leiden: Nederlands Instituut Voor Het Nabije Ossten.

Oberoi, Harjot (1994), *The Construction of Religious Boundaries: Culture, Identity, and Diversity in the Sikh Tradition*, Chicago: The University of Chicago Press.

O'Hanlon, Rosalind (1999), 'Gender in the British Empire', in Judith M. Brown and William Roger Louis (eds), *The Twentieth Century*, vol. IV of *The Oxford History of the British Empire*, Oxford: Oxford University Press, pp. 379–97.

Papanek, Hannah (1973), 'Purdah: Separate Worlds and Symbolic Shelter', *Comparative Studies in Society and History* 15, no. 3: 289–325.

Pernau, Margrit (2019), *Emotions and Modernity in Colonial India: From Balance to Fervor*, Oxford: Oxford University Press.

Pernau, Margrit (2015), 'Mapping Emotions, Constructing Feelings: Delhi in the 1840s', *Journal of the Economic and Social History of the Orient* 58, no. 5: 634–67.

Pernau, Margrit (2014), 'Space and Emotions: Building to Feel', *History Compass* 12, no. 7: 541–9.

Perry, Yaron (2010), 'Anglo-Judeo Confrontation: Jewish Antagonism towards the English Medical Mission in Nineteenth-Century Palestine', in Barbara Haider-Wilson and Dominique Trimbur (eds), *Europe and Palestine 1799–1948: Religion – Politics – Society*, Vienna: Austrian Academy of Science Press, pp. 299–313.

Pietsch, Tamson (2013), 'Rethinking the British World', *Journal of British Studies* 52, no. 2: 441–63.
Piggin, Stuart (1984), *Making Evangelical Missionaries, 1789–1858: The Social Background, Motives and Training of British Protestant Missionaries to India*, vol. 2 of *Evangelicals & Society from 1750*, Abingdon: Sutton Courtney Press.
Porter, Andrew (2004), *Religion versus empire? British Protestant missionaries and overseas expansion, 1700–1914*, Manchester: Manchester University Press.
Porter, Andrew (1999), 'Religion, Missionary Enthusiasm, and Empire', in Andrew Porter (ed.), *The Oxford History of the British Empire: Volume III: The Nineteenth Century*, Oxford: Oxford University Press, pp. 223–31.
Porterfield, Amanda (1997), *Mary Lyon and the Mount Holyoke Missionaries*, New York and Oxford: Oxford University Press.
Powell, Arvil A. (2009), 'Creating Christian Community in Early-nineteenth-century Agra', in Richard Fox Young (ed.), *India and the Indianness of Christianity: Essays on Understanding Historical, Theological, and Bibliographical – in Honour of Robert Eric Frykenberg*, Grand Rapids: William B. Eerdmans, pp. 82–107.
Pratt, Mary Louise (1992), *Imperial Eyes: Travel Writing and Transculturation*, London and New York: Routledge.
Prevost, Elizabeth E. (2010), *The Communion of Women: Missions and Gender in Colonial Africa and the British Metropole*, Oxford: Oxford University Press.
Prevost, Elizabeth (2008), 'Married to the Mission Field: Gender, Christianity, and Professionalization in Britain and Colonial Africa, 1865–1914', *Journal of British Studies* 47, no. 4: 797–826.
Price, Richard (2008), *Making Empire: Colonial Encounters and the Creation of Imperial Rule in Nineteenth-Century Africa*, Cambridge: Cambridge University Press.
Rageb, Ahmed (2015), *The Medieval Islamic Hospital: Medicine, Religion, and Charity*, Cambridge: Cambridge University Press.
Rajagopalan, Mrinalini (2016), *Building Histories: The Archival and Affective Lives of Five Monuments in Modern Delhi*, Chicago: The University Press of Chicago.
Ramanna, Mridula (2002), *Western Medicine and Public Health in Colonial Bombay, 1845–1895*, Hyderabad: Orient Longman.
Ranger, Terence O. (1981), 'Godly Medicine: The Ambiguities of Medical Mission in Southeast Tanzania, 1900–1945', *Social Science and Medicine, Part B: Medical Anthropology* 15, no. 3: 261–77.
Reckwitz, Andreas (2012), 'Affective Spaces: A Praxeological Outlook', *Rethinking History: The Journal of Theory and Practice* 16, no. 2: 241–58.

Reckwitz, Andrew (2002), 'Towards a Theory of Social Practices: A Development in Culturalist Theorizing', *European Journal of Social Theory* 5, no. 2: 243–63.

Reddy, William M. (2001), *The Navigation of Feeling: A Framework for the History of Emotions*, Cambridge: Cambridge University Press.

Reinarz. Jonathan (2012), 'Learning to Use Their Senses: Visitors to Voluntary Hospitals in Eighteenth-Century England', *Journal of Eighteenth-Century Studies* 35, no. 4: 505–20.

Reinders, Eric (2004), *Borrowed Gods and Foreign Bodies: Christian Missionaries Imagine Chinese Religion*, Berkeley, Los Angeles and London: University of California Press.

Renshaw, Michelle (2009), 'Family-Centred Care in American Hospitals in Late-Qing China', in Graham Mooney and Jonathan Reinarz (eds), *Permeable Walls: Historical Perspectives on Hospital and Asylum Visiting*, Amsterdam, New York: Rodopi, pp. 55–80.

Richardson, Harriet (ed.) (1998), *English Hospitals 1660–1948: A Survey of their Architecture and Design*, The Royal Commission on the Historical Monuments of England.

Risse, Guenter B. (1999), *Mending Bodies, Saving Souls: A History of Hospital*, New York and Oxford: Oxford University Press.

Robert, Dana Lee (2008), 'Introduction', in Dana Lee Robert (ed.), *Converting Colonialism: Visions and Realities in Mission History, 1706–1914*, Grand Rapids: William B. Eerdmans, pp. 1–20.

Robert, Dana Lee (1996), *American Women in Mission: A Social History of Their Thoughts and Practice. The Modern Mission Era, 1792–1992*, Macon, GA: Mercer University Press.

Rosenberg, Charles E. (1974), 'Social Class and Medical Care in Nineteenth-Century America: The Rise and Fall of the Dispensary', *Journal of the History of Medicine and Allied Sciences* XXIX, no. 1: 32–54.

Rosenwein, Barbara H. (2006), *Emotional Communities in the Early Middle Ages*, Ithaca and London: Cornell University Press.

Rosenwein, Barbara H. (2002), 'Worrying about Emotions in History', *The American Historical Review* 107, no. 3: 821–45.

Rosenwein, Barbara H. and Riccardo Cristiani (2018), *What is the History of Emotions?*, Cambridge: Polity.

Ross, Andrew C. (2006), *David Livingstone: Mission and Empire*, London and New York: Bloomsbury.

Ruggles, D. Fairchild (2008), *Islamic Gardens and Landscapes*, Philadelphia: University of Pennsylvania Press.

Şahin, Emrah (2018), *Faithful Encounters: Authorities and American Missionaries in the Ottoman Empire*, Montreal, Kingston, London and Chicago: McGill-Queen's University Press.

Sample, Rhonda Anne (2003), *Missionary Women: Gender, Professionalism and the Victorian Idea of Christian Mission*, Rochester: The Roydell Press.

Sandon, Emma (2013), 'Projecting Africa: two 1920s British travel films', in Elizabeth Hallam and Brian Street (eds), *Cultural Encounters: Representing Otherness*, London and New York: Routledge, pp. 108–48.

Scarce, Jennifer (2011), 'Isabella Bird Bishop (1831–1904) and her Travels in Persia and Kurdistan in 1890', *Iranian Studies* 44, no. 2: 243–50.

Scheer, Monique (2013), 'Feeling Faith: The Cultural Practice of Religious Emotions in Nineteenth Century German Methodism', in Monique Scheer, et al. (eds), *Out of the Tower: Essays on Culture and Everyday Life*, Tubingen: Tubinger Vereinigung fur Volkskunde, pp. 217–47.

Scheer, Monique (2012), 'Are Emotions a Kind of Practice (and is that what makes them have a history)? A Bourdieuian Approach to Understanding Emotion', *History and Theory* 51, no. 2: 193–220.

Scriver, Peter and Vikramaditya Prakash (2007), 'Between Materiality and Representation: Framing an Architectural Critique of Colonial South Asia', in Peter Scriver and Vikramaditya Prakash (eds), *Colonial Modernities: Building, dwelling and architecture in British India and Ceylon*, London and New York: Routledge, pp. 3–26.

Sentilles, Renée M. (2005), 'Toiling in the Archives of Cyberspace', in Antoinette Burton (ed.), *Archive Stories: Facts, Fictions, and the Writing of History*, Durham, NC and London: Duke University Press, pp. 136–56.

Seton, Rosemary (2013), *Western Daughters in Eastern Lands: British Missionary Women in Asia*, Santa Barbara, Denver and Oxford: Praeger.

Seymour, Mark (2012), 'Emotional Arenas: From Provincial Circus to National Courtroom in Late Nineteenth-century Italy', *Rethinking History: The Journal of Theory and Practice* 16, no. 2: 177–97.

Sharkey, Heather J. (2008), *American Evangelicals: Missionary Encounters in an Age of Empire*, Princeton and Oxford: Princeton University Press.

Siegel, Jennifer (2002), *Endgame: Britain, Russia and the Final Struggle for Central Asia*, London: I. B. Tauris.

Sohmer, Sara H. (1994), 'Christianity without Civilization: Anglican Sources for an Alternative Nineteenth-Century Mission Methodology', *Journal of Religious History* 18, no. 2: 174–97.

Sparke, Penny (2003), 'Introduction', in Brenda Martin and Penny Sparke (eds), *Women's Places: Architecture and Design 1860–1960*, London and New York: Routledge, pp. xi–xix.

Stevens Crawshaw, Jane L. (2012), *Plague Hospitals: Public Health for the City in Early Modern Venice*, Farnham: Ashgate.

Stevens Crawshaw, Jane L., Irena Benyovsky Latin and Kathleen Vongsathorn (eds) (2020), *Tracing Hospital Boundaries: Integration and Segregation in Southeastern Europe and Beyond, 1050–1970*, Leiden and Boston: Brill.

Stevenson, Christine (2000), *Medicine and Magnificence: British Hospital and Asylum Architecture, 1660–1815*, New Haven and London: Yale University Press.

Strong, Rowan (2007), *Anglicanism and the British Empire c. 1700–1850*, Oxford: Oxford University Press.

Stuart, John (2008), 'Mission and Empire', *Social Sciences and Missions* 21, no. 1: 1–5.

Subrahmanyam, Sanjay (2012), *The Portuguese Empire in Asia, 1500–1700: A Political and Economic History*, Chichester: Wiley & Sons.

Sunderland, Willard (1996), 'Russians into Iakuts? "Going Native" and Problems of Russian National Identity in the Siberian North, 1870s–1914', *Slavic Review* 55, no. 4: 806–25.

Swartz, Rebecca (2017), 'Educating Emotions in Natal and Western Australia, 1854–65', *Journal of Colonialism and Colonial History* 18, no. 2. Doi: 10.1353/cch.2017.0022

Tarlow, Sarah (2012), 'The Archaeology of Emotion and Affect', *The Annual Review of Anthropology* 41, no. 1: 169–185.

Tatla, Darshan Singh (1995), 'Sikh free and military migration during the colonial period', in Robin Cohen (ed.), *The Cambridge Survey of World Migration*, Cambridge: Cambridge University Press, pp. 69–73.

Taylor, Jeremy (1997), *The Architect and the Pavilion Hospital: Dialogue and Design Creativity in England 1890-1914*, London and New York: Leicester University Press.

Taylor, Jeremy (1991), *Hospital and Asylum Architecture in England 1840–1914: Building for Health Care*, London and New York: Mansell Publishing Limited.

Thorp, Daniel (2003), 'Going native in New Zealand and America: Comparing Pakeha Maori and white Indians', *The Journal of Imperial and Commonwealth History* 31, no. 3: 1–23.

Titus, Paul (1998), 'Honor the Baloch, Buy the Pushtun: Strategies, Social Organization and History in Western Pakistan', *Modern Asian Studies* 32, no. 3: 657–87.

Touati, Houari (2010), *Islam and Travel in the Middle Ages*, Chicago and London: The University Press of Chicago.

Trigg, Stephanie (2014), 'Introduction: Emotional Histories – Beyond the Personalization of the Past and the Abstraction of Affect Theory', *Examplaria* 26, no. 1: 3–15.

Tucker, Ruth A. (1998), *Guardians of the Great Commission: The Story of Women in Modern Mission*, Grand Rapids: Zondervan.

Turner, Emily (2015), 'The Church Missionary Society and Architecture in the Mission Field: Evangelical Anglican Perspectives on Church Building Abroad. C. 1850–1900', *Architectural History* 58: 197–228.

Vallgårda, Karen (2016), 'Were Christian Missionaries Colonizers?', *Interventions: International Journal of Postcolonial Studies* 18, no. 6: 865–86.

Vallgårda, Karen (2015), 'Tying Children to God with Love: Danish Mission, Childhood, and Emotions in Colonial South India', *Journal of Religious History* 39, no. 4: 595–613.

Vallgårda, Karen, Kristine Alexander and Stephanie Olsen (2015), 'Emotions and the Global Politics of Childhood', in Stephanie Olsen (ed.), *Childhood, Youth and Emotions in Modern History*, Basingstoke: Palgrave Macmillan, pp. 12–34.

Van Gent, Jacqueline (2020), 'Global Protestant Missions and the Role of Emotions', in Ulinka Rublack (ed.), *Protestant Empires: Globalizing the Reformations*, Cambridge: Cambridge University Press, pp. 275–95.

Van Gent, Jacqueline (2017), 'Protestant Global Missions', in Susan Broomhall (ed.), *Early Modern Emotions: An Introduction*, Oxford and New York: Routledge, pp. 313–16.

Vander Werff, Lyle. L. (1977), *Christian Mission to Muslims: The Record: Anglican and Reformed Approaches in India and the Near East, 1800–1938*, Pasadena: William Carey Library.

Vaughan, Megan (1991), *Curing their Ills: Colonial Power and African Illness*, Cambridge: Polity Press.

Vaughn Cross, Carol Ann (2004), 'Missionary Returns and Cultural Conversions in Alabama and Shandong: The Latter Years of Madam Gao (Martha Foster Crawford)', in Wilbert R. Shenk (ed.), *North American Foreign Missions, 1810–1914: Theology, Theory, and Policy*, Grand Rapids: William B. Eerdmans, pp. 243–60.

Viswanatha, Gaui (1998), *Outside the Fold: Conversion, Modernity, and Belief*, Princeton: Princeton University Press.

Vogl-Bienek, Ludwig and Richard Crangle (eds) (2014), *Screen Culture and the Social Question 1880–1914*, London: Studies in Early Cinema, John Libbey Publishing.

Vongsathorn, Kathleen (2015), 'Teaching, Learning and Adapting Emotions in Uganda's Child Leprosy Settlement, *c.* 1930–1962', in Stephanie Olsen (ed.),

Childhood, Youth and Emotions in Modern History: National, Colonial and Global Perspectives, Basingstoke: Palgrave Macmillan, pp. 56–75.

Walcher, Heidi (2008), *In the Shadow of the Kind: Zill Al-Sultan and Isfahan under the Qajars*, London: Bloomsbury Academic.

Walker, Lynne (1989), 'Women and Architecture', in Judy Attfield and Pat Kirkham (eds), *A View from the Interior: Feminism, Women and Design*, London: The Women's Press.

Ward, Kevin (1999), 'The legacy of Eugene Stock', *International Bulletin of Missionary Research* 23, 2: 75–9.

Watson, Geoff (2009), 'The Ultimate Evangelical Away Game: British Missionary Endeavour in Central Asia, *c.* 1830–1930', in Ken Parry (ed.), *Art, Architecture and Religion Along the Silk Roads*, Turnhout: Brepols Publishers, pp. 127–52.

Weaver-Hightower, Rebecca (2007), *Empire Islands: Castaways, Cannibals, and Fantasies of Conquest*, Minneapolis and London: University of Minnesota Press.

Wenzlhuemer, Ronald (2020), *Doing Global History: An Introduction in 6 Concepts*, London and New York: Bloomsbury Academic.

Williams, C. Peter (1982), 'Healing and Evangelism: The Place of Medicine in later Victorian Protestant Missionary Thinking', in W. J. Sheils (ed.), *The Church and Healing, Studies in Church History 19*, Oxford: Basil Blackwell for the Ecclesiastical History Society, pp. 271–85.

Williams, C. Peter (1990), *The Ideals of the Self-Governing Church: A Study in Victorian Missionary Strategy*, Leiden: Brill.

Williams, C. Peter (2008), 'The Church Missionary Society and the Indigenous Church in the Second Half of the Nineteenth Century: The Defence and Destruction of the Venn Ideals', in Dana L. Robert (ed.), *Converting Colonialism: Visions and Realities in Mission History, 1706–1914*, Grand Rapids and Cambridge: William B. Eerdmans, pp. 86–111.

Wills, Julie, Philip Goad and Cameron Logan (2019), *Architecture and the Modern Hospital: Nosolomeion to Hygeia*, London and New York: Routledge.

Wilson, Linda (1998), 'Nonconformist Obituaries: How Stereotyped was their View of Women?', in Anne Hogan and Andrew Bradstock (eds), *Women of Faith in Victorian Culture: Reassessing the Angle in the House*, Basingstoke: Palgrave, pp. 145–58.

Winks, Robin W. (1999), 'The Future of Imperial History', in Robin W. Winks (ed.), *Historiography*, vol. V of *The Oxford History of the British Empire*, Oxford: Oxford University Press, pp. 653–68.

Withey, Alan (2016), 'Medicine and Charity in Eighteenth-century Northumberland: The Early Years of the Bamburgh Castle Dispensary and Surgery, *c.* 1772–1802', *Social History of Medicine* 29, no. 3: 467–89.

Wolfram, Kleiss (1993), 'Safavid Palaces', *Ars Orientalis: The Arts of Islam and the East* 23, 269–72.

Woodward, Catherine S. (2011), 'The Discourse and Experience of the Arabian Mission's Medical Missionaries: Part I 1920–39', *Middle Eastern Studies* 47, no. 5: 779–805.

Worboys, Michael (2000), *Spreading Germs: Disease Theories and Medical Practice in Britain, 1865–1900*, Cambridge: Cambridge University Press.

Worpole, Ken (2000), *Here Comes the Sun: Architecture and Public Space in Twentieth-century European Culture*, London: Reaktion Books.

Wytenbroek Lydia (2018), 'Generational Difference: American Medical Missionaries in Iran, 1834–1940', in Margaux Whiskin and David Bagot (eds), *Iran and the West: Cultural Perceptions from the Sasanian Empire to the Islamic Republic*, London: Bloomsbury, pp. 179–94.

Yapp, M. A. (2001), 'The Legend of the Great Game', *Proceedings of the British Academy* 111: 179–98.

Yapp, M. A. (1987), 'British Perception of the Russian Threat to India', *Modern Asian Studies* 21, no. 4: 647–65.

Yates, Nigel (2000), *Buildings, Faith and Worship: The Liturgical Arrangement of Anglican Churches, 1600–1900*, Oxford: Oxford University Press.

Young, Theron Kue-Hing (1973), 'A Conflict of Professions: The Medical Missionary in China, 1835–1890', *Bulletin of the History of Medicine* 47, no. 3: 250–72.

INDEX

Abdul Massih, 4, 154
Adams, Annmarie, 157
Adivasis, 36
affect theory, 15
affective bodies, saving souls, 6, 216
    based on the missionaries' gender, national affiliation and the country they worked in, 149
affective lives, 219–20
    based on gender, age, occupation, past experiences, 219, 221
    conformed to the expectations, 78
    lived-in architecture, 220–1
    see also social settings for interaction, 35
Afghan frontier, 195
Afghan soldier, 189
Afghanistan, 42, 55, 131, 185, 194, 200, 204
Africa, 1, 5, 68, 70, 73, 104, 137, 140, 199, 216
    East Africa, 137
    South Africa, 150, 157, 182
    see also southern Africa, 196
Afshār, Iraj, 221
Albert, Samul, 73
All Saints' Memorial Church, 83–84
Alvi, Seema, 49
American Board of Commission for Foreign Mission (ABCFM), 4, 7, 9–10, 35, 158
Amritsar, 9, 45, 51, 118, 154, 185, 194
Anantnag, 23, 120, 155–6; *see also* Islamabad

andarūni, 163
    courtyard house, 22, 85, 87, 100, 170–1
    privacy, 169–70
    protected and separated from the eyes of male stranger, 166
    purdah, 161–2, 164, 168
    purdah arrangement, 166–7, 171, 218
    purdah family, 168
    purdah hospital, 23, 149, 159, 161, 166, 168–9 187, 171, 218
    purdah-like, 169
    purdah system, 168, 172
    see also zenana, 39, 154
Anglo-Russian rivalry, 23, 180, 182–4, 186, 205; *see also* India' defence
Anglo-Afghan War, 194
Arabian mission, 129
architect, 91, 149
    McIntuyre, J., 85, 91, 93
Asia, 1, 68, 104, 195, 204, 204, 216
    Central Asia, 22, 131, 185, 194, 196, 200
    see also South Asia, 16, 78, 115, 161
attractive agencies, 104
    attractive place, 89
    found it attractive, 219
    find so attractive, 83
    see also make them as attractive as possible, 84

Baloch, 201–2, 204
Baluchistan, 194, 200

INDEX

Bannu, 9, 42, 45, 49, 77–8, 168, 187, 190, 195, 201–2, 205
Bannu Hospital, 74–5, 80, 128, 131, 159, 165, 182, 186, 191
Bannu medical mission, 45, 49
bazaar life in Persia, 220
Beresford Pite, Arthur, 73
Bird, Isabella Lucy,119–20, 157, 171;
   see also Mrs Bishop
Bird, Mary, 38–9, 52, 119–220, 154, 158
birūni, 163
Bishop, John, 120, 157
  John Bishop Memorial hospital, 155–7, 159, 161, 171
Bishop, Mrs, 119
Blackett, Arthur Russell, 125, 154
block system, 96
Boddice, Rob, 6, 11, 14, 18
Bolan Pass, 195, 204
Bombay, 40, 84, 118, 130
Boulos, Samir, 16, 36
Bourmand, Philippe, 40–1, 169
Bremner, G. A., 72, 78
Browne, Elizabeth Mary, 148 *see also* Mrs Clark
bungalow, 2, 78–9, 159
Burdett, Henry, 70, 78, 159

Cairo, 18, 79; *see also* Old Cairo
Calcutta, 151, 154, 185
Carless, Henry, 51, 194, 197–8
caravanserai, 22, 41, 52, 56, 114, 131, 134, 137, 141, 162, 171, 220
  caravan, 37
  commodious, 116
  family wards, 130–1, 186
  inn, 22, 116
  James serai, 85, 131, 133, 134
  serai building, 140
  serai hospital, 130, 133, 137, 140–1
  serai system, 22, 141, 148, 166
  see also Indian block, 137
Carr, Donald, 50–2, 85, 87, 117, 125, 154, 161
Central Asia, 22, 131, 185, 194, 196, 200
China, 35–6, 70, 120, 124, 128, 158, 190, 199
Chopra, Preeti, 84, 130
Church of England Zenana Missionary Society (CEZMS), 9, 118, 131, 149, 153–4, 157
Clark, Mrs, 2, 51, 148, 150–2, 154, 171

Clark, Robert, 1, 2, 9, 71, 148, 150–1, 185, 194–5, 197–8, 204
Cleall, Esme, 137
cleanliness, 103, 125, 127, 183
  hygiene, 69, 124, 165
  hygienic rules, 103
  sanitary, 70, 122, 140
  see also sanitary facilities, 87
climatic conditions, 82, 140
  fierce heat, 165
  heat outside, 96
  see also periods of oppressive heat, 130
close associates, 116, 123, 126–8, 130, 133, 141
  family and friends, 123–4, 126–8, 140–1
  relative, 114, 116, 124, 127, 129, 131, 166
  see also whole family, 125, 131
Cook, Albert, 38–9, 42
Cornford, Henrietta, 152–3
cottage hospital, 130, 159–60, 171
courtyard house, 22, 85, 87, 100, 170–1
Cox, Jeffrey, 148, 183, 184, 190, 195

Darmānū Mountains, 102; *see also* Dog-tooth hills
Delhi, 16, 158
Dera Ghazi Khan, 39, 187, 198, 202
disciplining gaze, 16
dispensary, 2, 3, 21, 34–7, 47–51, 57, 81, 87, 121, 123, 159, 161, 197, 205
  moving hospitals, 46
doctor's gaze, 102
Dodson, George Everard, 39–40, 42, 95, 99, 148, 158, 220
dog-tooth hills, 102
domestic sphere, 151
domestic-scale details, 160

East Africa, 137
East Indian Company (EIC), 7, 187, 194
ecclesiastical imperialism, 184
  ecclesiastical pathway to [Afghanistan] and Central Asia, 185
Edinburgh Missionary Conference, 155
Eger, Annie Wilhelmina, 40, 153, 161–2, 165–7
Egypt, 5, 7, 9, 18, 73, 153, 199
Elmslie, William Jackson, 2, 3, 40, 119, 148, 154, 161
emotional communities, 11

emotional formation, 13, 15
emotional frontier, 13
emotional practices, 11–12
emotional regime, 14
emotional scripts, 121
  narrative tropes, 121
emotional set-up, 12
emotional style, 14, 18
emotional tie, 5
Endfield, Georgina, 197
evangelical missionary movement, 150
evangelistic agency, 118
evangelistic work, 148, 152

family and friends, 123–4, 126–8, 140–1
family wards, 130–1, 186
fellow feeling, 13
  sympathy, 3, 18, 190–1
femininity, 150, 158
  ladylike qualities, 156
  masculinity, 150
  see also took on an extra shape for female missionaries, 149
First World War, 7, 10, 40, 151
Fitzgerald, Rosemary, 159
four-part garden, 22, 80
  four-part cross-axial Islamic garden, 83
  water canals, 83

Gaza, 73
Gierku medical mission, 140
Goffman, Erving, 119
Gomery, Minnie, 44, 153–6, 160, 171
Goodarz, Mehriban, 41
Gospel, 74, 90, 129
Gothic Revival Style, 84
gramophones, 89–90
  noise, 17, 90
  see also sound, 12, 68, 84, 90, 186, 217
Grodzins Gold, Ann, 168

Hammond, Cynthia Imogen, 130
Hardiman, David, 5, 36, 124
Heywood, W. B., 74, 117
Holland, Henry Tristram, 39, 44
hospital visiting, 22, 114–16, 217
house visitors, 116–20
Hume-Griffith, A., 38, 158
humped roofs, 102; *see also* Kermānī arch and Kermānī Adome

hygiene, 69, 124, 165
hygienic rules, 103

indigenous hospital, 133
Indo-Saracenic, 83
infection, 68, 124, 128
  aseptic barrier, 69
  aseptic joint case, 126
  aseptic precautions, 81
  aseptic surgery, 82
  septic cases, 82
  septic operating room, 82
Indian block, 137
Isfahan, 7, 37–8, 41, 50, 67, 85–7, 89, 91, 93, 95, 117, 120, 195
Isfahan hospital, 125, 165, 169
Isfahan women's hospital, 129
Islamabad, 23, 43–4, 120, 153, 156, 159–61, 171
Ironside, Catherine, 87, 128–9, 153
itinerant apothecaries, 46
itineration, 21, 35–7, 41–7, 57, 197

Jalal-ul-Dowlah, 121
James, F. M., 126, 129
James serai, 85, 131, 133, 134
Japan, 120, 157
Jennings, Michael, 70
Jerusalem, 73
John Bishop Memorial hospital, 155–9, 171
Jukes, Andrew, 39, 118, 197

Kashmir, 1–3, 40, 43, 46, 51, 71, 74, 120, 131, 148, 155, 157, 159, 171, 186, 196–7, 200, 219
Kashmir hospital, 71, 73, 82, 119, 125, 148, 157, 182, 217
Kashmir medical mission, 2, 5–7, 9, 73, 104, 120, 123, 148, 156, 158, 171, 186
Kent, Eliza, 46, 163, 164
Kerman, 1, 19, 37–40, 42–3, 45, 51–2, 93, 95–6, 100, 102, 118–20, 126, 130, 154; *see also* Kirman
Kerman hospital, 148, 158, 170; *see also* Morsalīn hospital
Kermānī arch, 22, 95
Kermānī vault, 99–100
Keys, Cathy, 130, 158
Khyber, 204
King, Anthony, 16

King of Persia, 121, 128
Kirman, 51, 195, 201
Kisacky, Jeanne, 69
Kūh Payeh Mountains, 102

ladylike qualities, 156
Lankester, Arthur, 38, 80, 82, 84, 131, 137, 202
Lankester, Cecil, 42, 52, 87
lantern slide, 46–7
Latham, Urania, 34, 153
Lee, Rachel, 18
Levine, Phillipa, 151
Livingston, David, 41, 199
Livingston, David N., 199
London Medical Missionary Association, 120
London Missionary Society (LMS), 35, 116, 121, 150, 156–7
London Society for Promoting Christianity amongst the Jews, 73
local chiefs, 119
   Amirs of Afghanistan, 194
   King of Persia, 121, 128
   Maharajah, 2, 40, 186, 196
   Mullah, 45, 85, 128–9, 187, 189
   nawab, 45
   Shahzada, 127
   see also Sultan of Oman, 41
local clothes, 190
local dress, 192
local garment, 191

MacIntyre, J., 85, 91, 93
McLisky, Clare, 186
Madagascar, 158
maharajah, 2, 40, 186, 196
Manktelow, Emily, 150
Martin, Henry, 7
masculinity, 150
mausoleum, 81
   Said Khan Tower, 81
   Shrine, 56
   tomb, 83
   see also ziarab, 56
Maxwell, Theodore, 3, 71, 131, 200
mechanical ventilation, 87, 96
Medical Mission Auxiliary (MMA), 5, 37, 131, 137, 202
Medical Sub-conference, 122

Mengo hospital, 38, 137, 141
Mengo medical mission, 140
Mercy and Truth, 73, 118, 123, 184
miasma, 104
   cross-ventilation, 69, 96, 100, 113, 218
Middle East, 35, 39, 70
Ministry of Cultural Heritage, Handicraft and Tourism of Iran, 219
Miran Baksh, 80, 84
Mooney, Graham, 114–16, 118, 128
Morsalīn hospital, 1, 19
mosque, 46, 196, 217
moving hospitals, 46
Mughal, 16, 22
Mullah, 45, 85, 128–9, 187, 189
Multan, 40, 67, 153, 161–2, 164, 166, 182
Multan hospital, 168, 169, 171

Nablus, 40, 73, 169
narrative tropes, 121
native city, 160, 191
Nath, Golak, 190
Nelson, Louis P., 72
Neve, 3, 43, 74, 197, 199–200
Neve, Arthur, 5, 46, 71, 123, 161, 186, 201, 206
Neve brothers, 159–60, 171
Nightingale, Florence, 69, 77–8
Nightingale ward, 130
North-western British India, 117
North-west Frontier, 137
North-west Frontier Province, 120
Note on Hospitals, 69
nursing staff, 115, 124–5, 130, 141

official visitors, 116, 122
Old Cairo, 153
Office des Cites Africaines, 220

Palestine, 9, 45, 73, 118
Palestine mission, 153
Pashtun, 201–2, 204–6; *see also* Pathan
Pathan, 54, 189, 190, 202
patients' visitors, 114, 116
patriarchal structure, 151
pavilion plan, 68, 71–4, 77, 82, 96, 104, 130, 140, 159
   block plan, 77
   block system, 96
   international standard, 69–70

pavilion plan (cont.)
  Nightingale ward, 130
  prevailing approaches, 70
  prevailing hospital design principles, 67
  standardisation and uniformity among hospitals, 123
Pennell, Theodore, 42, 45, 75, 125–6, 128, 130–1, 182, 185–8, 189–90, 191–2, 202, 204–6
Pernau, Margrit, 16
Persia mission, 50, 122, 130, 153, 194–5
Peshawar, 34, 38, 42–3, 52, 54, 55, 67, 80–3, 85, 87, 104, 114, 117, 118, 122, 127, 131, 134, 141, 182, 201
Peshawar hospital, 168
Peshawari khan, 189
Prevost, Elizabeth, 156, 158
privacy, 170
Protestant missionary influence, 185
providential discourse, 185
  providential gift of the empire, 185, 206
  providential purpose of the empire, 23
Public Work Department (PWD), 78, 159
public visitors, 116–19
Punjab, 9, 45, 74, 118–20, 184–5, 194
Punjab mission, 122, 153, 184
Punjab Model, 74
purdah, 162
purdah arrangement, 167, 171
purdah hospital, 23, 149, 159, 161, 166, 168, 171, 187
purdah system, 168

Quetta, 39, 123, 131, 194–5, 197–8, 201
Quetta mission, 195
Quetta medical mission, 196

Rajagopalan, Mrinalini, 220
Ramanna, Mridula, 49
Rāsikh, Abolghāsim, 220
regiments, 182, 185
relatives, 127
religion versus empire, 183
Renshaw, Michelle, 36, 115, 124
Roberts, Frederick, 182–3, 185–7, 189, 200, 206
Royal Infirmary, Edinburgh, 72
Royal Victorian hospital, 87
Russia, 182, 194–5
Russian empire, 188

sadhu or mendicant pilgrim, 187
Said Khan Tower, 81
Sample, Rhonda Ann, 154
Sanatīzādih Kermanī, Abdolhoseyn, 221
sanitary, 70, 122, 140
sanitary facilities, 87
seems to him like home, 54
sensibility, 5
  sensation, 35
  see also sensory relationship, 6, 12, 149, 191, 217
Sentilles, Renée M., 18
serai building, 140
serai hospital, 130, 133, 137, 140–1
serai system, 22, 141, 148, 166
Shahzada, 127
shrine, 56
Society for Promoting Female Education in China, India and the East (FES), 40, 151, 161–2
Society for the Propagation of the Gospel in Foreign Parts (SPG), 35, 55, 158, 184
South Africa, 150, 157, 182
southern Africa, 196
Stanley, John R., 36, 124
Stileman, Charles Harvey, 51–2
Strong, Rowan, 184–5
Stuart, Emmeline, 50, 85, 125, 152
Sudan and Upper Niger mission, 187
Sudan Pionier Mission (SPM), 35–6
Summerhayes, John Orlando, 39, 202
surveillance and control, 130
  doctor's gaze, 102
  see also disciplining gaze, 16
Sykes, Ella, 118–19, 121
Sykes, Percy Molesworth, 118, 120

tastes, 17
  cooking in the hospital, 12, 167, 218
  drinking tea, 12
  see also tea party, 90
Taylor, Jeremy, 69
Tochi Pass, 195
tomb, 83
touch, 68, 102, 128–9, 186, 217
  utensils, 15, 17, 91, 167, 191, 218
tuberculosis, 69, 87
traditional building practices, 131
  local to the region, 99
  see also local to the respective regions, 22
trans-frontier families, 133

traveller patients, 114, 127, 141

Uganda, 137, 141, 150, 153
Uganda Mission, 153

Vallgårda, Karen, 37, 186
Venn, Henry, 84
veranda, 2, 76, 78, 87, 96

Walcher, Heidi, 50
Walker, Lynne, 149, 157
water canals, 83
water pipe, 17
Watson, Geoff, 200

Westlake, Winfred, 39–40, 45, 95, 148, 150, 153, 158
White, Henry, 42, 51, 91, 121, 148
whole family, 125, 131
women's work for women, 39, 152
Wortley Montagu, Mary, 166
Wright, Gaskoin, 40

Yādigārhāyi Yazd, 221
Yazd, 34, 38, 41–2, 44, 51–2, 91, 93, 120, 127, 148, 195

zenana, 39, 154
Zill al Sultan, 41, 120

EU representative:
Easy Access System Europe
Mustamäe tee 50, 10621 Tallinn, Estonia
Gpsr.requests@easproject.com

www.ingramcontent.com/pod-product-compliance
Lightning Source LLC
Chambersburg PA
CBHW070323240426
43671CB00013BA/2350